Inorganic Nanoprobes for Biological Sensing and Imaging

Artech House Series
Engineering in Medicine & Biology

Series Editors

Martin L. Yarmush, Harvard Medical School
Christopher J. James, University of Southampton

Advanced Methods and Tools for ECG Data Analysis, Gari D. Clifford, Francisco Azuaje, and Patrick E. McSharry, editors

Advances in Photodynamic Therapy: Basic, Translational, and Clinical, Michael Hamblin and Pawel Mroz, editors

Biological Database Modeling, JakeChen and Amandeep S. Sidhu, editors

Biomedical Informaticsin Translational Research, Hai Hu, Michael Liebman, and Richard Mural

Biomedical Surfaces, Jeremy Ramsden

Genome Sequencing Technology and Algorithms, Sun Kim, Haixu Tang, and Elaine R. Mardis, editors

Inorganic Nanoprobes for Biological Sensing and Imaging, Hedi Mattoussi and Jinwoo Cheon, editors

Intelligent Systems Modeling and Decision Support in Bioengineering, Mahdi Mahfouf

Life Science Automation Fundamentals and Applications, Mingjun Zhang, Bradley Nelson, and Robin Felder, editors

Microscopic ImageAnalysis for Life Science Applications, Jens Rittscher, Stephen T. C. Wong, and Raghu Machiraju, editors

Next Generation Artificial Vision : Reverse Engineering the Human Visual System, Maria Petrou and Anil Bharath,editors

Systems Bioinformatics: An Engineering Case-Based Approach, Gil Alterovitz and Marco F. Ramoni, editors

Systems Engineering Approach to Medical Automation, Robin Felder.

Translational Approaches in Tissue Engineering and Regenerative Medicine, Jeremy Mao, Gordana Vunjak-Novakovic, Antonios G. Mikos, and Anthony Atala, editors

Inorganic Nanoprobes for Biological Sensing and Imaging

Hedi Mattoussi
Jinwoo Cheon

Editors

ARTECH HOUSE
BOSTON | LONDON
artechhouse.com

Library of Congress Cataloging-in-Publication Data
A catalog record for this book is available from the U. S. Library of Congress.

British Library Cataloguing in Publication Data
A catalogue record for this book is available from the British Library.

ISBN-13: 978-1-59693-196-1

Cover design by Igor Valdman

685 Canton Street
Norwood, MA 02062

10 9 8 7 6 5 4 3 2 1

Contents

CHAPTER 1

Colloidal Quantum Dots: Synthesis, Photophysical Properties, and Biofunctionalization Strategies

Kimihiro Susumu, Igor L. Medintz, and Hedi Mattoussi

1.1 Introduction

Fluorescence tagging of biological molecules is a commonly used approach in biotechnology that has relied on conventional organic fluorophores and fluorescent proteins [1–3]. All available organic fluorophores and fluorescent proteins, however, have some inherent limitations that reduce their effective use to develop biological sensing and imaging. Among these, the most limiting properties are narrow excitation spectral windows, broad photoluminescence (PL) spectra, and low resistance to chemical and photo-degradation [4, 5]. Luminescent semiconductor nanocrystals—often referred to as quantum dots (QDs), such as those made of CdSe and PbSe cores—in comparison offer several unique properties and promise significant advantages in certain bioanalytical and imaging applications [4–8]. Because they have broad absorption envelopes, extending from the ultraviolet (UV) to the band edge, it is possible to simultaneously excite QDs of different emission colors at a single wavelength, making them suitable for multiplexing applications. This promising feature is very difficult to achieve with conventional organic fluorophores. Depending on the materials used, QDs can emit light over a wide range of wavelengths from the visible to near infrared (NIR) regions of the optical spectrum [4, 5, 9–15]. Since the first reports on the use of QD in biology were published, there have been several demonstrations showing that QDs conjugated with biomolecular receptors (including peptides, proteins, and DNA) can be used in a range of biological applications, such as sensing, imaging, and diagnostics. However, successful integration of QDs in biotechnology necessitates a thorough understanding of the nanocrystals, namely their reproducible synthetic routes, surface treatment/functionalization, and biocompatibility.

In this chapter, we provide an overview of the most commonly used synthetic schemes to make colloidal nanocrystals, along with their photophysical and structural characterization. We will then describe some of the most effective schemes reported to date to promote water solubility of these nanocrystals and discuss the simplest conjugation techniques that can be reproducibly applied to colloidal QDs.

1.2 Chemistry and Physics of Semiconductor Quantum Dots

1.2.1 Basic Physical Properties of Semiconductor Quantum Dots

Semiconductor nanocrystals (or QDs) are small crystalline assemblies of a given material consisting of a few hundred to several thousand atoms. Their sizes range anywhere from 10Å to 1,000Å in radius; the exact range depends on the constituent elements used to make the nanocrystals. They can be divided into two main subgroups: (a) Self-assembled QDs are usually grown in vacuum via molecular beam epitaxy or other lithography techniques; these tend to be anisotropic in shape, "pancake like," and overall larger at least within the 2-D plane (see Figure 1.1) [10, 16]. (b) Solution grown nanocrystals are colloidal in nature, and they can be spherical with a radius of 10 ~ 200Å, as well as cubic, rod-like, triangular, and so on (see Figure 1.1) [17]. Their colloidal feature stems from the fact that they are surface-capped with organic ligands that promote their dispersion in the solution environment.

These nanoscale assemblies are neither wholly atomic nor bulk semiconductors. Instead, they exhibit novel electronic properties attributed to what is commonly referred to as quantum confinement effects: this is the spatial confinement of intrinsic electron and hole carriers to the physical dimensions of the nanocrystal material rather than to bulk length scales. Because they somewhat combine properties that are both bulk-like and atomic-like, they have often been described as "artificial atoms." These confinement effects manifest when the nanocrystal size becomes comparable to, or smaller than, the bulk Bohr exciton radius [10, 18, 19]. One of the best-known and -understood confinement effects is the widening of the energy band gap with decrease of nanocrystal size. This manifests itself as a blue shift of the first absorption peak and the photoluminescence maximum with decreasing particle size, along with the appearance of discrete energy states in both the valence and conduction bands (Figure 1.1). However, resolution in the excited state energy levels and separation between the valence and conduction band levels depends on the type of semiconducting materials used.

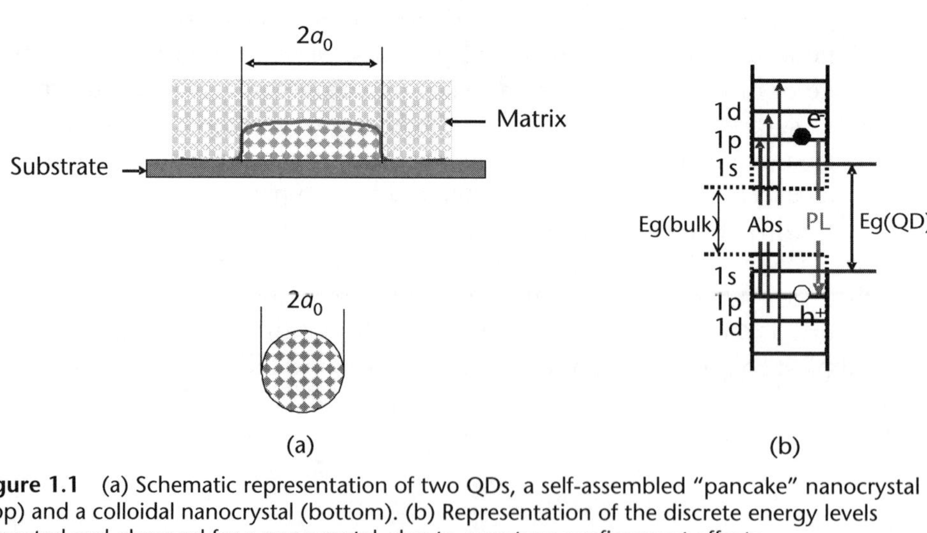

Figure 1.1 (a) Schematic representation of two QDs, a self-assembled "pancake" nanocrystal (top) and a colloidal nanocrystal (bottom). (b) Representation of the discrete energy levels expected and observed for a nanocrystal, due to quantum confinement effects.

This phenomenon can be understood by a simple extension or adaptation of the expected behavior of a quantum mechanical particle confined in a one-dimensional box of length L to a three-dimensional box (or sphere) of radius a_0, where the potential minimum represents the QD and the barrier to escape originates from the abrupt termination of the semiconducting material at the QD surface (boundary conditions) [10, 18, 19]. In this model/description, a carrier is localized within a potential minimum between two infinite barriers. For a one-dimensional box, effects of carrier confinement manifest in quantization of the carrier energies to discrete values that exhibit inverse square dependence on the length of the box ($E_n \propto n^2/L^2$, with $n = 1,2,3,...$).

For a spherical QD with a radius a_0 treated within the conditions of an infinite potential barrier, the electron and hole energy levels in the particle can be written using the following expression:

$$E_{l,n}^{e,h} = \frac{\hbar^2 \beta_{l,n}^2}{2m_{e,h} a_0^2} \tag{1.1}$$

Here $\beta_{l,n}$ is the nth root of the spherical Bessel function of order l (solution obeying the boundary conditions), $m_{e,h}$ is the effective mass of the electron (e) or hole (h), and a_0 is the radius of the QD. This treatment predicts discrete (quantized) electron-hole (exciton) transitions, along with an increase in the effective band gap energy (or HOMO-LUMO transition) with decreasing particle size, which can also be expressed as:

$$E_g(QD) = E_g(bluk) + \frac{\hbar^2 \pi^2}{2m_{e,h} a_0^2} \tag{1.2}$$

Conversely, (1.1) and (1.2) also predict a decrease in the energy spacing between states with increasing nanocrystal size. It should be noted that the physical behavior of these nanocrystals is also affected by the Coulomb interactions between the confined carriers (these are charged). However, because this contribution/term has a weaker dependence on size (scales as $1/a_0$ compared to $\sim 1/a_0^2$ shown in (1.1)), it is small and is often treated as perturbation to the overall energy values. For the interested readers, there are several excellent review articles on the subject published in the past decade, including those recently assembled by Yoffe [16, 19], Gaponenko [18], Efros [10], and Kippeny [20].

Earlier work probing the optical properties of QDs was primarily focused on understanding the correlation between size and spectral shifts in absorption and luminescence based on confinement effects. Today, the absorption properties of CdSe as well as other QDs are relatively well understood with up to 10 excited states in the absorption assigned and theoretical avoided crossings observed [22]. A representative experimental example of absorption spectra for II–VI colloidal QDs is shown in Figure 1.2.

There is a unique spectroscopic property registered primarily for colloidal QDs, but rarely reported for their self-assembled nanocrystal counterparts. Bawendi and coworkers reported in 1996 that under CW laser excitation, the emission of isolated TOP/TOPO-capped single-particle CdSe and CdSe-ZnS QDs was not continuous.

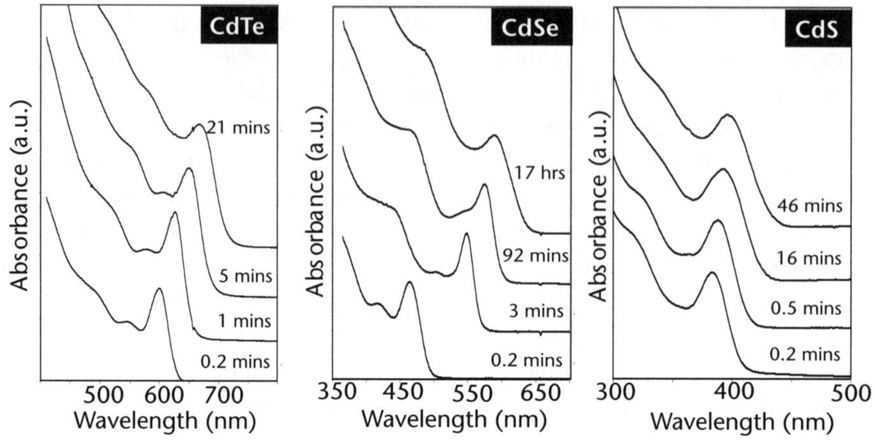

Figure 1.2 Representative absorption spectra for CdS, CdSe, and CdTe QDs prepared using high-temperature solution reaction. The spectra are shown at successive time intervals of nanocrystal growth. The shift in the position of the first absorption peak reflects an increase in the nanocrystal size. Reproduced from [21], with permission from the American Chemical Society.

Instead, they observed that QDs underwent intermittent on/off photoluminescence, now widely identified as the PL "blinking" of single QDs [23]. Blinking of single QD photoluminescence has since been widely reported in a variety of conditions, including extremely dilute dispersions in polymeric films, surface tethered nanocrystals, and more recently cellular media [24]. In particular, there is a nonvanishing probability for a QD to enter a long dark period. The on/off intermittency in QD emission was attributed to Auger ionization of the QD [23, 25, 26]. Despite the remarkable progress made, this phenomenon is still not fully understood.

1.2.2 Synthesis, Characterization, and Capping Strategies

1.2.2.1 Growth of Colloidal Nanocrystals in Doped Glasses

A range of experimental techniques such as e-beam lithography, X-ray lithography, molecular beam epitaxy (MBE), ion implantation, and growth in size-restricted environments has been reported for making small nanocrystallites not only of semiconductors but also of metals; colloidal QDs are a subset of those semiconducting nanocrystals. However, the first reported discovery of QDs by Ekimov and Onuschenko used doped silicate glasses [27–34]. The authors showed that if a supersaturated solution of copper and chlorine in glass was heated at high temperatures, controlled precipitation of CuCl within the glass matrix could take place. They further demonstrated that additional heating and annealing of the glass melt systematically creates collections of nano-scale particulates of crystalline CuCl containing a finite number of atoms, ranging from tens to hundreds of angstroms; the authors initially denoted these structures as *quantum droplets*. Following those remarkable demonstrations, growth of QDs made of II–VI semiconductors (e.g., CdS and CdSe) in glass was achieved by doping the melt with salts of the desired materials/precursors [27, 29, 35]. When the temperature of the glass rapidly decreases, small nuclei of the semiconductor are generated. Following heat treatment over temperatures ranging from 400 to 1,000 degrees C, nucleation and growth culminate in the formation of small spherical crystalline particles of semiconductor dispersed in the amorphous glass matrices. This technique provided highly crystalline nanoparticles in glass host samples that can support very large (a few hundred angstroms) QDs. However, because the QDs remain trapped within a solid glass matrix, these nanocrystals cannot be easily manipulated to alter surface chemistry or improve their size distribution.

1.2.2.2 Synthetic Routes of Dispersible and Highly Luminescent QDs

Solution-phase growth of semiconductor nanoparticles carried out within inverse micelles was demonstrated shortly after the first realization of carrier confinements in semiconductor crystallites using doped silicate glasses by Ekimov and coworkers [28–31, 36–38]. This "wet chemistry" route allows preparation of functionalized, and thus dispersible, nanocrystals, by essentially exploiting the natural geometrical structures created by water-in-oil mixtures upon adding an amphiphilic surfactant such as sodium dioctyl sulfosuccinate (AOT), cetyltrimethylammonium bromide (CTAB), and tetraoctylammonium bromide (TOAB) (see schematics in Figure 1.3). This route was in fact demonstrated for a variety of other inorganic nanoparticles. In this technique, one can vary the water content of the mixture to control the size of the water droplets (nanoscale reaction pools) suspended in the oil phase. Addition of appropriate metal salts to the solution, which naturally migrate to the water pools, initiates nucleation and growth of colloidal nanocrystals. This technique has a few advantages including the fact that the reactions are carried out at room temperature. Furthermore, it provides one the unique ability to perform postsynthesis processing of these materials from solutions. This approach, however, was not able to provide QDs that have good crystalline structure and high photoluminescence quantum yields necessary for potential transition to technological use.

A major breakthrough took place in 1993, when Bawendi and coworkers showed that high quality nanocrystals of CdSe QDs with crystalline cores, narrow size distribution (~10 percent), and relatively high quantum yields can be prepared using an *organometallic synthesis* based on the "pyrolysis" of metal-organic precursors [9, 39]. This rationale was confirmed shortly thereafter by other groups including Alivistaos and coworkers [40]. This reaction scheme initially employed

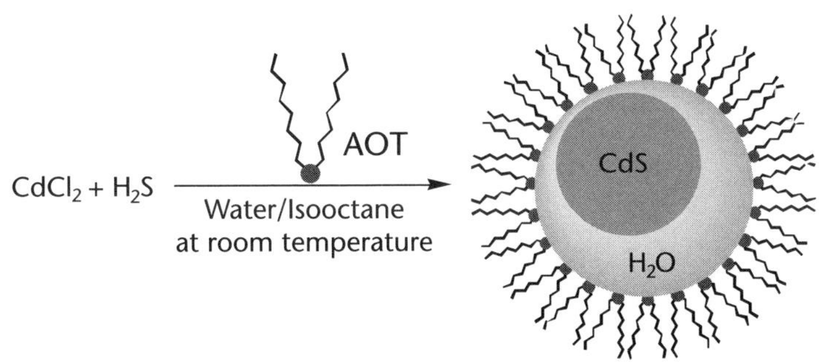

Figure 1.3 Schematic representation of the growth of CdS semiconductor nanocrystals in inverse micelles. Other materials such as CdSe and CdTe have also been prepared using the inverse micelles approach.

dimethylcadmium ($CdMe_2$) and trioctylphosphine selenide (TOP:Se), diluted in trioctylphosphine (TOP), and their rapid injection into a hot (280–300 degrees C) coordinating solution of trioctylphosphine oxide (TOPO) (see schematics in Figure 1.4) [39]. They also demonstrated that size distribution can be further improved by postreaction processing. Following this breakthrough, colloidal QDs could be made with quantum yields (QYs) on the order of 5 to 10 percent at room temperature, making fluorescence-based studies of QDs viable and raising the potential for use in technological applications. The QYs of these nanocrystals can reach near unity at low temperature.

Subsequently, Peng and coworkers further refined the reaction scheme and showed that additional precursors that are less volatile and less pyrophoric than $CdMe_2$ could effectively be employed to prepare high-quality colloidal nanocrystals [21, 43]. In those studies, they and other groups have eventually outlined the importance of impurities—usually acids coordinating to the metal precursors, such as hexylphosphonic acid (HPA) and tetradecylphosphonic acid (TDPA)—in the reaction progress, and showed that these impurities can be externally controlled. They also applied this rationale to making other types of colloidal nanocrystals, including CdTe and CdS as well as Pb-based QDs. In this route, high purity TOPO and controlled amounts of metal coordinating ligands and metal precursors such as CdO, cadmium acetate ($Cd(OAc)_2$), and cadmium acetylacetonate ($Cd(acac)_2$) were used for preparing Cd-based nanocrystals. The high temperature synthetic route was extended to making near-IR emitting QDs by Murray and coworkers (and further confirmed by other groups), using oleic acid and Lead(II) acetate trihydrate or lead oxide for PbSe QDs [14, 44, 45]. In most reported methods the selenium precursor still relies on TOP:Se [14, 21, 43, 46, 47].

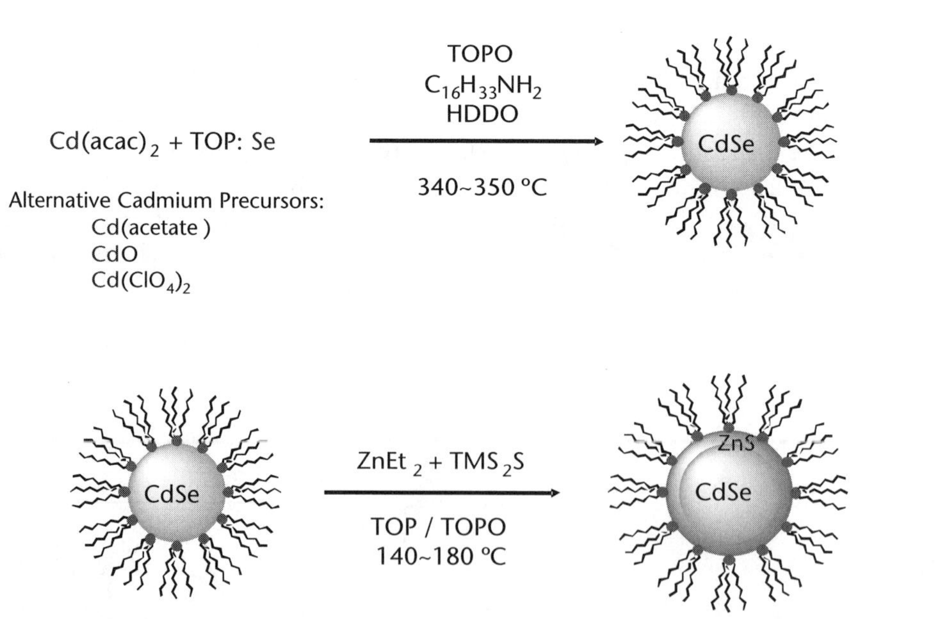

Figure 1.4 (top) Schematic depiction of the high-temperature organometallic reaction and growth method used for colloidal CdSe nanocrystals. (bottom) Reaction scheme for the overcoating CdSe quantum dots with ZnS using the same high-temperature solution route. Additional details can be found in [41, 42].

In these high-temperature reaction schemes, it has been demonstrated that applying size selective precipitation using polar solvents such as methanol or ethanol following nanocrystal growth could reduce the particle size distribution/polydispersity of the nanocrystals. In addition to reducing polydispersity, this procedure also removes impurities and precipitated metals from the reaction solution [9, 39]. This cleaning step is crucial for nanocrystals made using less reactive precursors and the various metal-coordinating molecules, since larger amounts of unreacted metals, acids, and amines can be left in the final QD crude samples. Available techniques to characterize nanocrystals include high- and low-resolution transmission electron microscopy (TEM), wide angle X-ray diffraction (XRD), small angle X-ray scattering (SAXS), and absorption and fluorescence spectroscopy, which extract information such as size, distribution width, crystal structure, band edge value and emission energy level (see Figures 1.5 and 1.6 and Table 1.1) [9, 11, 21, 39, 41–43, 46–50]. TEM tends to provide slightly smaller values for the inorganic core than SAXS, for example, because TEM does not take into account the amorphous outermost atomic layer on the nanocrystal surface [51].

Additional details on the synthetic routes, structural characterization, physics of quantum confinements effects, and their implications on the electronic and spectroscopic properties of colloidal QDs can be found in these thorough reviews [17, 52]. A summary of the reported synthetic methods for making colloidal QDs is provided in Table 1.2, with particular emphasis on preparations yielding colloidal QDs

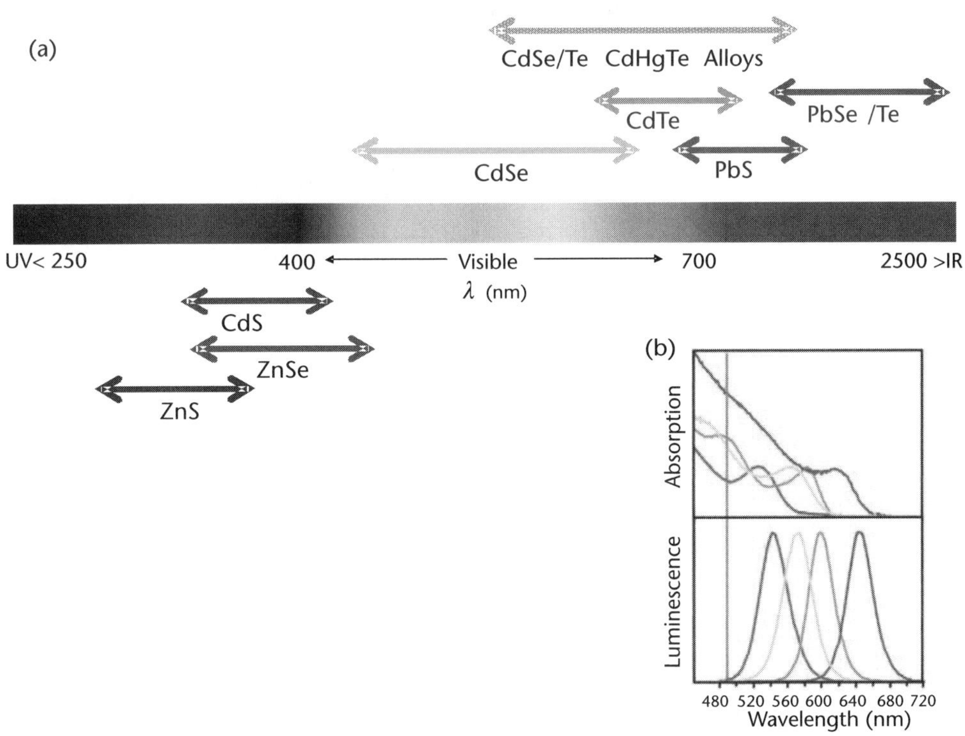

Figure 1.5 (a) Representative set of emission spectral windows for several types of QD materials. Core materials of II–VI, III–V and hybrid "III–VI" are shown. Partially reproduced from [5], with permission from NPG. (b) A representative example of absorption and normalized emission spectra collected for solutions of CdSe-ZnS QDs. Partially reproduced from [4], with permission from AAS. Other materials not represented here include InP and InAs QDs. (See Color Plate 1.)

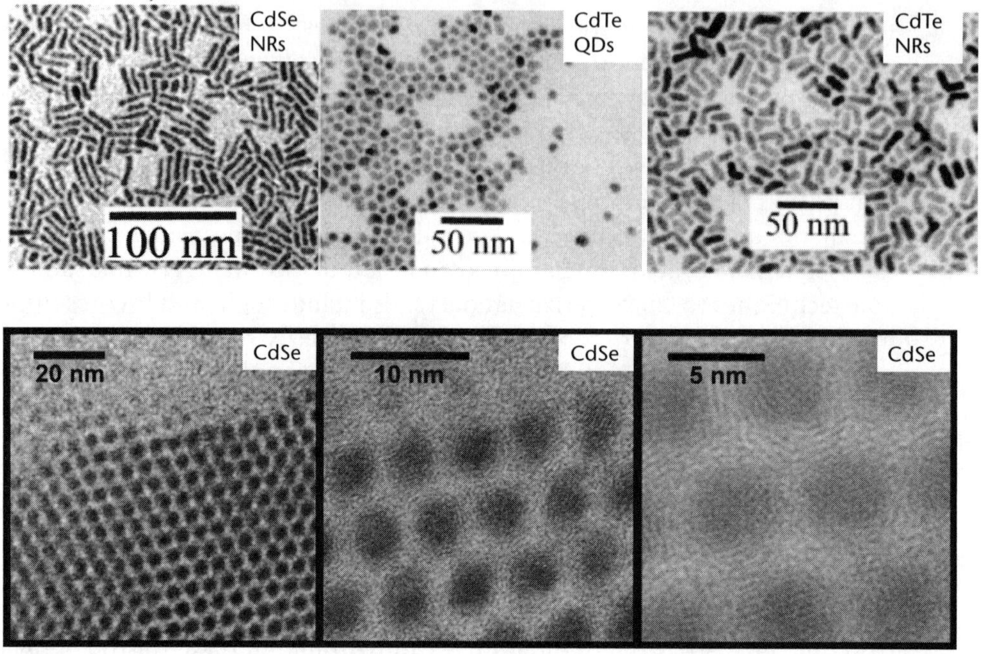

Figure 1.6 (top) Three panels showing high TEM images collected from CdSe nanorods (left), CdTe spherical dots (center), and CdTe nanorods. Reproduced from [46], with permission from the American Chemical Society. (bottom) TEM images of ordered CdSe nanocrystals (diameter 3.6 nm), prepared by solvent evaporation of a colloidal solution in toluene. The nanocrystals were synthesized using high temperature reaction of air-stable (and air sensitive) organometallic precursors.

Table 1.1 Radii of CdSe Nanocrystals Extracted from SAXS Measurements on Solution Samples, Together with the Corresponding Location of the First Absorption Peak*

Location of the First Absorption Peak λ_M	a_0(Å)
622-TBP/TBPO in hexane	29.7
600-TOP/TOPO in hexane	24.9
586-PIC in butanol	22.0
564-TOP/TOPO in hexane	21.3
562-TBP/TBPO in hexane	20.6
560-PYR in pyridine	19.7
550-TOP/TOPO in hexane	19.3
540-TOP/TOPO in hexane	18.8
520-TOP/TOPO in hexane	17.4
510-TOP/TOPO in hexane	14.5

*The type of ligands and solvent used are also shown. In addition to TOP/TOP discussed in the text, TBP, TBPO, PIC, and PYR designate tributylphosphine, tributylphosphine oxide, picoline, and pyridine cap, respectively. Reproduced partially from [51], with permission from the American Institute of Physics.

Table 1.2 Major Types of Colloidal Semiconductor QDs (Group II–VI) Prepared via Wet Chemistry Along with the Method of Preparation and Representative References

Nanocrystal Type	*Preparation Method*	*Literature Citation*
CdS	Silica glass	[32, 54–56]
	Aqueous solutions, inverted micelles	[13, 37, 38, 57]
	Polymer and high-temperature coordinating solutions	[39, 58–60]
	Sol-gel glass, zeolite	[61–65]
	High-temperature coordinating solutions using air-stable precursors	[21]
CdSe	Silica glass	[32, 35, 66]
	High-temperature coordinating solutions	[39]
	Polycrystalline films	[67]
	High-temperature coordinating solutions using air-stable precursors	[21, 46]
CdTe	Silicate glass	[68, 69]
	Semiconductor-glass composite films	[70]
	High-temperature coordinating solutions	[39]
	High-temperature coordinating solutions using air-stable precursors	[21]
ZnSe	High-temperature coordinating solutions	[12, 71]
	High-temperature coordinating solutions using air-stable precursors	[72]
PbSe	High-temperature coordinating solutions	[14, 45, 47]
CdSe-overcoating with wider band semiconductors	ZnSe using hybrid micelle/organometallics	[73]
	ZnS using high-temperature coordinating solutions	[41, 42]
	CdS using high-temperature coordinating solutions	[49]
	ZnSe using high-temperature coordinating solutions using air-stable organometallic precursors	[46]

that have surface capping/passivating ligands. The fluorescence windows allowed by these various colloidal nanocrystals spanning the full region from UV to NIR regions of the optical spectrum are schematically depicted in Figure 1.5. The absorption and PL spectra for the particular example of QDs having CdSe cores is also shown in Figure 1.5.

In the following section we will provide a detailed description of two typical laboratory scale organometallic preparations used to make CdSe-based QDs. We will first describe the synthetic route using dimethylcadmium ($CdMe_2$) and trioctylphosphine selenide (TOP:Se) precursors, diluted in trioctylphosphine (TOP), and follow that by detailing the steps involved in more recent routes using air-stable organometallic precursors.

Synthesis of CdSe Nanocrystals Using Highly Reactive $CdMe_2$ Precursor

1. Load a 100-ml three-neck flask with ~20–30g of TOPO (90 percent) and heat the contents to 150–180 degrees C for 2–3 hours under vacuum using a

Schlenk line, while stirring. This allows removal of residual water and oxygen.

2. In parallel or before, prepare a 1M stock solution of trioctylphosphine selenide (TOP:Se) by adding 7.9g of amorphous Se (99.99 percent) shot to 100 ml of trioctylphosphine (TOP, 90 to 95 percent). It is recommended that this stock solution is prepared in an inert atmosphere (e.g., in a glove box, under nitrogen). Higher concentration (1.5 or 2M) stock solutions could also be used.
3. An injection solution is usually made by diluting ~170–250 μl of $CdMe_2$ with 3.5–4 ml of 1M TOP:Se and ~15 ml of TOP. If 1.5M or 2M TOP:Se stock solutions were used, volumes of the TOP used will have to be adjusted so that the total volume of the Se precursor solution stays the same. This step must also be handled in an inert atmosphere (glove box).
4. The reagents are thoroughly mixed and then loaded into a syringe equipped with a large gauge needle for rapid injection.
5. After 2–3 hours heating and degassing (TOPO content is "dry"), the flask is backfilled with inert gas (N_2 or Ar) and the temperature is raised to ~300 degrees C.
6. Remove the loaded syringe from the dry box and quickly inject the contents into the flask containing TOPO, while vigorously stirring.
7. Upon injection, there is a rapid color change of the solution to light yellow, and the temperature falls to ~250 degrees C. The absorption spectrum is collected and should how sharp features with the peak of the first transition usually located between 470 and 490 nm, similar to what is shown in Figure 1.2.
8. Raise the temperature slowly to 290–300 degrees C to promote growth and annealing of the nanocrystals.
9. To verify the quality of the materials during growth, aliquots from the reaction solution are periodically retrieved and their absorption spectra are collected. The location of the first absorption peak gives an estimate of the nanocrystal size as checked by TEM and small angle X-ray scattering (SAXS) (see Figure 1.6 and Table 1.1) [50]. Furthermore, the relative width of the transition peak gives a measure of size distribution of the sample. Occasionally there is a decrease in the growth rate accompanied by an increase in the relative size distribution. To overcome this growth bottleneck, the temperature is raised by several degrees.
10. When the first absorption peak reaches a wavelength maximum indicative of a desired size, lower the temperature to below 100 degrees C to stop the crystal growth.

Synthetic Routes Using Air-Stable Cd-Based Precursors

The procedure described here represents one of several variations developed and used by various research groups. This protocol is optimized for the condition described earlier. However, other comparable precursors, including CdO and cadmium acetate, can also be used as Cd precursors.

1. Prepare 1M stock solution of trioctylphosphine selenide (TOP:Se) by dissolving 7.9g of Se (99.99 percent) into 100 mL of TOP (90–95 percent). A 1.5 or 2M solution of TOP:Se could also be used, but this higher concentration must be taken into account when adding Se precursors to the reaction mixture.
2. Load TOPO (20g), hexadecylamine (10g), and TOP (5 mL) into 100-mL three-neck round bottom flask, fitted with a thermocouple temperature sensor, condenser, and a nitrogen/vacuum inlet adapter, and heat to 120–140 degrees C under vacuum for 1 to 2 hours. This step removes water and oxygen from the solution.
3. As the content of the round bottom flask is degassed, mix $Cd(acac)_2$ (620 mg), 1,2-hexadecanediol, HDDO, (1.2g), and TOP (10 mL) in a separate 20 mL vial, and heat to 100 degrees C under vacuum. The solution should become homogeneous after ~30 minutes.
4. Let the mixture cool to approximately 80 degrees C and add 10 mL of 1 M TOP:Se (or 5 mL of 2 M TOP:Se) and mix thoroughly.
5. Switch the atmosphere in the three-neck flask to nitrogen and raise the temperature to 340–350 degrees C.
6. Transfer the TOP:Se mixture to a syringe equipped with a large gauge needle, and rapidly inject the solution mixture of cadmium and selenium precursors into the hot flask containing the coordinating solvent; then quickly cool the mixture down to ~100–200 degrees C. This prevents further growth of the nanoparticles.
7. The resulting nanoparticles can be either collected for subsequent processing and use or further grown to larger sizes with additional heating to 250–280 degrees C for several minutes.
8. The solution is then cooled to 60–80 degrees C, mixed with toluene (or hexane) and butanol, and centrifuged to remove any unreacted metal salts and other impurities.
9. Purification is carried out using a solution mixture with excess methanol or ethanol followed by centrifugation and removal of the supernatant.

Overcoating the Native Cores with a Thin Layer of ZnS

Following the initial progress made in high temperature QD synthesis, it was demonstrated that passivating the native QD cores with a layer of wider band gap material(s) could dramatically enhance the PL quantum yield of the resulting core-shell nanocrystals. Although the concept was previously known from work on band gap engineering in semiconductors [73, 74], the optimal set of conditions for creating strongly fluorescent overcoated QDs was not realized until 1996, when Hines and Guyot-Sionnnest showed that overcoating CdSe QDs with ZnS could improve the PL quantum yields to values of 30 percent or higher [41]. The complete reaction conditions for preparing a series of core-shell nanoparticles that are strongly fluorescent and stable were further detailed in two comprehensive reports by Dabbousi et al. [42], and Peng et al. [49]. We should also stress the fact that as for core-only synthesis, air-stable precursors were used for the overcoating reactions by various groups (e.g., see [46]), following the reports by Peng and coworkers on the synthesis of CdS, CdSe nanocrystals [21, 43]. Here we describe the reactions used in [41, 42].

For overcoating CdSe with a thin layer of ZnS or CdS, the temperature of a solution containing CdSe QDs mixed with TOPO is raised to ~150 degrees C but kept lower than 200 degrees C to prevent further growth of the QDs. A dilute solution of Zn (or Cd) and S precursors is then slowly introduced into the hot stirring QD solution (see schematics in Figure 1.4). The amount of Zn and S precursors added varies depending on the size of the CdSe QD and is calculated to yield a 2–6 atomic monolayer coverage on the nanoparticle surface. The high dilution and relatively low temperature of the mixture prevent separate nucleation of ZnS or CdS quantum dots. Once the precursors have been added, the temperature is lowered to ~80 degrees C. The reaction vessel can be left undisturbed for several hours, as this annealing was shown to produce noticeable improvements in the PL quantum yield [42].

A typical laboratory scale ZnS overcoating process for CdSe QDs includes the following steps [42]:

1. Mount a round-bottom flask (100 or 250 mL) with a pressure equalizing addition funnel.
2. Load 20–30g of TOPO into the round bottom flask and dry/degas at 120–140 degrees C for two to three hours under vacuum.
3. Add purified CdSe QD solution (dispersed in hexane or toluene) at 70–80 degrees C to a final Cd concentration of ~0.1–0.5 mM.
4. Evaporate the solvent under vacuum.
5. Increase the temperature of the QD/TOPO solution to between 140 degrees C and 180 degrees C, depending on the initial core radius (lower temperatures are used for smaller core sizes).
6. Separately, to a vial containing 4–5 mL of TOP, add equimolar amounts of diethylzinc ($ZnEt_2$) and hexamethyldisilathiane (TMS_2S) precursor that correspond to the desired overcoating layer for the appropriate CdSe nanocrystal radius. Use an inert atmosphere (e.g., glove box) to carry out this step since $ZnEt_2$ is highly reactive with oxygen and water.
7. Load the Zn and S precursor solution from step 6 into a syringe (inside the glove box) and transfer the content to the addition funnel.
8. Slowly add the Zn and S precursor solution to the QD/TOPO solution at a rate of about 0.3–0.5 mL/min.
9. Once the addition is complete, lower the solution temperature to 80 degrees C and leave the mixture stirring for several hours.
10. Cool down the flask content, then add ~10 mL of butanol and hexanes and precipitate the ZnS-overcoated QDs with methanol to recover the QD product by centrifugation.

We should remark that an extra annealing step carried out postovercoating is recommended, as this often produces an improvement in the quality, stability, and PL quantum yield of the final core-shell nanocrystals.

Purification of the Nanocrystals

Size selective precipitation can be applied to core-only as well as to core-shell nanocrystals as a means of removing extra unreacted metals and ligands and obtaining narrow size distribution. This involves adding a nonsolvent (bad solvent) mixture for the TOP/TOPO-capped nanocrystals [39, 51]. This method is widely employed for polymers and colloids to reduce polydispersity after synthesis. The absorption spectra of core-shell QDs are usually not as well resolved as those measured for core only, in particular for samples using thick overcoating shells. Furthermore, the photoluminescence experiences a slight red shift combined with slight broadening compared with what is measured for the initial core-only nanocrystals. Shifts of the emission are usually more pronounced for lower band gap overcoating materials, such as CdS and ZnSe versus ZnS. A smaller mismatch between the crystal structures of the core and shell presumably allow smoother surface structures and potentially more epitaxial growth of the shell layer [42]. These changes are expected and often attributed to leakage of the exciton wavefunction outside the native core to within the overcoating shell. It is also caused by a slight broadening of the size distributions of the initial nanocrystals since overcoating is carried at relatively high temperatures.

1.3 Strategies for Surface-Functionalization and Conjugation to Biomolecules

1.3.1 Water-Solubilization Strategies

The easiest and most obvious approach to prepare water-soluble QDs is to grow the nanocrystals directly in aqueous environments using inverse micelles or coprecipitation as reported for some CdTe nanocrystals [75]. However, most highly luminescent QDs that have found effective use in biological studies are prepared using high-temperature solution routes and are essentially capped with TOP/TOPO ligands mixed with small fractions of amine and carboxyl molecules. They thus require use of water solubilization strategies to make them compatible with biological environments. Several strategies aimed at achieving this goal have been developed since the first reports on developing colloidal QDs as biological labels were published [76–78]. These strategies can essentially be loosely divided in two main categories: ligand-exchange and encapsulation (see Table 1.3) [5].

1.3.1.1 Ligand Exchange

This method involves the replacement of the original hydrophobic surface ligands (TOP/TOPO and such) with bi- and/or multifunctional hydrophilic ligands. The hydrophilic ligands are usually comprised of anchor group(s) for binding to the inorganic nanocrystal surface (typically via a thiol group) at one end. At the other end the ligands present hydrophilic groups (carboxyl, amine, or poly(ethylene glycol)) that promote affinity to aqueous solutions.

Cap exchange with molecular-scale ligands has been attempted by several groups in the past decade, because of its ease of implementation. The most commonly reported examples used monothiol-terminated alkyl carboxylic acids, including mercaptoacetic acid (MAA) [77, 79], mercaptopropionic acid (MPA) [79, 80], mercaptoundecanoic acid (MUA) [79, 81], poly(ethylene glycol) derivatives [82–85], and cysteine [86, 87]; most of these ligands are commercially available. Though the cap exchange strategy with these ligands is straightforward, the stabil-

Table 1.3 Surface-Functionalization Methods Reported in the Literature

Surface Capping Strategies	*Preparation Method*	*Literature Citation*
Ligand exchange	(i) Single thiol	
	Mercaptoacetic acid (MAA)	[77, 79]
	Mercaptopropionic acid (MPA)	[79, 80]
	Mercaptoundecanoic acid (MUA)	[79, 81]
	PEG derivatives	[82–85]
	Cysteine	[86, 87]
	Dendron	[88, 89]
	(ii) Multiple thiols	
	Dihydrolipoic acid (DHLA)	[78]
	DHLA–PEG conjugates	[90, 92, 93]
	(iii) Peptides	[94, 95]
	(iv) Oligomeric phosphine (oxide)	[96, 97]
	(v) Amines	[98–100, 112]
	(vi) Silica coating	[76, 101, 113]
Encapsulation	(i) Di- or triblock copolymers	[102–106, 114, 115]
	(ii) Phospholipids	[107, 108]
	(iii) Calixarene derivatives	[109–111, 116]

ity of the resulting QDs in buffer solutions is often poor. For instance, with MAA, MPA, and MUA, the nanocrystals tend to progressively aggregate in physiological conditions within a relatively short period of time concomitant with a decrease of fluorescence quantum yield. This is most likely due to desorption of the ligands from the QD surface [5]. Peng and coworkers tried to resolve this problem by preparing hydroxyl-terminated dendron ligands that were also end-fucntionalized with thiol groups to promote anchoring on the QD surface [88]. In a subsequent study, they used amine-terminated dendrimers for cap exchange, which allowed cross-linking of the ligands to form "dendron-boxed" QDs [89]. Another approach to addressing the long-term stability of QDs prepared via cap exchange relied on the use of bidentate thiol ligands such as dihydrolipoic acid (DHLA) [78]. These bidentate-thiol ligands have significantly improved the stability of the QDs in aqueous environments, as DHLA-capped nanocrystals could reproducibly be made stable in aqueous buffer solutions with usable lifetimes of several months. Most of the thiol-terminated ligands mentioned earlier (e.g., MAA, MPA, MUA, and DHLA) have carboxyl terminal groups, and water-solubility of the QDs relies on deprotonation of the carboxyl groups, which has limited the ability of preparing homogeneously dispersed solutions of QDs in acidic pHs [5, 78]. To overcome these pH limitations, we have recently developed a new set of DHLA ligand derivatives, where poly(ethylene glycol) (PEG) segments with variable chain-lengths were appended onto dihydrolipoic acid via an ester linkage [90]. Our results showed that QDs capped with DHLA–PEG ligands are well dispersed in aqueous media and stable over an extended period of time and over a relatively broad pH range from weakly acidic to strongly basic conditions. The DHLA-PEG-capped nanocrystals additionally benefited from the strong anchoring provided by the dithiol end groups, and were also compact in size [91]. PEGs are known for low toxicity and also minimize nonspecific binding with biological molecules [2]. The physiological compatibility of PEG-coated QDs is thus very promising for various cellular assays. Moreover, the long-term stability of the QDs has a significant impact not only for in vitro biological assays but also for cellular tracking experiments.

More recently, the terminal groups of DHLA–PEG ligands were further improved by functionalization with additional bioreactive groups, such as biotin, amine, and carboxyl groups to promote bioconjugation of the QDs capped with DHLA–PEG ligands [92, 93]. Overall, this design provided modular ligand structures, containing a PEG single chain with variable size to promote water solubility, a DHLA at one end of the PEG chain for strong anchoring onto the QD surface, and a biological functional group at the other end of the PEG (see Figure 1.7). These QDs have indeed demonstrated easy access to biological molecules through avidin-biotin binding or EDC (1-ethyl-3-(3-dimethylaminopropyl)carbodiimide) coupling [92, 93].

In a somewhat different rationale that utilizes a similar process, Weiss and coworkers have used phytochelatin-related peptides having multiple terminal-repeats of cysteines for anchoring on QDs [94, 95]. This strategy has a few unique advantages. Similar to DHLA, it relies on the multidentate thiol interactions with the inorganic surface of the nanocrystals, which improves the stability of the ligand/QD system. In addition, using peptides as the actual ligands makes it possible

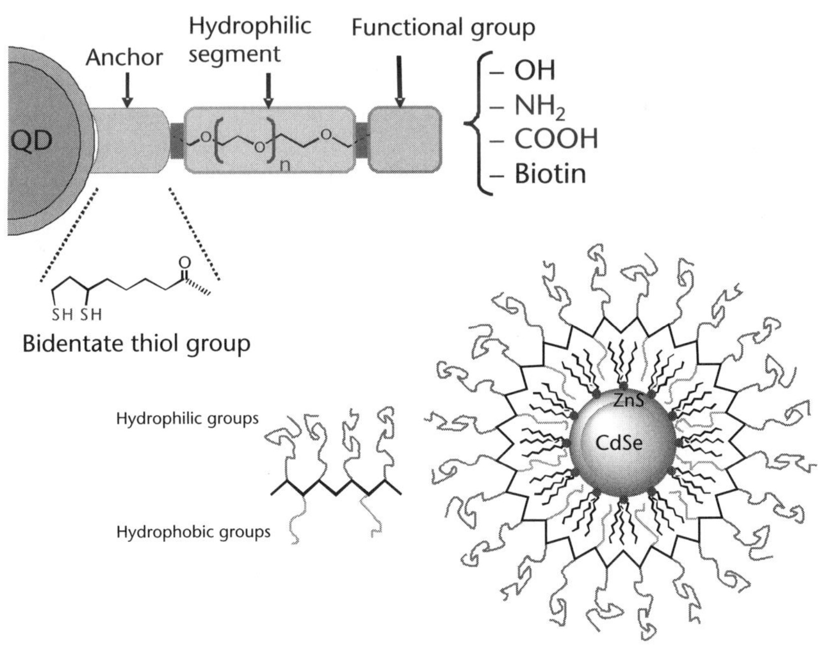

Figure 1.7 (top) Schematic representation of a QD capped with modular hydrophilic ligands based on the DHLA motif. Each ligand molecule has a central tunable length PEG segment, an anchoring dithiol head, and a terminal functional group that can be chemically modified. Reproduced from [92], with permission from the American Chemical Society. (bottom) Schematic representation of the strategy based on encapsulation of QDs with di-block copolymer shell. The polymer chain contains hydrophobic and hydrophilic blocks. The hydrophobic block is expected to strongly interact with the TOP/TOPO cap while the hydrophilic block promotes compatibility with aqueous environments. (See Color Plate 2.)

to combine improved affinity to aqueous media and potential biological targeting. Peptide structure and length can potentially be modified and controlled. The authors have applied these peptide-coated nanocrystals in various functional assays ranging from live cell imaging to FRET (see Chapter 3 by Bentolia et al.). One of the potential limitations, however, is the need for rather large amounts of peptide ligands to carry out an effective cap exchange, as this process is mass-action driven and necessitates a large excess of ligands for effective cap exchange. Preparation of large amounts of peptides is time consuming and can be rather costly.

Another attempt aimed at improving the stability of hydrophilic QDs prepared via cap-exchange strategy was reported by Bawendi and coworkers, who have described the synthesis of oligomeric phosphine (oxide) ligands comprised of an inner phosphine layer, a linking layer between the phosphines and an outer functionalized "network" [96, 97]. The inner phosphine layer served to passivate and protect the QD surface, while the outer layer was functionalized with carboxyl or PEG groups to promote water solubility. Though this approach uses phosphine anchoring groups, which are similar to the native TOP/TOPO, synthesis and purification of the ligands is tedious. In other studies, several groups used amine-rich polymers to functionalize the QD surfaces. Nann showed phase transfer of QDs into water using amphiphilic hyperbranched polyethyleneimine [98]. Nie and coworkers suggested that poly(ethylene glycol)-grafted polyethylenimine could provide the ability to realize endosome-disrupting surface coatings for QDs [99]. Winnik and coworkers used a poly(ethylene glycol-*b*-2-*N*,*N*-dimethylaminoethyl methacrylate) (PEG-*b*-PDMA) diblock copolymer, in which the DMA groups served as multidentate anchoring sites on core only CdSe QDs [100]. These examples rely on the availability of multiple amine groups for anchoring on the QD surface, due to weak binding of single amine groups. In both cases the authors concluded that the polymer removes the native TOP/TOPO shell due to the affinity of amines groups to inorganic ZnS and CdS surfaces, which makes their approach in essence a cap-exchange method.

The first reported study introducing the use of QDs in biology by Alivisatos and coworkers used QDs cap-exchanged with thiol-terminated silane ligands, followed by further cross-linking to form a silica shell coating as a means to enhance stability and promote hydrophilicity of CdSe-CdS(ZnS) core-shell nanocrystals [76, 101]. The "silica-shell coating" method is conceptually a very effective method for surface passivation due to the robustness of silica; it also provides the option of adding functional groups onto the shell for further functionalization. This strategy is, however, time consuming and control of the shell growth is difficult.

Studies with the DHLA-PEG-amine and DHLA-PEG-carboxyl ligands indicate that thiol-binding to the QD surface is stronger than amine and carboxyl groups when both end groups are presented on the same ligands [92, 93]. With this strategy, the nature of the anchoring group to the QD surface (e.g., monodentate versus multidentate) can make a substantial difference in terms of the long-term stability of the hydrophilic QDs; stability of the QD-ligand interactions is substantially improved with multidentate capping molecules. The cap exchange strategy maintains the QD size compact, and this is especially true for molecular-scale ligands. This can be crucial for fluorescence resonance energy transfer (FRET) assays with

QDs since close proximity between energy donor and acceptor is directly correlated to the energy transfer efficiency (see Chapter 4).

1.3.1.2 Encapsulation within Block Copolymer Shells and Phospholipid Micelles

This method uses bifunctional amphiphilic molecules having distinct hydrophobic and hydrophilic segments (Figure 1.7). The hydrophobic units selectively interact and interdigitate with the native TOP/TOPO shell, while the hydrophilic units interact with the aqueous environment, thus promoting dispersion of the QD in aqueous media. Water solubility of the resulting QDs is mostly ensured by the presence of charged groups (such as amine or carboxyl groups) and/or poly(ethylene glycol) (PEG) chains within the hydrophilic units.

Di- and triblock copolymers have been widely used as the amphiphilic coating shell for QDs coated with original hydrophobic ligands [102–105]. Generally, these polymers have a poly(acrylic acid) main chain, where substitution of some of the carboxyl groups with alkyl chains allows a controlled balance of hydrophobic and hydrophilic blocks within the polymers. This balance is crucial for stabilization of the polymer coating on the TOP/TOPO-cap and promotion of water solubility of the resulting QDs. Wu and coworkers used a block copolymer shell consisting of 40 percent octylamine-modified polyacrylic acid [102]. The latter is currently used with commercial QDs offered by Invitrogen (www.invitrogen.com). Pellegrino and coworkers used poly(maleic anhydride alt-1-tetradecene) for QD encapsulation [106]. Following adsorption on the TOP/TOPO QDs, further addition of bis(6-aminohexyl)amine formed cross-linked polymers on the QDs. Hydrolysis of the unreacted anhydride units made the QDs water soluble. The use of block copolymers can take advantage of the wealth of knowledge about block copolymers gained over the years and the ability to form sophisticated phases and structures that can be controlled on the nanoscale. Nonetheless, the resulting hydrophilic nanoparticles inevitably have rather large sizes [4, 5]. Further, the affinity for the QD surface may not be very strong, as the polymer shell could swell or shrink depending on natural paramaters such pH and ionic strength of the surrounding media.

The second encapsulation method employed phospholipid derivatives, which formed micelles. In particular, the first demonstration of this strategy was reported by Dubertret and coworkers, who used phospholipids containing 40 percent 1,2-dipalmitoyl-*sn*-glycero-3-phosphoethanolamine-N-[methoxy(polyethylene glycol)-2000] (mPEG-2000 PE) and 60 percent of 1,2-dipalmitoylglycero-3-phosphocholine (DPPC) to carry out encapsulation of CdSe-ZnS QDs and their transfer to buffer solutions. This technique is simple to implement, as most phopholipids are commercially available (though not reasonably cheap) [107, 108]. Nanocrystals prepared via this route were stable in embryonic cells and did not show measurable toxicity effects. However, this strategy has some of the stability issues at very low concentrations encountered by micelles in general. In addition, it is possible that more than a single nanocrystal could be contained within each micelle.

Cyclic molecules such as calixarene have also been demonstrated as potential compact surface coating materials. Jin et al. used calix[4]arene with carboxylic acid groups for QD coating, and successfully prepared compact CdSe-ZnS QDs (<10 nm in diameter) [109]. They also reported that the emission peaks of QDs can be shifted to longer wavelengths with increasing the ring size of the calix[*n*]arene used ($n = 4$, 6, 8) [110]. CdSe QDs coated with calixarene analogues with alkyl chains and saccharide moieties were also employed as endosome markers [111].

Each surface-functionalization strategy has both inherent advantages and disadvantages. In particular, the cap exchange approach is simple and can be versatile in light of recently developed reproducible methods for the synthesis of modular ligands such as DHLA–PEG–FN motifs, where the PEG chain length can be tuned and the terminal functional groups (FN) can be varied (see Figure 1.7). It also provides compact-size nanocrystals. It does, however, tend to produce QDs with decreased PL quantum yields compared to the native TOP/TOPO-capped nanocrystals. Encapsulation approaches on the other hand can produce nanocrystals with higher quantum yields, because it is expected that this method keeps the native ligands attached to the QD surface. This method, however, tends to produce rather large nanocrystals and does not allow for control over the number of encapsulating chains wrapped around a given QD and the number of reactive groups available for further functionalization. Thus, when applied, the advantages of each strategy need to be carefully balanced against potential drawbacks.

1.3.2 Methods for Conjugating QDs with Biomolecular Receptors

Strategies reported thus far for conjugating hydrophilic QDs to biomolecular receptors can essentially be divided into three groups (see Figure 1.8): (1) The first employs the common EDC (1-ethyl-3-(3-dimethylaminopropyl)carbodiimide) coupling of carboxyl groups on the QD surface and target amines on biological entities such as peptides, proteins, and antibodies [92, 93, 99, 102]. (2) The second employs metal-affinity driven self-assembly using either thiolated peptides or polyhistidine (His)-appended tracts and noncovalent self-assembly using engineered proteins [94, 117]; metal-affinity driven self-assembly is versatile and has a high binding constant ($K_{Dissociation} \sim 10^{-10}$-$10^{-8}$ M) [117]. (3) Avidin-biotin binding, which involves the use of an avidin (or streptavidin) bridge between two biotinylated biomolecules (peptides and proteins), can benefit from the strong avidin-biotin binding ($K_{Dissociation} \sim 10^{-15}$ M) [2]. Each conjugation technique has certain advantages but also a few limitations, as remarked earlier for water-solubilization strategies. For example, EDC condensation applied to QDs capped with thiol-alkyl-COOH ligands often produces intermediate aggregates due to poor QD stability in neutral and acidic buffers [5, 78]. However, insertion of a PEG segment between the thiol anchoring group and COOH groups (modular ligands) has successfully allowed EDC coupling to QDs [92]. This constraint can also be removed by using QDs capped with functional peptides, where solubility is now driven by the peptide ligands [94]. EDC coupling has also been applied to QDs encapsulated with polymeric shells bearing COOH groups [102]. It can however produce large conjugates with less control over the number of biomolecules per QD-bioconjugate. This approach has been used by Invitrogen to prepare QD-Streptavidin conjugates having ~20 proteins per QD. Due to the rather large number of charges on these QD-conjugates, care must be paid to the fact that they can bind all biotinylated proteins in the sample and may result in

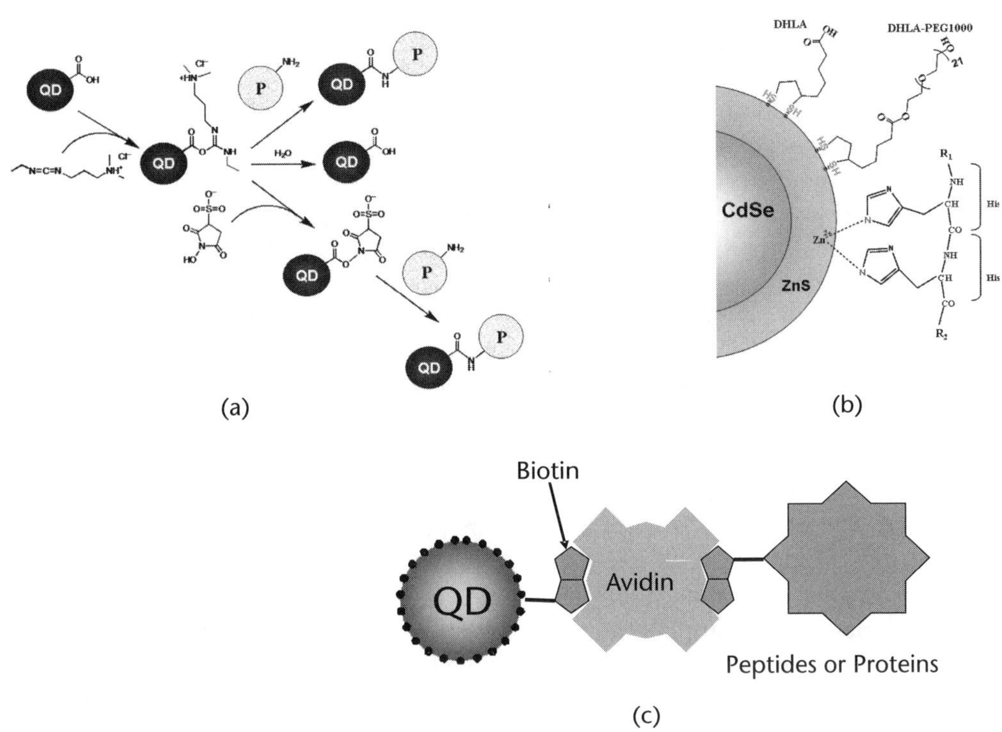

Figure 1.8 Schematic representations of three conjugation techniques described in this chapter: (a) EDC coupling between carboxyl terminal groups on the QD coating and amines on target biomolecules. (b) Self-assembly driven by metal-histidine interactions. For the metal-His conjugation DHLA and DHLA-PEG ligands are shown on the QD surface; R_1 or R_2 designate the N- or C-termini of a peptide or a protein. (c) Avidin–biotin bridging through avidin between biotin-functionalized QDs and biotinylated target protein and peptides. Reproduced partially from [117], with permission from the American Chemical Society.

aggregate formation. Self-assembly of peptides/proteins onto the QD using, for example, metal-histidine driven interactions can reduce aggregation and permit control over the bioconjugate valence. However, it still requires that the bioreceptor is engineered with the desired His-tag before use. Furthermore, we have shown in a recent study that this conjugation strategy also requires that the His tract is extended/exposed laterally for direct interactions with the nanocrystal surface [117]. For instance, QDs capped with DHLA-PEG (MW ~600 and ~1000) could not allow self-assembly of QDs with His_5-appended proteins, due to steric hindrance, even though conjugation to peptides was effective regardless of the His-tag length [117].

1.4 Concluding Remarks and Future Outlook

In their early days, quantum dots were somewhat of a novelty in the field of low-dimensional semiconductor physics. The last two decades have witnessed a tremendous scientific interest and progress in understanding the fundamental properties of these materials and in developing techniques to make them better. This was prompted by the realization that these materials are of great conceptual and technological interests. There has also been a drive to develop and commercialize various technological applications.

Advances in the synthesis and characterization of luminescent and nonluminescent QDs have provided a wide array of nanocrystals with a range of unique properties (optical and spectroscopic, metallic, and magnetic properties). In particular, there has been a clear progress in developing reproducible synthetic routes for making high-quality luminescent QDs emitting over a broad range of wavelengths and dispersible in solution phases. The high temperature solution reaction route (originally developed by Bawendi and coworkers but rapidly expanded by his and other groups including Alivisatos and his groups, Murray and coworkers and Peng and coworkers) was shown to be extremely versatile. The reaction scheme and variation of that scheme have now allowed making of QDs with a wide range of material combinations. It has been further expanded to making magnetic nanoparticles (e.g., see Chapter 2, Chapter 10, and Chapter 11).

Development of luminescent QDs as biological probes, for example, has rapidly grown in the past decade. Clearly these materials offer a great potential for use in a whole array of applications such as in vivo cellular and tissue imaging. Fluorescence-based cellular and tissue imaging and sensing using direct one- and two-photon excitation, or FRET, are the areas where QDs should experience substantial development and expansion. For example, multiplexed and two-photon driven FRET have been explored in proof-of-concept demonstrations, but applications in real in vivo set have been rather scarce.

Despite the remarkable progress made for QD use in biology (described, for example, in Chapter 3 by Bentolia et al., Chapter 4 by Medintz et al., and Chapter 6 by Pons et al.), there still remain several issues that are not fully solved yet, and understanding and eventually solving them will increase their utility in biology. These issues can be summarized in the following order: (1) Still needed are improvement and likely consolidation of most available water-solubilization strategies into a simple scheme able to provide QDs that are stable in a wide range of biologically relevant conditions (acidic and basic pHs, excess salt, and so on). (2) Still needed are improvement and simplification of the conjugation strategies reported by various groups. This will require a coordinated effort to develop simple and reproducible conjugation schemes, capable of providing compact multifunctional conjugates. (3) Due to the unavailability of a simple and general strategy that allows effective translocation of QDs across the cell membrane and into the cytoplasm, more effort geared toward developing easy-to-implement approaches for intracellular delivery is needed.

Acknowledgments

The authors acknowledge the NRL and the Office of Naval Research, the Army Research Office, and the DTRA for support.

References

[1] Schröck, E., et al., "Multicolor Spectral Karyotyping of Human Chromosomes," *Science*, Vol. 273, 1996, pp. 494–497.

[2] Hermanson, G. T., *Bioconjugate Techniques*, San Diego: Academic Press, 1996.

[3] Roederer, M., et al., "8 Color, 10-parameter flow cytometry to elucidate complex leukocyte heterogeneity," *Cytometry*, Vol. 29, 1997, pp. 328–339.

[4] Michalet, X., et al., "Quantum Dots for Live Cells, in vivo Imaging, and Diagnostics," *Science*, Vol. 307, 2005, pp. 538–544.

[5] Medintz, I. L., et al., "Quantum dot bioconjugates for imaging, labelling and sensing," *Nat. Mater.*, Vol. 4, 2005, pp. 435–446.

[6] Mattoussi, H., et al., *Colloidal Semiconductor Quantum Dot Conjugates in Biosensing*, In: *Optical Biosensors: Present and Future.* Edited by Ligler, F. S. and C. A. Rowe Taitt. Amsterdam, The Netherlands: Elsevier: 2002, 537–569.

[7] Hotz, C. Z. and M. Bruchez (eds.): Quantum Dots: Applications in Biology. Totowa, NJ: Humana Press, 2007.

[8] Alivisatos, P., "The use of nanocrystals in biological detection," *Nat. Biotechnol.*, Vol. 22, 2004, pp. 47–52.

[9] Murray, C. B., C. R. Kagan and M. G. Bawendi, "Synthesis and Characterization of Monodisperse Nanocrystals and Close-Packed Nanocrystal Assemblies," *Annu. Rev. Mater. Sci.*, Vol. 30, 2000, pp. 545–610.

[10] Efros, A. L. and M. Rosen, "The Electronic Structure of Semiconductor Nanocrystals," *Annu. Rev. Mater. Sci.*, Vol. 30, 2000, pp. 475–521.

[11] Klimov, V. I., "Mechanisms for Photogeneration and Recombination of Multiexcitons in Semiconductor Nanocrystals: Implications for Lasing and Solar Energy Conversion," *J. Phys. Chem. B*, Vol. 110, 2006, pp. 16827–16845.

[12] Hines, M. A. and P. Guyot-Sionnest, "Bright UV-Blue Luminescent Colloidal ZnSe Nanocrystals," *J. Phys. Chem. B*, Vol. 102, 1998, pp. 3655–3657.

[13] Weller, H., et al., "Photochemistry of colloidal semiconductors. Onset of light absorption as a function of size of extremely small CdS particles," *Chem. Phys. Lett.*, Vol. 124, 1986, pp. 557–560.

[14] Murray, C. B., et al., "Colloidal synthesis of nanocrystals and nanocrystal superlattices," *IBM J. Res. Dev.*, Vol. 45, 2001, pp. 47–56.

[15] Pietryga, J. M., et al., "Pushing the Band Gap Envelope: Mid-Infrared Emitting Colloidal PbSe Quantum Dots," *J. Am. Chem. Soc.*, Vol. 126, 2004, pp. 11752–11753.

[16] Yoffe, A. D., "Low-dimensional systems: quantum size effects and electronic properties of semiconductor microcrystallites (zero-dimensional systems) and some quasi-two-dimensional systems," *Adv. Phys.*, Vol. 42, 1993, pp. 173–262.

[17] Peng, X. and J. Thessing, *Controlled Synthesis of High Quality Semiconductor Nanocrystals*, In: *Semiconductor Nanocrystals and Silicate Nanoparticles,* Vol. 118, Berlin: Springer Berlin / Heidelberg: 2005, 79–119.

[18] Gaponenko, S. V., *Optical Properties of Semiconductor Nanocrystals*, Vol. 23, Cambridge: Cambridge University Press, 1998.

[19] Yoffe, A. D., "Semiconductor quantum dots and related systems: electronic, optical, luminescence and related properties of low dimensional systems," *Adv. Phys.*, Vol. 50, 2001, pp. 1–208.

[20] Kippeny, T., L. A. Swafford and S. J. Rosenthal, "Semiconductor Nanocrystals: A Powerful Visual Aid for Introducing the Particle in a Box," *J. Chem. Educ.*, Vol. 79, 2002, pp. 1094–1100.

[21] Peng, Z. A. and X. Peng, "Formation of High-Quality CdTe, CdSe, and CdS Nanocrystals Using CdO as Precursor," *J. Am. Chem. Soc.*, Vol. 123, 2001, pp. 183–184.

[22] Norris, D. J. and M. G. Bawendi, "Measurement and assignment of the size-dependent optical spectrum in CdSe quantum dots," *Phys. Rev. B*, Vol. 53, 1996, pp. 16338–16346.

[23] Nirmal, M., et al., "Fluorescence intermittency in single cadmium selenide nanocrystals," *Nature*, Vol. 383, 1996, pp. 802–804.

[24] Dahan, M., et al., "Diffusion Dynamics of Glycine Receptors Revealed by Single-Quantum Dot Tracking," *Science*, Vol. 302, 2003, pp. 442–445.

[25] Chepic, D. I., et al., "Auger ionization of semiconductor quantum drops in a glass matrix," *J. Lumin.*, Vol. 47, 1990, pp. 113–127.

[26] Efros, A. L. and M. Rosen, "Random Telegraph Signal in the Photoluminescence Intensity of a Single Quantum Dot," *Phys. Rev. Lett.*, Vol. 78, 1997, pp. 1110–1113.

[27] Ekimov, A. I., A. A. Onushchenko and V. A. Tsekhomskii, "Exciton absorption by copper(I) chloride crystals in a glassy matrix," *Fiz. Khim. Stekla*, Vol. 6, 1980, pp. 511–512.

[28] Ekimov, A. I. and A. A. Onushchenko, "Quantum size effect in three-dimensional microscopic semiconductor crystals," *JETP Lett.*, Vol. 34, 1981, pp. 345–349.

[29] Ekimov, A. I. and A. A. Onushchenko, "Quantum Size Effect in the Optical-Spectra of Semiconductor Micro-Crystals," *Sov. Phys. Semicond.*, Vol. 16, 1982, pp. 775–778.

[30] Ekimov, A. I. and A. A. Onushchenko, "Size quantization of the electron energy spectrum in a microscopic semiconductor crystal," *JETP Lett.*, Vol. 40, 1984, pp. 337–340.

[31] Ekimov, A. I., et al., "Size quantization of excitons and determination of their energy spectrum parameters in cuprous chloride," *Sov. Phys. JETP*, Vol. 88, 1985, pp. 1490–1501.

[32] Ekimov, A. I., A. L. Efros and A. A. Onushchenko, "Quantum size effect in semiconductor microcrystals," *Solid State Commun.*, Vol. 56, 1985, pp. 921–924.

[33] Ekimov, A. I., et al., "Absorption and intensity-dependent photoluminescence measurements on CdSe quantum dots: Assignment of the first electronic transitions," *J. Opt. Soc. Am. B*, Vol. 10, 1993, pp. 100–107.

[34] Ekimov, A., "Growth and optical properties of semiconductor nanocrystals in a glass matrix," *J. Lumin.*, Vol. 70, 1996, pp. 1–20.

[35] Borrelli, N. F., et al., "Quantum confinement effects of semiconducting microcrystallites in glass," *J. Appl. Phys.*, Vol. 61, 1987, pp. 5399–5409.

[36] Henglein, A., "Photodegradation and fluorescence of colloidal cadmium sulfide in aqueous solution," *Ber. Bunsen-Ges. Phys. Chem.*, Vol. 86, 1982, pp. 301–305.

[37] Rossetti, R., S. Nakahara and L. E. Brus, "Quantum size effects in the redox potentials, resonance Raman spectra, and electronic spectra of CdS crystallites in aqueous solution," *J. Chem. Phys.*, Vol. 79, 1983, pp. 1086–1088.

[38] Rossetti, R., et al., "Size effects in the excited electronic states of small colloidal CdS crystallites," *J. Chem. Phys.*, Vol. 80, 1984, pp. 4464–4469.

[39] Murray, C. B., D. J. Norris and M. G. Bawendi, "Synthesis and Characterization of Nearly Monodisperse CdE (E=S, Se, Te) Semiconductor Nanocrystallites," *J. Am. Chem. Soc.*, Vol. 115, 1993, pp. 8706–8715.

[40] Bowen Katari, J. E., V. L. Colvin and A. P. Alivisatos, "X-ray Photoemission Spectroscopy of CdSe Nanocrystals with Applications to Studies of the Nanocrystal Surface," *J. Phys. Chem.*, Vol. 98, 1994, pp. 4109–4117.

[41] Hines, M. A. and P. Guyot-Sionnest, "Synthesis and Characterization of Strongly Luminescing ZnS-Capped CdSe Nanocrystals," *J. Phys. Chem.*, Vol. 100, 1996, pp. 468–471.

[42] Dabbousi, B. O., et al., "(CdSe)ZnS Core-Shell Quantum Dots: Synthesis and Characterization of a Size Series of Highly Luminescent Nanocrystallites," *J. Phys. Chem. B*, Vol. 101, 1997, pp. 9463–9475.

[43] Qu, L., Z. A. Peng and X. Peng, "Alternative Routes toward High Quality CdSe Nanocrystals," *Nano Lett.*, Vol. 1, 2001, pp. 333–337.

[44] Du, H., et al., "Optical Properties of Colloidal PbSe Nanocrystals," *Nano Lett.*, Vol. 2, 2002, pp. 1321–1324.

[45] Yu, W. W., et al., "Preparation and Characterization of Monodisperse PbSe Semiconductor Nanocrystals in a Noncoordinating Solvent," *Chem. Mater.*, Vol. 16, 2004, pp. 3318–3322.

[46] Reiss, P., J. Bleuse and A. Pron, "Highly Luminescent CdSe/ZnSe Core/Shell Nanocrystals of Low Size Dispersion," *Nano Lett.*, Vol. 2, 2002, pp. 781–784.

[47] Wehrenberg, B. L., C. Wang and P. Guyot-Sionnest, "Interband and Intraband Optical Studies of PbSe Colloidal Quantum Dots," *J. Phys. Chem. B*, Vol. 106, 2002, pp. 10634–10640.

[48] Gaponenko, S. V. and U. Woggon, *ZnSe, HgS, CdS, (Zn,Cd)S, (Zn,Mn)S, ZnS, CdO, ZnO quantum dots-nanocrystals: II-VI Quantum dots I - Nanocrystals*, In: *Optical Properties, Part 2,* Vol. 34C2, Berlin: Springer Berlin Heidelberg: 2004, 284–347.

[49] Peng, X., et al., "Epitaxial Growth of Highly Luminescent CdSe/CdS Core/Shell Nanocrystals with Photostability and Electronic Accessibility," *J. Am. Chem. Soc.*, Vol. 119, 1997, pp. 7019–7029.

[50] Mattoussi, H., et al., "Characterization of CdSe Nanocrystallite Dispersions by Small Angle X-ray Scattering," *J. Chem. Phys.,* Vol 105, 1996, pp. 9890–9896

[51] Mattoussi, H., et al., "Properties of CdSe nanocrystal dispersions in the dilute regime: Structure and interparticle interactions," *Phys. Rev. B*, Vol. 58, 1998, pp. 7850–7863.

[52] Gublin, S. P., N. A. Kataeva and G. B. Khomutov, "Promising avenues of research in nanoscience: chemistry of semiconductor nanoparticles," *Russ. Chem. Bull., Int. Ed.*, Vol. 54, 2005, pp. 827–852.

[53] Peng, Z. A. and X. Peng, "Mechanisms of the Shape Evolution of CdSe Nanocrystals," *J. Am. Chem. Soc.*, Vol. 123, 2001, pp. 1389–1395.

[54] Potter Jr., B. G. and J. H. Simmons, "Quantum size effects in optical properties of CdS-glass composites," *Phys. Rev. B*, Vol. 37, 1988, pp. 10838–10845.

[55] Liu, L.-C. and S. H. Risbud, "Quantum-dot size-distribution analysis and precipitation stages in semiconductor doped glasses," *J. Appl. Phys.*, Vol. 68, 1990, pp. 28–32.

[56] Zhao, X. S., et al., "Resonant-Raman-scattering and photoluminescence studies in glass-composite and colloidal CdS," *Phys. Rev. B*, Vol. 43, 1991, pp. 12580–12589.

[57] Woggon, U., et al., "Electro-optic properties of CdS embedded in a polymer," *Phys. Rev. B*, Vol. 48, 1993, pp. 11979–11986.

[58] Artemyev, M. V., et al., "Irreversible photochemical spectral hole burning in quantum-sized CdS nanocrystals embedded in a polymeric film," *Chem. Phys. Lett.*, Vol. 243, 1995, pp. 450–455.

[59] Misawa, K., et al., "Superradiance quenching by confined acoustic phonons in chemically prepared CdS microcrystallites," *J. Chem. Phys.*, Vol. 94, 1991, pp. 4131–4140.

[60] Wang, Y., et al., "Linear- and nonlinear-optical properties of semiconductor clusters," *J. Opt. Soc. Am. B*, Vol. 6, 1989, pp. 808–813.

[61] Nogami, M., k. Nagasaka and M. Takata, "CdS microcrystal-doped silica glass prepared by the sol-gel process," *J. Non-Cryst. Solids*, Vol. 122, 1990, pp. 101–106.

[62] Minti, H., M. Eyal and R. Reisfeld, "Quantum dots od cadmium sulfide in thin glass films prepared by sol-gel technique," *Chem. Phys. Lett.*, Vol. 183, 1991, pp. 277–282.

[63] Spanhel, L., E. Arpac and H. Schmidt, "Semiconductor clusters in the sol-gel process: synthesis and properties of CdS nanocomposites," *J. Non-Cryst. Solids*, Vol. 147–148, 1992, pp. 657–662.

[64] Mathieu, H., et al., "Quantum confinement effects of CdS nanocrystals in a sodium borosilicate glass prepared by the sol-gel process," *J. Appl. Phys.*, Vol. 77, 1995, pp. 287–293.

[65] Herron, N., et al., "Structures and Optical Properties of CdS Superclusters in Zeolite Hosts," *J. Am. Chem. Soc.*, Vol. 111, 1989, pp. 530–540.

[66] Gaponenko, S. V., et al., "Nonlinear-optical properties of semiconductor quantum dots and their correlation with the precipitation stage," *J. Opt. Soc. Am. B*, Vol. 10, 1993, pp. 1947–1954.

[67] Hodes, G., et al., "Three-dimensional quantum-size effect in chemically deposited cadmium selenide films," *Phys. Rev. B*, Vol. 36, 1987, pp. 4215–4221.

[68] Potter Jr., B. G. and J. H. Simmons, "Quantum-confinement effectsin CdTe-glass composite thin films produced using rf magnetron sputtering," *J. Appl. Phys.*, Vol. 68, 1990, pp. 1218–1224.

[69] Liu, L. C., et al., "High-resolution electron microscopy and microanalysis of cadmium sulfide and cadmium telluride quantum dots in glass matrixes," *Philos. Mag. B*, Vol. 63, 1991, pp. 769–776.

[70] Ochoa, O. R., et al., "Quantum confinement effects on the photoluminescence spectra of CdTe nanocrystallites," *Solid State Commun.*, Vol. 98, 1996, pp. 717–721.

[71] Chestnoy, N., R. Hull and L. E. Brus, "Higher excited electronic states in clusters of ZnSe, CdSe, and ZnS: Spin-orbit, vibronic, and relaxation phenomena," *J. Chem. Phys.*, Vol. 85, 1986, pp. 2237–2242.

[72] Li, L. S., et al., "High Quality ZnSe and ZnS Nanocrystals Formed by Activating Zinc Carboxylate Precursors," *Nano Lett.*, Vol. 4, 2004, pp. 2261–2264.

[73] Kortan, A. R., et al., "Nucleation and Growth of CdSe on ZnS Quantum Crystallite Seeds, and Vice Versa, in Inverse Micelle Media," *J. Am. Chem. Soc.*, Vol. 112, 1990, pp. 1327–1332.

[74] Steigerwald, M. L., et al., "Surface Derivatization and Isolation of Semiconductor Cluster Molecules," *J. Am. Chem. Soc.*, Vol. 110, 1988, pp. 3046–3050.

[75] Mamedova, N. N., et al., "Albumin–CdTe Nanoparticle Bioconjugates: Preparation, Structure, and Interunit Energy Transfer with Antenna Effect," *Nano Lett.*, Vol. 1, 2001, pp. 281–286.

[76] Bruchez Jr., M., et al., "Semiconductor Nanocrystals as Fluorescent Biological Labels," *Science*, Vol. 281, 1998, pp. 2013–2016.

[77] Chan, W. C. W. and S. Nie, "Quantum Dot Bioconjugates for Ultrasensitive Nonisotopic Detection," *Science*, Vol. 281, 1998, pp. 2016–2018.

[78] Mattoussi, H., et al., "Self-Assembly of CdSe–ZnS Quantum Dot Bioconjugates Using an Engineered Recombinant Protein," *J. Am. Chem. Soc.*, Vol. 122, 2000, pp. 12142–12150.

[79] Aldana, J., Y. A. Wang and X. Peng, "Photochemical Instability of CdSe Nanocrystals Coated by Hydrophilic Thiols," *J. Am. Chem. Soc.*, Vol. 123, 2001, pp. 8844–8850.

[80] Mitchell, G. P., C. A. Mirkin and R. L. Letsinger, "Programmed Assembly of DNA Functionalized Quantum Dots," *J. Am. Chem. Soc.*, Vol. 121, 1999, pp. 8122–8123.

[81] Breus, V. V., C. D. Heyes and G. U. Nienhaus, "Quenching of CdSe-ZnS Core-Shell Quantum Dot Luminescence by Water-Soluble Thiolated Ligands," *J. Phys. Chem. C*, Vol. 111, 2007, pp. 18589–18594.

[82] Åkerman, M. E., et al., "Nanocrystal targeting in vivo," *Proc. Natl. Acad. Sci.*, Vol. 99, 2002, pp. 12617–12621.

[83] Hong, R., et al., "Control of Protein Structure and Function through Surface Recognition by Tailored Nanoparticle Scaffolds," *J. Am. Chem. Soc.*, Vol. 126, 2004, pp. 739–743.

[84] Derfus, A. M., W. C. W. Chan and S. N. Bhatia, "Intracellular Delivery of Quantum Dots for Live Cell Labeling and Organelle Tracking," *Adv. Mater.*, Vol. 16, 2004, pp. 961–966.

[85] Kang, E. C., et al., "Preparation of Water-soluble PEGylated Semiconductor Nanocrystals," *Chem. Lett.*, Vol. 33, 2004, pp. 840–841.

[86] Shi, L., N. Rosenzweig and Z. Rosenzweig, "Luminescent Quantum Dots Fluorescence Resonance Energy Transfer-Based Probes for Enzymatic Activity and Enzyme Inhibitors," *Anal. Chem.*, Vol. 79, 2007, pp. 208–214.

[87] Liu, W., et al., "Compact Cysteine-Coated CdSe(ZnCdS) Quantum Dots for in Vivo Applications," *J. Am. Chem. Soc.*, Vol. 129, 2007, pp. 14530–14531.

[88] Wang, Y. A., et al., "Stabilization of Inorganic Nanocrystals by Organic Dendrons," *J. Am. Chem. Soc.*, Vol. 124, 2002, pp. 2293–2298.

[89] Guo, W., et al., "Conjugation Chemistry and Bioapplications of Semiconductor Box Nanocrystals Prepared via Dendrimer Bridging," *Chem. Mater.*, Vol. 15, 2003, pp. 3125–3133.

[90] Uyeda, H. T., et al., "Synthesis of Compact Mutidentate Ligands to Prepare Stable Hydrophilic Quantum Dot Fluorophores," *J. Am. Chem. Soc.*, Vol. 127, 2005, pp. 3870–3878.

[91] Pons, T., et al., "Hydrodynamic Dimensions, Electrophoretic Mobility, and Stability of Hydrophilic Quantum Dots," *J. Phys. Chem. B*, Vol. 110, 2006, pp. 20308–20316.

[92] Susumu, K., et al., "Enhancing the Stability and Biological Functionalities of Quantum Dots via Compact Multifunctional Ligands," *J. Am. Chem. Soc.*, Vol. 129, 2007, pp. 13987–13996.

[93] Liu, W., et al., "Compact Biocompatible Quantum Dots Functionalized for Cellular Imaging," *J. Am. Chem. Soc.*, Vol. 130, 2008, pp. 1274–1284.

[94] Pinaud, F., et al., "Bioactivation and Cell Targeting of Semiconductor CdSe/ZnS Nanocrystals with Phytochelatin-Related Peptides," *J. Am. Chem. Soc.*, Vol. 126, 2004, pp. 6115–6123.

[95] Iyer, G., et al., "Solubilization of Quantum Dots with a Recombinant Peptide from Escherichia coli," *Small*, Vol. 3, 2007, pp. 793–798.

[96] Kim, S. and M. G. Bawendi, "Oligomeric Ligands for Luminescent and Stable Nanocrystal Quantum Dots," *J. Am. Chem. Soc.*, Vol. 125, 2003, pp. 14652–14653.

[97] Kim, S.-W., et al., "Phosphine Oxide Polymer for Water-Soluble Nanoparticles," *J. Am. Chem. Soc.*, Vol. 127, 2005, pp. 4556–4557.

[98] Nann, T., "Phase-transfer of CdSe@ZnS quantum dots using amphiphilic hyperbranched polyethylenimine," *Chem. Commun.*, Vol., 2005, pp. 1735–1736.

[99] Duan, H. and S. Nie, "Cell-Penetrating Quantum Dots Based on Multivalent and Endosome-Disrupting Surface Coatings," *J. Am. Chem. Soc.*, Vol. 129, 2007, pp. 3333–3338.

[100] Wang, M., et al., "Water-Soluble CdSe Quantum Dots Passivated by a Multidentate Diblock Copolymer," *Macromolecules*, Vol. 40, 2007, pp. 6377–6384.

[101] Gerion, D., et al., "Synthesis and Properties of Biocompatible Water-Soluble Silica-Coated CdSe/ZnS Semiconductor Quantum Dots," *J. Phys. Chem. B*, Vol. 105, 2001, pp. 8861–8871.

[102] Wu, X., et al., "Immunofluorescent labeling of cancer marker Her2 and other cellular targets with semiconductor quantum dots," *Nature Biotechnol.*, Vol. 21, 2003, pp. 41–46.

[103] Ballou, B., et al., "Noninvasive Imaging of Quantum Dots in Mice," *Bioconjugate Chem.*, Vol. 15, 2004, pp. 79–86.

[104] Gao, X., et al., "In vivo cancer targeting and imaging with semiconductor quantum dots," *Nat. Biotechnol.*, Vol. 22, 2004, pp. 969–976.

[105] Yu, W. W., et al., "Forming Biocompatible and Nonaggregated Nanocrystals in Water Using Amphiphilic Polymers," *J. Am. Chem. Soc.*, Vol. 129, 2007, pp. 2871–2879.

[106] Pellegrino, T., et al., "Hydrophobic Nanocrystals Coated with an Amphiphilic Polymer Shell: A General Route to Water Soluble Nanocrystals," *Nano Lett.*, Vol. 4, 2004, pp. 703–707.

[107] Dubertret, B., et al., "In Vivo Imaging of Quantum Dots Encapsulated in Phospholipid Micelles," *Science*, Vol. 298, 2002, pp. 1759–1762.

[108] Fan, H., et al., "Surfactant-Assisted Synthesis of Water-Soluble and Biocompatible Semiconductor Quantum Dot Micelles," *Nano Lett.*, Vol. 5, 2005, pp. 645–648.

[109] Jin, T., et al., "Calixarene-coated water-soluble CdSe–ZnS semiconductor quantum dots that are highly fluorescent and stable in aqueous solution," *Chem. Commun.*, Vol., 2005, pp. 2829–2831.

[110] Jin, T., et al., "Control of the Optical Properties of Quantum Dots by Surface Coating with Calix[n]arene Carboxylic Acids," *J. Am. Chem. Soc.*, Vol. 128, 2006, pp. 9288–9289.

[111] Osaki, F., et al., "A Quantum Dot Conjugated Sugar Ball and Its Cellular Uptake. On the Size Effects of Endocytosis in the Subviral Region," *J. Am. Chem. Soc.*, Vol. 126, 2004, pp. 6520–6521.

[112] Nikolic, M. S., et al., "Tailor-Made Ligands for Biocompatible Nanoparticles," *Angew. Chem. Int. Ed.*, Vol. 45, 2006, pp. 6577–6580.

[113] Jana, N. R., C. Earhart and J. Y. Ying, "Synthesis of Water-Soluble and Functionalized Nanoparticles by Silica Coating," *Chem. Mater.*, Vol. 19, 2007, pp. 5074–5082.

[114] Gao, X., et al., "In vivo molecular and cellular imaging with quantum dots," *Curr. Opin. Biotechnol.*, Vol. 16, 2005, pp. 63–72.

[115] Luccardini, C., et al., "Size, Charge, and Interactions with Giant Lipid Vesicles of Quantum Dots Coated with an Amphiphilic Macromolecule," *Langmuir*, Vol. 22, 2006, pp. 2304–2310.

[116] Jin, T., et al., "Amphiphilic p-sulfonatocalix[4]arene-coated CdSe/ZnS quantum dots for the optical detection of the neurotransmitter acetylcholine," *Chem. Commun.*, Vol., 2005, pp. 4300–4302.

[117] Sapsford, K. E., et al., "Kinetics of Metal-Affinity Driven Self-Assembly between Proteins or Peptides and CdSe-ZnS Quantum Dots," *J. Phys. Chem. C*, Vol. 111, 2007, pp. 11528–11538.

CHAPTER 2

Colloidal Chemical Synthesis of Organic-Dispersible Uniform Magnetic Nanoparticles

Soon Gu Kwon and Taeghwon Hyeon

For the past 30 years, the synthesis of nanoparticles with size ranging from 1 nm to 50 nm has been intensively pursued, not only for their fundamental scientific interest, but also for their many technological applications [1]. Nanoparticles exhibit very interesting size-dependent electrical, optical, magnetic, and chemical properties that cannot be achieved by their bulk counterparts. For many future applications, the synthesis of uniform-sized nanoparticles (monodisperse with a size distribution of relative standard deviation, σ_r, less than 5 percent) is of key importance, because the electrical, optical, and magnetic properties of these nanoparticles are strongly dependent on their dimensions [2]. Among various nanoparticles, magnetic nanoparticles have been intensively studied for their many (potential) applications. For example, regular array of uniform-sized magnetic nanoparticles have been proposed as multiterabit/in^2 magnetic storage media [3–7]. Magnetic nanoparticles have found various biomedical applications including contrast enhancement agents for magnetic resonance imaging (MRI), magnetic carriers for drug delivery system (DDS), biosensors, and bioseparation [3–7]. In this chapter, we would like to summarize the colloidal chemical synthesis of uniform-sized magnetic nanoparticles. In the first section, magnetism in nanometer-scale will be briefly summarized. In the following sections, synthesis of uniform-sized magnetic nanoparticles using various colloidal chemical methods will be described.

2.1 Magnetism of Nanoparticles

Below the Curie temperature (T_c), the volume of a bulk magnetic (ferromagnetic or ferrimagnetic) material is divided into many magnetic domains to reduce the magnetostatic energy [8]. This energy is proportional to the volume, D^3, where D is the dimension of the magnetic materials. However, the extent of the reduced magnetostatic energy by the multidomain structure is offset by the energy of the interface between domains, which is called domain wall. The domain wall energy is proportional to the wall area (D^2). As a result, below some critical size, namely, D_c, the domain wall energy surpasses the stabilization energy by the multidomain structure, and the material becomes single domain (Figure 2.1) [8]. The magnetism of a multidomain material is the result of the collective behavior of many domains in its body. Thus, its magnetic property can be regarded as independent of the size. On the other hand, for a single domain particle, in which only one domain is confined in the particle volume, the magnetic property is strongly dependant on the particle size.

In a single domain particle, all magnetic spins are aligned parallel composing a single "giant spin." This giant spin, or, equivalently, the magnetization of the particle, tends to lie in the "easy direction" of the particle at which the potential energy is the minimum. The easy directions are separated by the energy barrier of height KV, where K is the anisotropy constant and V is the particle volume (Figure 2.2). As V gets smaller, it becomes easier to flip the magnetization from one direction to another because of the low energy barrier. In other words, the coercive field, H_c, for a single domain particle decreases with its size. When V is so small that KV is comparable to the thermal energy, kT, the magnetization direction is subjected to ran-

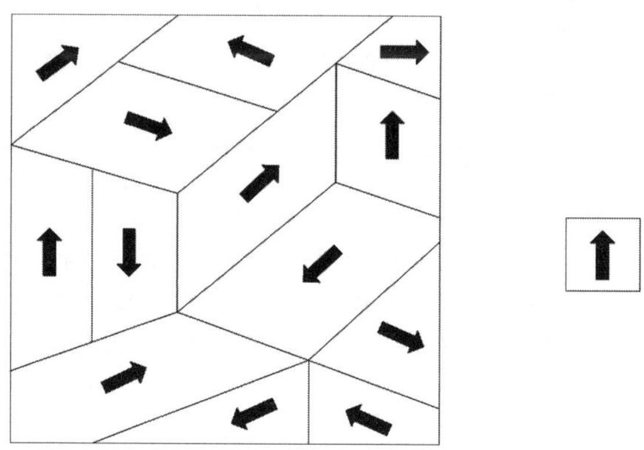

Figure 2.1 Schematic illustrations of the mutidomain (left) and single domain structures (right).

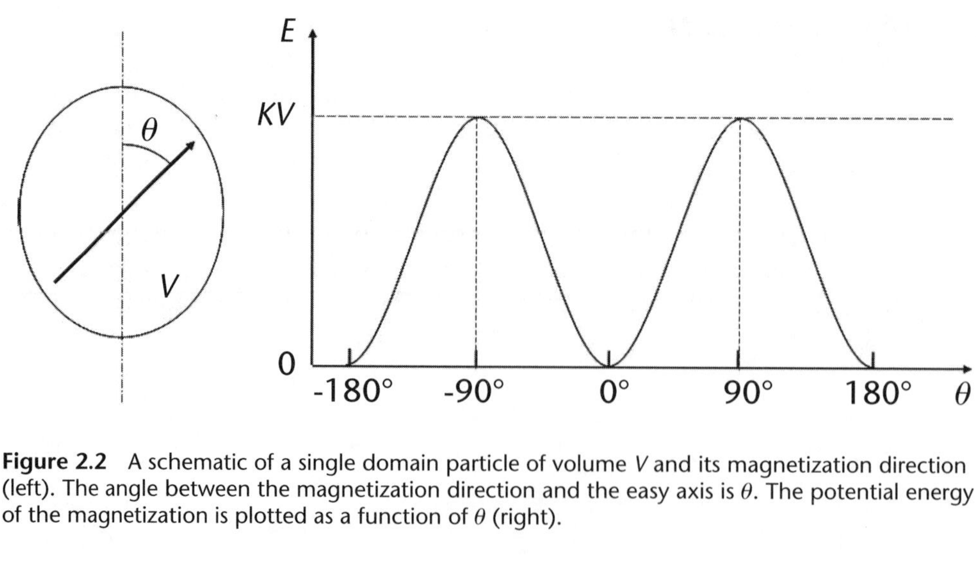

Figure 2.2 A schematic of a single domain particle of volume V and its magnetization direction (left). The angle between the magnetization direction and the easy axis is θ. The potential energy of the magnetization is plotted as a function of θ (right).

dom thermal fluctuation. This phenomenon is called superparamagnetism [9, 10]. In this condition, H_c is zero (no hysteresis) and the particle has no stable magnetization direction (Figure 2.3). For a particle of a fixed volume, the minimum temperature required to make it superparamagnetic is called the blocking temperature, T_B, which is expressed in terms of K and V as:

$$T_B = KV/25k \tag{2.1}$$

This shows how T_B varies with V when the particle is superparamagnetic ($V < V_p$). Conversely, (2.1) can be rearranged as $V_p = 25kT/K$, where V_p is the maximum volume of the superparamagnetic particle for a given T. When the particle is of single domain but $V > V_p$, the size dependency of H_c can be written as:

$$H_c/H_{c,o} = 1-(V_p/V)^{1/2} = 1-(D_p/D)^{3/2} \tag{2.2}$$

where $H_{c,o}$ is the coercive field of bulk material and D_p is the particle diameter that corresponds to V_p [8]. Note that, when $V = V_p$ (or $D = D_p$), H_c is zero in that equation as it should be.

For a single domain particle, H_c is strongly dependant not only on the size but also on the shape. In a magnetic material, the magnetic spin lying along the long axis has lower energy than along the shorter one because of weak demagnetizing field in that direction. Thus, the shape anisotropy of a particle contributes to its magnetic anisotropy, K. As a result, the height of the energy barrier, KV, and, in turn, H_c depend on the shape. When the particle shape is totally symmetric, namely, a sphere, the shape anisotropy contribution is zero. As the degree of the shape symmetry decreases, both K and H_c increase. For example, for a fixed V, the value of H_c increases in the order of sphere, cube, and rod. Another major contribution to the magnetic anisotropy is the magnetocrystalline anisotropy. In a magnetic material, there are easy directions of magnetization with respect to the crystallographic axis. The interaction between electron spin and the crystal lattice is mediated by the spin-orbit coupling between electron spin and the "orbital" of the crystal lattice. This anisotropy varies largely in different substances and crystal structures.

For nanoparticles, the surface state is also an important factor affecting their magnetic property. Because of their size, NPs have very high surface-to-volume ratio that the number of the atoms on the surface is comparable to that in the core. The surface is where the crystal symmetry is broken, and the high surface-free

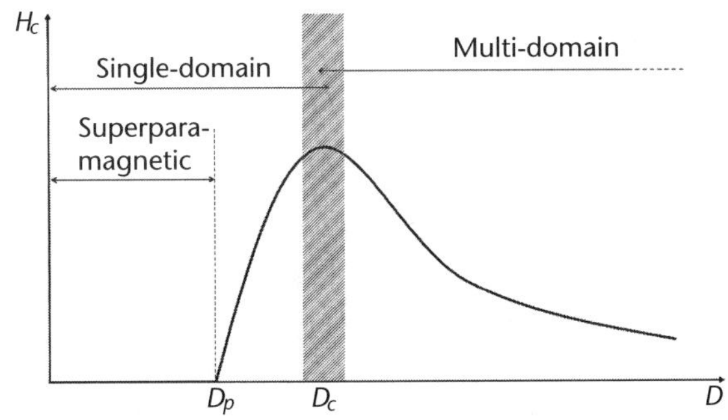

Figure 2.3 Change of the coercive field H_c with particle diameter D.

energy of nanoparticles leads to the surface relaxation that distorts the crystal structure on the surface. Those factors lead to the surface anisotropy that contributes to the magnetic anisotropy of nanoparticles to a considerable extent [11, 12]. As shown in (2.3), the surface anisotropy term is proportional to the surface curvature, 1/D:

$$K = K_V + 6K_S / D \tag{2.3}$$

where K_V and K_s are the anisotropy constants for the volume and the surface, respectively [12]. Moreover, the atoms on the surface have many dangling bonds, various coordinated ligands, and, sometimes, oxidation numbers different from that of the core atoms. They result in the change of the number of magnetic spins per atom and the disorder of the surface spins. For example, antiferromagnetic nanoparticles could have small net magnetization because of the broken symmetry at the surface and the surface spin disorder [11].

The discussions so far reveal that there are four critical factors in the synthesis of magnetic nanoparticles of controlled properties, namely, the size and shape uniformity, crystal structure, and the surface state. In the following sections, we discuss various synthetic methods of magnetic nanoparticles to control those factors.

2.2 Transition Metal Nanoparticles

The main problem in the synthesis of nanoparticles is to find an appropriate reaction system, in which the precipitation reaction is perfectly controlled to yield nanometer-sized particles of high uniformity as well as good quality in terms of, for example, crystallinity, purity, and surface state. For this purpose, many synthetic methods have been devised for various materials ranging from II–VI and III–V semiconductors to metals, metal alloys, and metal oxides. Among them, to date, the synthetic systems utilizing the high-temperature organic solution as the precipitation medium have been the most successful. The organic-solution medium enables us to use various molecular precursors that afford high versatility for the design of the nanoparticle synthetic system. Furthermore, the organic-solution methods utilize the surfactant molecules that are very effective in both controlling the nucleation and growth process and stabilizing the nanoparticles in the colloidal dispersion. Consequently, each synthetic method is characterized by its specific precursors, the surfactants, and the solvent. In the following sections, the synthetic methods are categorized according to their similarities in chemistry. There are several review articles on the magnetic nanoparticles [3–7].

2.2.1 Cobalt Nanoparticles

Co is the most intensely investigated material in the synthesis of magnetic metal nanoparticles, and, thus, it is worth discussing this material in detail. The synthesis of Co nanoparticles can be categorized in three methods. The first one utilizes the reduction of $CoCl_2$ in the solution by $LiBEt_3H$ [13]. The formation of NPs in the reaction solution was induced by the rapid injection of highly reactive reductant

($LiBEt_3H$) into the hot solution (~200 degrees C) containing Co^{2+} ions. The extremely rapid nucleation and growth process in this condition leads to the uniform Co NPs. It is an adaptation of the "hot injection" technique, which was originally devised for the synthesis of CdSe nanoparticles [14]. The second method is the reduction of cobalt(II) acetate [$Co(Ac)_2$] by the polyol process [15, 16]. In this method, 1,2-hexadecanediol (HDD), a mild reductant, is injected into a solution containing $Co(Ac)_2$ and the surfactant molecules at high temperature. This method yielded moderate size uniformity (σ_r ~ 10 percent). In the third, Co NPs are synthesized by the thermal decomposition of $Co_2(CO)_{10}$ in the solution. When it was firstly introduced in 1999, the size uniformity was not so good (σ_r ~ 15 percent) [17]. However, this method had been widely adopted and largely improved in the successive papers. In 2001, the Alivisatos group reported the synthesis of highly uniform Co NPs ($\sigma_r < 10$ percent) using $Co_2(CO)_{10}$ as the precursor [18]. To improve the size uniformity, they adopted the hot injection method and used oleic acid (OLEA) and alkylamines as the surfactants. The Chaudret group reported the thermal decomposition method using another organometallic precursor, $[Co(\eta^3\text{-}C_8H_{13})(\eta^4\text{-}C_8H_{12})]$ [19]. In this compound, the oxidation number of Co is –1 and the thermal decomposition reaction proceeded under the reductive atmosphere (3 bar H_2).

In addition to the size uniformity, the size control is also an important issue in the NP synthesis. However, in most cases, the technique for the size control is so subtle and complex that a general and systematic size control technique is not yet available. Control over size depends on several parameters (e.g., the bulkiness of the surfactant molecule, precursor to surfactant ratio, reaction temperature, and reaction time). Roughly speaking, bulkier surfactant molecules tend to produce smaller nanoparticles [13, 15]. It was suggested that the steric effect of bulk molecules on the surface of NP control the growth rate of NP [15]. In some cases, increasing the precursor to surfactant ratio produced larger NPs [15, 16, 20]. However, little is known about the mechanism of how these factors work for the size control.

The air sensitivity is an important problem in the synthesis of transition metal NPs. Moisture and oxygen dissolved in the solvent can oxidize metal NPs to metal oxide. It was reported that a simple washing of trioctylphosphine oxide (TOPO)-capped Co NPs with organic solvent could result in surface oxidation [17]. This result showed that TOPO is weakly bound to the surface of Co NP. It turned out that OLEA provided stable protection of Co NP surface [13, 21]. Fourier transform infrared and X-ray photoelectron spectroscopies revealed that the carboxylate group can anchor to the surface of Co NP by the formation of O–Co bond [21]. The Alivisatos group reported that when OLEA was used as the capping molecules, Co NPs were stable for months without oxidation.

An interesting feature in the synthesis of Co NPs is that, by varying reaction conditions, they can be prepared in a number of different phases (i.e., hcp, fcc, and ε-Co). Among them, ε-Co is an interesting phase because it has never been observed in bulk state. Dinega and Bawendi synthesized ε-Co NPs by the thermal decomposition of $Co_2(CO)_{10}$ in toluene containing TOPO as the surfactant [17]. They proposed that the coordination of bulky TOPO molecules on the surface of NPs could alter their precipitation kinetics and lead to the formation of that unusual phase. With the same precursor, ε-Co NPs were prepared by using fatty acid and alkylphosphines as the surfactants [18]. The hot injection method using $CoCl_2$ as the precursor also produced ε-Co NPs [13]. The Murray group reported that hcp-Co NPs and multiply twinned fcc-Co NPs were synthesized by the polyol method and the thermal decomposition of $Co_2(CO)_{10}$, respectively. Alivisatos et al. observed that in the very early stage of the precipitation in the hot solvent, hcp-Co nanorods were formed in the solution and then transformed to spherical ε-Co NPs, which suggests that in that reaction condition ε-Co is more energetically favored than hcp-Co. Epsilon-Co has a saturation magnetization similar to those of hcp- and fcc-Co but weaker magnetic anisotropy. This phase is metastable and transformed to hcp phase irreversibly after annealed at 500 degrees C [13].

2.2.2 Iron and Nickel Nanoparticles

The thermal decomposition of $Fe(CO)_5$ is the most widely adopted method for the synthesis of Fe NPs. In the earliest contributions, $Fe(CO)_5$ was decomposed thermally [22] or sonochemically [23] in the organic solution containing polymers as the capping molecules. As was in the case of the synthesis of Co NPs, adopting the hot injection technique greatly improved the quality of Fe NPs in terms of the size and shape uniformity and the size controllability. In 2000, Hyeon et al. reported the synthesis of highly uniform Fe NPs (σ_r < 6 percent) by the injection of the $Fe(CO)_5$ solution into hot TOPO (340 degrees C) [24]. Similarly, Murray et al. synthesized Fe NPs by the hot injection of $Fe(CO)_5$ into the solution containing OLEA and alkylphosphine as the surfactants [16]. In both cases, Fe NPs were amorphous or of disordered structure. In 2001, the Hyeon group reported a new synthetic method other than the hot injection yielding monodisperse Fe NPs [25]. In this method, $Fe(CO)_5$ was mixed with OLEA in the solution to form iron-oleate complex. Then, the solution was heated to decompose the as-synthesized iron-oleate complex. Unlike the other simple heating methods, heating of this metal-surfactant complex resulted in highly uniform NPs. With its simplicity, this method showed a possibility for the mass production of high-quality NPs. The precursors other than $Fe(CO)_5$ were also utilized for the synthesis of Fe NPs. In 2004, Chaudret et al. reported the synthesis of Fe nanocubes by the thermal decomposition of $Fe[N(SiMe_3)_2]_2$ under the reductive atmosphere [26]. Interestingly, Fe nanocubes were self-assembled in cubic superlattice in their as-synthesized form. Hyeon et al. synthesized Fe nanocubes and nanoframes using iron-stearate as the precursor. Note that they used Fe(II) species, rather than Fe(0). The spontaneous reduction of Fe(II) occurred in the thermal decomposition of iron-stearate at high temperature (~380 degrees C) [27]. The addition of sodium oleate resulted in the etching of the nanocubes to nanoframes, which was attributed to the molten salt corrosion by Na^+ ions.

The synthesis of Ni NPs was reported by Murray et al. in 2001 [16]. They used the same method as in the synthesis of Co NPs, the polyol reduction of metal acetate. The thermal decomposition method was also adopted using nickel(II) 1, 5-cyclooctadiene [$Ni(COD)_2$] as the precursor [28]. This method was successful in the synthesis of nanorods. The uniform spherical Ni NPs were synthesized using $Ni(acac)_2$ as the precursor [29, 30]. Similar to the synthesis of Fe NPs in [25], the precursor was coordinated with the surfactant molecules, oleylamine (OAm) or TOPO, at the lower temperature, and then thermally decomposed by heating. Interestingly, the thermal decomposition and reduction proceeded simultaneously in this reaction.

The techniques for the size control in the synthesis of Fe and Ni NPs were similar to those for Co NPs. In [25], it was reported that the larger NPs were obtained by decreasing the precursor to surfactant ratio. It is interesting that this trend is the opposite of the case for the synthesis of Co NPs. In the synthesis of Ni NPs, the use of bulkier surfactant resulted in the smaller NPs, as was in the case of Co NPs [29]. Majetich et al. reported the synthesis of highly uniform Fe NPs by the seed mediated growth using gold clusters as the heterogeneous seed [31].

2.3 Metal Alloy Nanoparticles

2.3.1 FePt Nanoparticles

The synthesis of FePt NPs has been very intensely studied over the past years for application in magnetic data storage media. For high areal data density (> 1 $Tbit/in^2$), the magnetic recording medium with fine grains as small as few nanometers is required [32, 33]. FePt in fct (or $L1_0$) phase has high magnetic anisotropy ($6.6\text{-}10 \times 10^7$ erg/cm^3) compared to the other transition metals (for example, 0.45×10^7 erg/cm^3 of Co). As a result, FePt particles can retain its ferromagnetism at room temperature even in the size of ~3 nm, making it a strong candidate material for high-density data storage medium [32].

Regarding application in data storage media, some issues had emerged in the synthesis of FePt NPs [7]. First, the size and shape uniformity has much greater importance with regard to signal-to-noise ratio (SNR). As mentioned earlier, the size and shape of a single domain particle largely affect the magnetic properties (i.e., the coercive field and the remanence magnetization). If those properties vary from particle to particle, read/write error frequency increases. Second, the crystal phase of FePt NPs should be controlled. As-synthesized FePt NPs are of disordered fcc structure whose magnetic anisotropy is low. Annealing at temperature over 540 degrees C turns the NPs into desired fct phase. However, the high annealing temperature results in agglomeration, which increases the grain size and broadens the size distribution. Thus, decreasing the annealing temperature is also an important problem. Third, the composition distribution of NPs should be uniform. The composition of metal alloy affects its magnetic property and, just as with the size and shape uniformity, has influence on SNR. In addition, it also affects the phase transition behavior from fcc to fct structure, as discussed later.

Sun et al. reported on the synthesis of FePt NPs by the simultaneous thermal decomposition of $Fe(CO)_5$ and the polyol reduction of $Pt(acac)_2$ [34, 35]. Those two precursors were added to the solution containing OLEA, OAm, and 1,2-hexadecanediol (HDD) at lower temperature. Then, this solution was heated to ~300 degrees C to produce FePt NPs. The NPs synthesized were so highly uniform that they formed a self-assembled superlattice. Interestingly, it is another case of NP synthesis in which the simple heating procedure resulted in very narrow size distribution. The FePt NP assemblies of various compositions were annealed at 540 degrees C and it turned out that only the composition near $Fe_{55}Pt_{45}$ was completely transformed to fct phase at that temperature. By varying the ratio between the Fe and Pt precursors, they prepared Fe_xPt_{100-x} NPs ,where x ranged from 30 to 80. They found that the composition of Fe in FePt NPs was systematically lower than the mole fraction of the Fe precursor. This mismatch was problematic for the precise composition control of FePt alloy, and some modified synthetic methods were introduced to solve this problem.

Sun et al. used $FeCl_2$ as the Fe precursor instead of $Fe(CO)_5$ [36]. This precursor was reduced by the dropwise addition of $LiBEt_3H$ solution during the reaction. They reported that the composition of FePt NPs synthesized by this method well matched to the molar ratio of Fe/Pt precursor. Liu et al. substituted $Fe(CO)_5$ with $Fe(acac)_2$, and both the Fe and Pt precursors were reduced by the polyol method [37]. However, they did not provide the atomic composition data of the product. Evans et al. reported the use of $Pt(acac)_2$ and $Na_2[Fe(CO)_4]$ as the precursors [38]. The synthetic reaction proceeded by the reduction/oxidation between Fe^{2-} and Pt^{2+} ($Fe^{2-} + Pt^{2+} \rightarrow$ FePt), which assures the exact compositional control. However, the size and shape uniformity of the product was not so good.

The synthetic method discussed so far has little size controllability, and the size of FePt NPs synthesized were almost fixed in the range of 3–4 nm. It was found that, by excluding HDD from the synthetic scheme introduced by Sun et al. [34, 35], the size control was possible [39]. Varying the heating rate, 6 nm (~15 degrees C/min) and 9 nm (~5 degrees C/min) FePt NPs were obtained. It was suggested that fast reduction of Pt^{2+} by HDD might be responsible for the incapability of the size control in the original scheme. The Yang group introduced an alternative method for the size control. They synthesized Pt/Fe_2O_3 core/shell NPs [40] and then converted them to fct-FePt NPs by the annealing in 5 percent H_2 atmosphere [41]. The mean size was 17 nm, which was unprecedentedly large in the synthesis of FePt NPs.

The composition distribution of FePt NPs is very hard to characterize, and there are only few papers dealing with this matter. Moreover, there are even some controversies between them. Sun et al. studied the composition analysis of FePt NPs by inductively coupled plasma atomic emission spectroscopy (ICP-AES), energy dispersive X-ray spectroscopy (EDS), and electron energy loss spectroscopy (EELS) [35]. ICP-AES measures the net composition of an ensemble of FePt NPs. EDS and EELS was used to analyze the composition of the small region of FePt NP assembly and the individual NPs, respectively. According to their report, the compositions measured by those techniques were all consistent with each other, indicating that the composition distribution is very narrow. However, in another paper adopting the similar technique to analyze the composition of individual NPs, it was reported that the distribution is so broad that only 30 percent of Fe_xPt_{100-x} NPs are in the range of $40 < x < 60$ [42]. Because the NPs out of that range do not transform to fct structure by the annealing process, the broad composition distribution lowers the quality of FePt NP assembly.

2.3.2 Other Metal Alloy Nanoparticles

The syntheses of other metal alloy NPs of $L1_0$ or related structures were also reported. Chaudret et al. synthesized Co_xPt_{1-x} NPs by the decomposition of $[Co(\eta^3\text{-}C_8H_{13})(\eta 4\text{-}C_8H_{12})]$ and $Pt_2(dba)_3$ (dba = bis-dibenzylidene acetone) in the solution containing polyvinyl- pyrrolidone (PVP) as the capping reagent [43]. Cheon et al. reported a synthetic method that yielded both Co/Pt core/shell and CoPt alloy NPs [44]. They used $Co_2(CO)_8$ and $Pt(hfac)_2$ (hfac = hexafluroacetylacetonate) as the precursors and no additional reductant was added for the reduction of the Pt precursor. They conjectured that the transmetalation between Co core and the Pt precursors resulted in the transformation of $Co_{core}Pt_{shell}$ to Co_xPt_y. The Weller group obtained $CoPt_3$ NPs using $Co_2(CO)_8$ and $Pt(acac)_2$ as the precursors [45]. This method resembles that for the synthesis of FePt NPs introduced by Sun et al. [34, 35]. The size control was accomplished by adjusting the reaction temperature and time, varying the nature of the surfactants, and the additional precursor injection. A detailed mechanistic study on the nucleation and growth process of this synthetic system was reported by the same group [46]. They found that the nucleation and growth was terminated at the early stage of the synthetic reaction and that there was no Ostwald ripening process. Also, they observed that the slower nucleation and the faster growth yielded the larger NPs. They showed that the balance between the nucleation and growth rate can be utilized to control the mean size of NPs reproducibly. Similarly, Chen and Nikles prepared CoPt NPs by the thermal decomposition of $Co(CO)_3NO$ and the polyol reduction of $Pt(acac)_2$. They also obtained FePd NPs using $Fe(CO)_5$ and $Pd(acac)_2$ as the surfactants under the same condition [47].

There are relatively few papers on the synthesis of ternary metal alloy NPs. $Fe_xCo_yPt_{100-x-y}$ NPs were synthesized by using $Pt(acac)_2$, $Co(acac)_2$, and $Fe(CO)_5$ as the precursors [48]. Using the same method, except for substituting $Co(acac)_2$ with the Cu precursor, copper bis(2,2,6,6-tetramethyl-3,5-heptanedionate), FePtCu NPs were also synthesized [49]. In both cases, the transition from fcc to fct ($L1_o$) structure occurred at the annealing temperature in the range of 550–600 degrees C. Interestingly, it was observed that FePtAg NPs, synthesized by using Ag(Ac) as the Ag precursor, had much lower transition temperature (~400 degrees C) [50]. This phenomenon was attributed to the vacancies in the FePt lattice formed by the sublimation of Ag atoms during the annealing process, which afforded the higher mobility of Fe and Pt atoms and enhanced the transformation.

2.4 Metal Oxide Nanoparticles

2.4.1 Monometallic Oxide Nanoparticles

Transition metal oxides have inferior magnetic properties compared to their metal counterparts (e.g., the saturation magnetization of iron and Fe_3O_4 at 300 K are 218 and 92 emu/g, respectively [8]). However, because of their good chemical stability, magnetic transition metal oxide NPs have been extensively used for various applications. For example, they can be used for the magnetic separation of the water pollutants [51]. The high affinity of metal ions exposed on the surface of NPs to biomolecules was utilized for the bioassay and separation [30]. Recently, the use of monodisperse magnetic metal oxide NPs as the MRI contrasting agent is gaining much interest because of their advantages of size uniformity and the availability of multiple functionalization compared to conventional contrasting agents such as superparamagnetic iron oxide particles [52, 53].

Traditionally, microstructured metal oxides are synthesized by the sol-gel process. However, in many cases, this process is not appropriate for the synthesis of highly uniform NPs. A significant advance in the synthesis of highly uniform metal oxide NPs was accomplished by the postoxidation method, which was introduced by the Hyeon group in 2001 [25]. It took the advantage of the well-controlled metal NP synthesis. The as-prepared highly uniform Fe NPs were oxidized by $(CH_3)_3NO$ to yield iron oxide (γ-Fe_2O_3 and Fe_3O_4) NPs. In another paper, it was reported that, in the same condition as in [25], hot injection rather than the simple heating yielded uniform iron oxide NPs and the addition of the oxidant was not necessary [54]. This study also revealed that in the presence of OLEA, the nucleation of NPs was retarded for a few minutes after the injection of $Fe(CO)_5$.

The direct thermal decomposition of the precursors containing M–O bonding was employed to synthesize metal oxide nanoparticles. In 1999, the Alivisatos group reported on the general synthesis of metal oxide NPs from the thermal decomposition of metal cupferronates, $M^x(Cup)_y$ where M^x was Fe^{3+}, Cu^{2+}, and Mn^{2+} [55]. The cupferronate precursor solutions were injected into hot alkylamine (250–300 degrees C) to generate NPs of metal oxides such as γ-Fe_2O_3, Cu_2O, and Mn_3O_4. However, the size uniformity of the products was not that good ($\sigma_r \sim 15$ percent). In 2002, Sun and Zeng reported the synthesis of iron oxide NPs by the thermal decomposition of $Fe(acac)_3$ in the solution containing HDD, OLEA, and OAm [56]. The reaction proceeded by simple heating instead of hot injection and resulted in good size uniformity. Similarly, manganese oxide NPs were synthesized by the thermal decomposition of $Mn(Ac)_2$ [57] and $Mn(acac)_2$ [58] in the organic solution.

In 2004, three different research groups reported independently that the thermal decomposition of metal-oleate complex in the organic solution at high temperature (300–365 degrees C) produced highly uniform metal oxide NPs [59–61]. Although the synthetic procedure was strikingly simple (i.e., mixing metal-oleate precursor with the organic solvent and then heating the solution to reflux), the size uniformity of the resulting nanoparticles was extremely good. Under the optimized synthetic conditions, the relative standard deviation (σ_r) of the NP size distribution was as good as < 5 percent, which is comparable to that of the best-quality NPs synthesized by the hot injection method. Figure 2.4 shows TEM image of uniform-sized magnetite nanoparticles synthesized from thermal decomposition of iron-oleate complex. This method was quite general and can be applied to the synthesis of NPs of iron oxide, Cr_2O_3, MnO, Co_3O_4, CoO, and NiO. Because of its simplicity, this method could be easily scaled up to produce the product in tens of grams by a single lab-scale reaction. A detailed structural analysis of iron-oleate complex used in this method was reported in [62]. When metal-oleate complexes were substituted with metal formates, which are of much simpler structure, NPs of similar quality were obtained [63], suggesting that the nature of the metal carboxylate precursor does not affect that much the synthetic reaction. CoO NPs synthesized by the thermal decomposition of cobalt-oleate complex had wurtzite structure, which has not been observed in bulk state [64]. It was found that some metal ions in metal-oleate complex were reduced during the thermal decomposition reaction, which resulted in metal oxide NPs of mixed phases. In the case of iron oxide NPs, X-ray absorption spectrascopy (XAS), and X-ray magnetic circular dichrosim (XMCD) analysis revealed that they were composed of γ-Fe_2O_3 and Fe_3O_4 [60, 65], indicating that some Fe^{3+} ions were

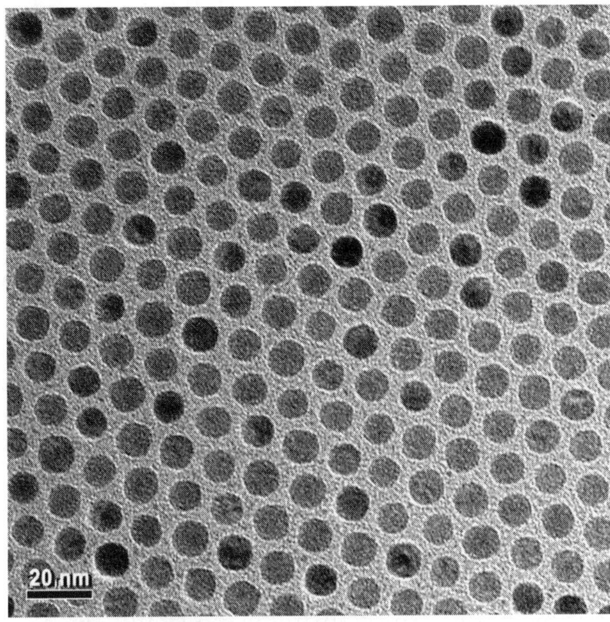

Figure 2.4 TEM image of uniform-sized magnetite nanoparticles synthesized from thermal decomposition of iron-oleate complex.

reduced to Fe^{2+} during the reaction. It seems that the trace amount of H_2 and carbon, the byproducts of the thermal decomposition, are responsible for the reduction. When the decomposition reaction was conducted at higher temperatures (> 380 degrees C), all Fe^{3+} ions were transformed to Fe^0 and Fe metal NPs were obtained [27, 60].

A notable study on the synthesis of iron oxide NPs was reported in 2004, in which NPs of γ-Fe_2O_3, Fe_3O_4, and Fe_xO ($0.84 < x < 0.95$) were prepared [66]. Fe_xO is a nonstoichiometric phase based on an fcc array of oxygen atoms. In this study, $Fe(Ac)_2$, $Fe(acac)_2$, $Fe(acac)_3$, and $Fe(CO)_5$ were used as the precursors, and a wide range of synthetic schemes, from the postoxidation to the thermal decomposition, were investigated systematically.

The technique for the size control of metal oxide NPs are the same as in the synthesis of metal and metal alloy NPs, namely, the seed mediated growth and the additional precursor injection, varying reaction temperature and time, and using different surfactants. A notable case of the size control by the seed mediated growth and the additional injection was reported in [65]. In this study, using the appropriate combination of uniform-sized as-synthesized NP seed dispersion and the precursor solution, the size control in one-nanometer scale was archived in the size range of 4–15 nm while the size distribution was kept narrow. When using the hot injection method, higher precursor to surfactant ratio resulted in the faster nucleation and smaller size [54]. Various size control techniques were available in the thermal decomposition method using metal oleate precursors. Lowering the precursor-to-surfactant ratio tended to increase the mean size of NPs [59–61]. Using Fe(II) precursor instead of Fe(III) also resulted in larger NPs [59]. When the precursor was decomposed by refluxing in the higher boiling point solvent, the larger NPs were obtained [60]. For example, the mean size of 5 nm, 9 nm, and 12 nm were obtained by using 1-hexadecene (b.p. 274 degrees C), octyl ether (b.p. 287 degrees C), 1-octadecene (b.p. 317 degrees C), and 1-eicosene (b.p. 330 degrees C), respectively. The influence of different surfactant and solvent molecules on the size of the nanoparticles was reported in [66]. The size-dependent magnetic property was well demonstrated by the variation of the blocking temperature according to the mean size of the iron oxide NPs (Figure 2.5).

An interesting point in the synthesis of metal oxide NPs is that the simple heating up of the reaction solution can yield highly uniform nanoparticles. In 2007, a study on the kinetics of this "heating up" method was reported [67]. By studying the synthetic reaction of iron oxide NPs introduced in [60], it was revealed that the size distribution control mechanism of the heating-up method is similar to that of the hot injection method, which is characterized by a sudden increase in the number concentration of the nanoparticles (burst of nucleation) and rapid narrowing of the size distribution accompanied by a high growth rate.

2.4.2 Bimetallic Ferrite Nanoparticles

The synthetic methods for monometallic oxide NPs can be extended to the synthesis of bimetallic ferrite NPs. Hyeon et al. synthesized cobalt ferrite ($CoFe_2O_4$) NPs using the post-oxidation method [68]. By the decomposition of (η^5-C_5H_5)$CoFe_2(CO)_9$, CoFe alloy NPs were produced first and then they were oxidized by $(CH_3)_3NO$ to yield $CoFe_2O_4$ NPs. Similarly, manganese ferrite ($MnFe_2O_4$) NPs were synthesize using $Fe(CO)_5$ and $Mn_2(CO)_{10}$ as the precursors by the same research group [69]. Sun et al. modified their synthetic scheme for ion oxide NPs [56] to produce MFe_2O_4 (M = Fe, Co, Mn) NPs. $Fe(acac)_3$, $Co(acac)_2$, and $Mn(acac)_2$ were used as the precursors. $CoFe_2O_4$ (or $MnFe_2O_4$) NPs were obtained by heating the solution containing

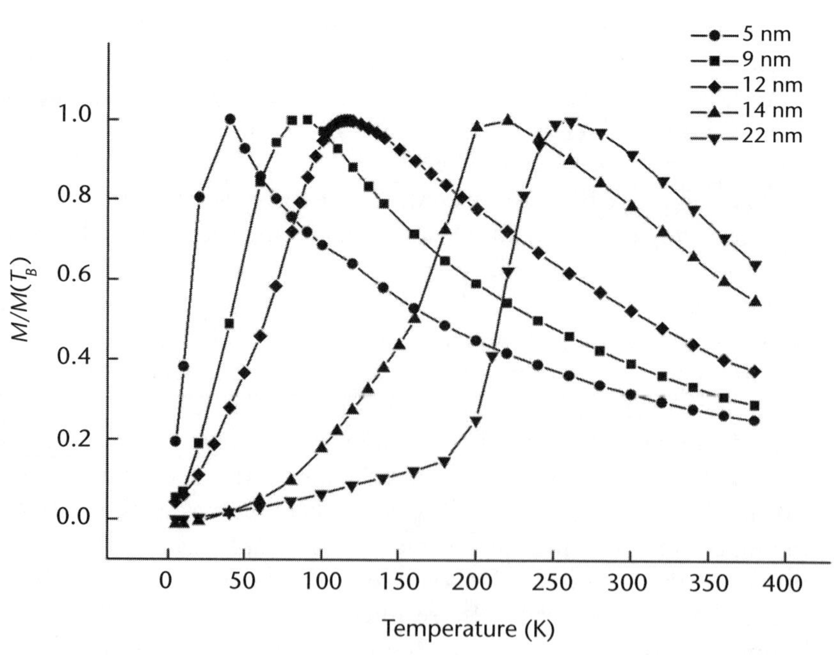

Figure 2.5 Zero-field cooling magnetization curves for iron oxide NPs of various mean size.

Fe and Co (or Mn) precursor in a 2:1 ratio [70]. A generalized thermal decomposition method using metal salts and carboxylic acid as the starting materials was studied by the Cheon group. They synthesized iron oxide NPs by heating the solution containing iron nitrate, lauric acid, and lauryl amine. By mixing iron nitrate and $MnCl_2$ or $CoCl_2$, $NiCl_2$ in the ration of 2:1, $MnFe_2O_4$, $CoFe_2O_4$, and $NiFe_2O_4$ NPs were obtained [52]. Fe_3O_4/$CoFe_2O_4$ core/shell structure was synthesized by the same group by annealing the binary superlattice of Co and Fe_3O_4 NPs [71].

A unique approach for the synthesis of iron oxide and various metal ferrite NPs was reported by Li et al. in 2005 [72]. In this method, the heterogeneous synthetic system was utilized for the size control in the nanometer scale. Liquid-solid-solution (LSS) was obtained by combining linoleic acid dissolved in ethanol (liquid), sodium linoleate (solid), and water-ethanol mixture (solution). When the metal ions were introduced in the aqueous solution, a phase transfer process led to the formation of metal linoleate in separated solid phase. Subsequent dehydration reaction at the interface between metal linoleate and the aqueous solution phase produced metal oxide NPs. This LSS method yielded MFe_2O_4 (M = Fe, Co, Mn) NPs of moderate size uniformity.

Markovich et al. pointed out an important problem in the synthesis of bimetallic ferrite NPs [73]. The phase segregation of single metal oxide could impede the formation of the homogeneous bimetallic ferrite structure. They analyzed cobalt ferrite NPs by MCD spectroscopy to probe the exact position of Co^{2+} ions in the crystal structure. It was found that cobalt ferrite NPs synthesized by the coprecipitation, sol-gel like, and the thermal decomposition methods are not of the stoichiometric structure, which is supposedly due to the phase segregation of cobalt oxide phase. In the same paper, they introduced a modified synthetic method. In this method, $Fe(acac)_3$, iron(III) ethoxide [$Fe(OEt)_3$], and cobalt(II) isopropoxide [$Co(O^iPr)_2$] were used as the precursors. It was intended that the condensation reaction between $Fe(acac)_3$ and $Co(O^iPr)_2$ ensures the formation of Co–O–Fe link and prevents the segregation of cobalt oxide. By the MCD spectroscopy analysis, they showed that this method actually worked for the synthesis of cobalt ferrite NPs of the exact structure.

2.5 Representative Synthetic Procedures for Magnetic Nanoparticles

2.5.1 Iron Nanoparticles

In a typical synthesis, spherical iron NPs are obtained as follows [24]: 0.2 mL of $Fe(CO)_5$ is injected into 5.0g of TOPO at 340 degrees C under argon atmosphere, and the resulting solution is aged for 30 min at 320 degrees C. The reaction mixture is added into excess acetone to separate iron NPs as a black precipitate. After collecting the precipitate and drying under vacuum, the powder is well dispersed in various organic solvents, such as pyridine, chloroform, and hexane.

As mentioned earlier, this method is a direct adaptation of the hot injection method for the synthesis of CdSe nanoparticles. Upon the injection of the precursor, $Fe(CO)_5$, it decomposes instantaneously releasing CO gas. The decomposition reaction is so violent that some iron-containing solution evaporates together with gas evolved. Fe^0 atoms liberated from carbonyl ligands are then coordinated by the solvent molecules. However, TOPO is not a good ligand to stabilize Fe^0 atoms in high concentration. As a result, Fe^0 atoms get aggregated to form macromolecular clusters. These clusters act as nuclei on which more Fe^0 atoms bind and clusters grow to NPs.

As evident in this description, choosing appropriate coordinating ligands (surfactants) in the reaction mixture is very important when designing the NP synthetic procedure. If coordinating species bind to metal atoms too strongly, nucleation will not occur. On the other hand, weak binding might lead to uncontrolled growth of NPs due to the instability of metal atoms, which results in particles of micrometer size and/or broad size distribution. The surface of iron NPs synthesized is covered with TOPO, whose polar head (O=P) is coordinated to Fe atoms on the surface, while the hydrophobic tails ($-(CH_2)_7CH_3$) face the solvent molecules. Those surface-coordinated molecules yield the good dispersibility in nonpolar solvent and high colloidal stability of NPs. Because of their size, iron NPs are vulnerable to oxidation. In ambient condition, iron NPs dispersed in organic solvent are readily oxidized within days to form iron oxide nanoparticles.

2.5.2 Iron Oxide Nanoparticles

Thermal decomposition of metal carboxylate has been utilized as a versatile way for the synthesis of metal oxide NPs, as discussed earlier [60].

Iron-oleate complex is synthesized via a two-phase reaction. First, 10.8g of hydrated iron chloride ($FeCl_3 \cdot 6H_2O$, 40 mmol) and 36.5 g of sodium oleate (120 mmol) was dissolved in a mixture of 80 ml ethanol, 60 ml distilled water, and 140 ml hexane. Sodium oleate molecules act as phase transfer agent. They diffuse from organic phase into water phase and react with Fe^{3+} ions. Then, iron-oleate complex molecules transfer back to the organic phase, leaving sodium chloride in the aqueous phase as a byproduct. After reflux for 12h, organic phase containing iron-oleate complex is collected and washed several times with water. Finally, solvent is evaporated under vacuum.

The following is a typical synthetic procedure of iron oxide NPs: 36g (40 mmol of Fe) of the iron-oleate complex and 5.7g of OLEA (20 mmol) are dissolved in 200g of 1-octadecene. The reaction mixture was heated to 320 degrees C at a rate of 3.3 degrees C min^{-1}, and then kept at that temperature for 30 min. After the reaction stops, the reaction mixture is cooled and excess ethanol is added to precipitate the product. Iron oxide NPs synthesized are of mixed phase of Fe_3O_4 and γ-Fe_2O_3, containing both Fe^{3+} to Fe^{2+} ions. In the course of heating procedure, carboxylate group of iron-oleate complex decomposes into CO_2, CO, and hydrocarbon chains. Some oxygen atoms in carboxylate group remain bound to iron ions, which seem to form oxo-bridges between iron ions. Due to the high reaction temperature, some hydrocarbons decompose yielding H_2 and a trace amount of carbon, which might be responsible for the reduction of Fe^{3+} to Fe^{2+}. The color changes abruptly from brown to turbid black when the temperature reaches 320 degrees C, demonstrating the formation of NPs.

The most appealing point in this procedure is its simplicity. The only operation needed for the synthesis is just heating the reaction mixture. As a result, this procedure is very easy to scale-up without deterioration in the product quality, in terms of size and shape uniformity.

References

[1] Schmid, G., *Nanoparticles: From Theory to Application*, Weinheim: Wiley-VCH, 2004.

[2] Park, J., et al., "Synthesis of Monodisperse Spherical Nanocrystals," *Angew. Chem. Int. Ed.* Vol. 46, 2007, 4630–4660.

[3] Hyeon, T., "Chemical synthesis of magnetic nanoparticles," *Chem. Commun.*, 2003, pp. 927–934.

[4] Green, M., "Organometallic based strategies for metal nanocrystal synthesis," *Chem. Commun.*, 2005, pp. 3002–3011.

[5] Jeong, U., et al., "Superparamagnetic Colloids: Controlled Synthesis and Niche Applications," *Adv. Mater.*, Vol. 19, 2007, pp. 33–60.

[6] Lu, A. H., E. L. Salabas and F. Schüth, "Magnetic Nanoparticles: Synthesis, Protection, Functionalization, and Application," *Angew. Chem. Int. Ed.*, Vol. 46, 2007, pp. 1222–1244.

[7] Sun, S., "Recent Advances in Chemical Synthesis, Self-Assembly, and Applications of FePt Nanoparticles," *Adv. Mater.*, Vol. 18, 2006, pp. 393–403.

[8] Cullity, L. C., *Introduction to Magnetic Materials*, Reading, MA: Addison-Wesley, 1972.

[9] Bean, C. P. and J. D. Livingston, "Superparamagnetism," *J. Appl. Phys.*, Vol. 30, 1959, pp. S120–S129.

[10] Batlle, X. and A. Labarta, "Finite-size effects in fine particles: Magnetic and transport properties," *J. Phys. D: Appl. Phys.*, Vol. 35, 2002, pp. R15–R42.

[11] Kodama, R. H., "Magnetic nanoparticles," *J. Magn. Magn. Mater.*, Vol. 200, 1999, pp. 359–372.

[12] Bødker, F., S. Mørup and S. Linderoth, "Surface effects in metallic iron nanoparticles," *Phys. Rev. Lett.*, Vol. 72, 1994, pp. 282–285.

[13] Sun, S. and C. B. Murray, "Synthesis of monodisperse cobalt nanocrystals and their assembly into magnetic superlattices," *J. Appl. Phys.*, Vol. 85, 1999, pp. 4325–4330.

[14] Murray, C. B., D. J. Norris and M. G. Bawendi, "Synthesis and Characterization of Nearly Monodisperse CdE (E = S, Se, Te) Semiconductor Nanocrystallites," *J. Am. Chem. Soc.*, Vol. 115, 1993, pp. 8706–8715.

[15] Murray, C. B., et al., "Colloidal synthesis of nanocrystals and nanocrystal superlattices," *IBM J. Res. Dev.*, Vol. 45, 2001, pp. 47–56.

[16] Murray, C. B., et al., "Monodisperse 3d Transition-Metal (Co, Ni, Fe) Nanoparticles and Their Assembly into Nanoparticle Superlattices," *Mater. Res. Bull.*, Vol. 26, 2001, pp. 985–991.

[17] Dinega, D. P. and M. G. Bawendi, "A Solution-Phase Chemical Approach to a New Crystal Structure of Cobalt," *Angew. Chem. Int. Ed.*, Vol. 38, 1999, pp. 1788–1791.

[18] Puntes, V. F., K. M. Krishnan and A. P. Alivisatos, "Synthesis, self-assembly, and magnetic behavior of a two-dimensional superlattice of single-crystal å-Co nanoparticles," *Appl. Phys. Lett.*, Vol. 78, 2001, pp. 2187–2189.

[19] Dumestre, F., et al., "Shape Control of Thermodynamically Stable Cobalt Nanorods through Organometallic Chemistry," *Angew. Chem. Int. Ed.*, Vol. 41, 2002, pp. 4286–4289.

[20] Samia, A. C. S., et al., "Ligand Effect on the Growth and the Digestion of Co Nanocrystals," *J. Am. Chem. Soc.*, Vol. 127, 2005, pp. 4126–4127.

[21] Wu, N., et al., "Interaction of Fatty Acid Monolayers with Cobalt Nanoparticles," *Nano Lett.*, Vol. 4, 2004, pp. 383–386.

[22] Griffiths, C. H., M. P. O. Horo and T. W. Smith, "The structure, magnetic characterization, and oxidation of colloidal iron dispersions," *J. Appl. Phys.*, Vol. 50, 1979, pp. 7108–7115.

[23] Suslick, K. S., M. Fang and T. Hyeon, "Sonochemical Synthesis of Iron Colloids," *J. Am. Chem. Soc.*, Vol. 118, 1996, pp. 11960–11961.

[24] Park, S. J., et al., "Synthesis and Magnetic Studies of Uniform Iron Nanorods and Nanospheres," *J. Am. Chem. Soc.*, Vol. 122, 2000, pp. 8581–8582.

[25] Hyeon, T., et al., "Synthesis of Highly Crystalline and Monodisperse Maghemite Nanocrystallites without a Size-Selection Process," *J. Am. Chem. Soc.*, Vol. 123, 2001, pp. 12798–12801.

[26] Dumestre, F., et al., "Superlattices of Iron Nanocubes Synthesized from $Fe[N(SiMe_3)_2]_2$," *Science*, Vol. 303, 2004, pp. 821–823.

[27] Kim, D., et al., "Synthesis of Hollow Iron Nanoframes," *J. Am. Chem. Soc.*, Vol. 129, 2007, pp. 5812–5813.

[28] Cordente, N., et al., "Synthesis and Magnetic Properties of Nickel Nanorods," *Nano Lett.*, Vol. 1, 2001, pp. 565–568.

[29] Kang, E., et al., "Monodisperse Nanoparticles of Ni and NiO: Synthesis, Characterization, Self-Assembled Superlattices, and Catalytic Applications in the Suzuki Coupling Reaction," *Adv. Mater.*, Vol. 17, 2005, pp. 429–434.

[30] Lee, I. S., et al., "Ni/NiO Core/Shell Nanoparticles for Selective Binding and Magnetic Separation of Histidine-Tagged Proteins," *J. Am. Chem. Soc.*, Vol. 128, 2006, pp. 10658–10659.

[31] Farrell, D., S. A. Majetich and J. P. Wilcoxon, "Preparation and Characterization of Monodisperse Fe Nanoparticles," *J. Phys. Chem. B*, Vol. 107, 2003, pp. 11022–11030.

[32] Weller, D., et al., "High K_u Materials Approach to 100 Gbits/in2," *IEEE Trans. Magn.*, Vol. 36, 2000, pp. 10–15.

[33] Moser, A., et al., "Magnetic recording: advancing into the future," *J. Phys. D Appl. Phys.*, Vol. 35, 2002, pp. R157–R167.

[34] Sun, S., et al., "Monodisperse FePt Nanoparticles and Ferromagnetic FePt Nanocrystal Superlattices," *Science*, Vol. 287, 2000, pp. 1989–1992.

[35] Sun, S., et al., "Compositionally Controlled FePt Nanoparticle Materials," *IEEE Trans. Magn.*, Vol. 37, 2001, pp. 1239–1243.

[36] Anders, S., et al., "Controlled Synthesis and Assembly of FePt Nanoparticles," *J. Phys. Chem. B*, Vol. 107, 2003, pp. 5419–5425.

[37] Liu, C., et al., "Polyol Process Synthesis of Monodispersed FePt Nanoparticles," *J. Phys. Chem. B*, Vol. 108, 2004, pp. 6121–6123.

[38] Howard, L. E. M., et al., "A Synthetic Route to Size-Controlled fcc and fct FePt Nanoparticles," *J. Am. Chem. Soc.*, Vol. 127, 2005, pp. 10140–10141.

[39] Chen, M., J. P. Liu and S. Sun, "One-Step Synthesis of FePt Nanoparticles with Tunable Size," *J. Am. Chem. Soc.*, Vol. 126, 2004, pp. 8394–8395.

[40] Teng, X., et al., "Platinum-Maghemite Core-Shell Nanoparticles Using a Sequential Synthesis," *Nano Lett.*, Vol. 3, 2003, pp. 261–264.

[41] Teng, X. and H. Yang, "Synthesis of Face-Centered Tetragonal FePt Nanoparticles and Granular Films from Pt@Fe2O3 Core-Shell Nanoparticles," *J. Am. Chem. Soc.*, Vol. 125, 2003, pp. 14559–14563.

[42] Yu, A. C. C., et al., "Atomic Composition Effect on the Ordering of Solution-phase Synthesized FePt Nanoparticle Films," *Appl. Phys. Lett.*, Vol. 85, 2004, pp. 6242–6244.

[43] Ely, T. O., et al., "Nanoscale Bimetallic Co_xPt_{1-x} Particles Dispersed in Poly(vinylpyrrolidone): Synthesis from Organometallic Precursors and Characterization," *J. Phys. Chem. B*, Vol. 104, 2000, pp. 695–702.

[44] Park, J. I. and J. Cheon, "Synthesis of "Solid Solution" and "Core-Shell" Type Cobalt-Platinum Magnetic Nanoparticles via Transmetalation Reactions," *J. Am. Chem. Soc.*, Vol. 123, 2001, pp. 5743–5746.

[45] Shevchenko, E. V., et al., "Colloidal Synthesis and Self-Assembly of $CoPt_3$ Nanocrystals," *J. Am. Chem. Soc.*, Vol. 124, 2002, pp. 11480–11485.

[46] Shevchenko, E. V., et al., "Study of Nucleation and Growth in the Organometallic Synthesis of Magnetic Alloy Nanocrystals: The Role of Nucleation Rate in Size Control of $CoPt_3$ Nanocrystals," *J. Am. Chem. Soc.*, Vol. 125, 2003, pp. 9090–9101.

[47] Chen, M. and D. E. Nikles, "Synthesis of Spherical FePd and CoPt Nanoparticles," *J. Appl. Phys.*, Vol. 91, 2002, pp. 8477–8479.

[48] Chen, M. and D. E. Nikles, "Synthesis, Self-Assembly, and Magnetic Properties of $Fe_xCo_yPt_{100-x-y}$ Nanoparticles," *Nano Lett.*, Vol. 2, 2002, pp. 211–214.

[49] Sun, X., et al., "Synthesis, Chemical Ordering, and Magnetic Properties of FePtCu Nanoparticle Films," *J. Appl. Phys.*, Vol. 93, 2003, pp. 7337–7339.

[50] Kang, S., J. W. Harrell and D. E. Nikles, "Reduction of the fcc to $L1_0$ Ordering Temperature for Self-Assembled FePt Nanoparticles Containing Ag," *Nano Lett.*, Vol. 2, 2002, pp. 1033–1036.

[51] Yavuz, C. T., et al., "Low-Field Magnetic Separation of Monodisperse Fe_3O_4 Nanocrystals," *Science*, Vol. 314, 2006, pp. 964–967.

[52] Lee, J. H., et al., "Artificially Engineered Magnetic Nanoparticles for Ultra-sensitive Molecular Imaging," *Nature Med.*, Vol. 13, 2007, pp. 95–99.

[53] Na, H. B., et al., "Development of a T_1 Contrast Agent for Magnetic Resonance Imaging Using MnO Nanoparticles," *Angew. Chem. Int. Ed.*, Vol. 46, 2007, pp. 5397–5401.

[54] Casula, M. F., et al., "The Concept of Delayed Nucleation in Nanocrystal Growth Demonstrated for the Case of Iron Oxide Nanodisks," *J. Am. Chem. Soc.*, Vol. 128, 2006, pp. 1675–1682.

[55] Rockenberger, J., E. C. Scher and A. P. Alivisatos, "A New Nonhydrolytic Single-Precursor Approach to Surfactant-Capped Nanocrystals of Transition Metal Oxides," *J. Am. Chem. Soc.*, Vol. 121, 1999, pp. 11595–11596.

[56] Sun, S. and H. Zeng, "Size-Controlled Synthesis of Magnetite Nanoparticles," *J. Am. Chem. Soc.*, Vol. 124, 2002, pp. 8204–8205.

[57] Yin, M. and S. O'Brien, "Synthesis of Monodisperse Nanocrystals of Manganese Oxides," *J. Am. Chem. Soc.*, Vol. 125, 2003, pp. 10180–10181.

[58] Seo, W. S., et al., "Size-Dependent Magnetic Properties of Colloidal Mn_3O_4 and MnO Nanoparticles," *Angew. Chem. Int. Ed.*, Vol. 43, 2004, pp. 1115–1117.

[59] Jana, N. R., Y. Chen and X. Peng, "Size- and Shape-Controlled Magnetic (Cr, Mn, Fe, Co, Ni) Oxide Nanocrystals via a Simple and General Approach," *Chem. Mater.*, Vol. 16, 2004, pp. 3931–3935.

[60] Park, J., et al., "Ultra-large-scale Syntheses of Monodisperse Nanocrystals," *Nature Mater.*, Vol. 3, 2004, pp. 891–895.

[61] Yu, W. W., et al., "Synthesis of Monodisperse Iron Oxide Nanocrystals by Thermal Decomposition of Iron Carboxylate Salts," *Chem. Commun.*, 2004, pp. 2306–2307.

[62] Bronstein, L. M., et al., "Influence of Iron Oleate Complex Structure on Iron Oxide Nanoparticle Formation," *Chem. Mater.*, Vol. 19, 2007, pp. 3624–3632.

[63] Sun, X., et al., "Metal (Mn, Co, and Cu) Oxide Nanocrystals from Simple Formate Precursors," *Small*, Vol. 1, 2005, pp. 1081–1086.

[64] An, K., et al., "Synthesis, Characterization, and Self-Assembly of Pencil-Shaped CoO Nanorods," *J. Am. Chem. Soc.*, Vol. 128, 2006, pp. 9753–9760.

[65] Park, J., et al., "One-Nanometer-Scale Size-Controlled Synthesis of Monodisperse Magnetic Iron Oxide Nanoparticles," *Angew. Chem. Int. Ed.*, Vol. 44(19), 2005, pp. 2872–2877.

[66] Redl, F. X., et al., "Magnetic, Electronic, and Structural Characterization of Nonstoichiometric Iron Oxides at the Nanoscale," *J. Am. Chem. Soc.*, Vol. 126, 2004, pp. 14583–14599.

[67] Kwon, S. G., et al., "Kinetics of Monodisperse Iron Oxide Nanocrystal Formation by Heating-Up Process," *J. Am. Chem. Soc.*, Vol. 129, 2007, pp. 12571–12584.

[68] Hyeon, T., et al., "Synthesis of Highly Crystalline and Monodisperse Cobalt Ferrite Nanocrystals," *J. Phys. Chem. B*, Vol. 106, 2002, pp. 6831–6833.

[69] Kang, E., et al., "Direct Synthesis of Highly Crystalline and Monodisperse Manganese Ferrite Nanocrystals," *J. Phys. Chem. B*, Vol. 108, 2004, pp. 13932–13935.

[70] Sun, S., et al., "Monodisperse MFe_2O_4 (M = Fe, Co, Mn) Nanoparticles," *J. Am. Chem. Soc.*, Vol. 126, 2004, pp. 273–279.

[71] Cheon, J., et al., "Magnetic Superlattices and Their Nanoscale Phase Transition Effects," *Proc. Natl. Acad. Sci. USA*, Vol. 103, 2006, pp. 3023–3027.

[72] Wang, X., et al., "A General Strategy for Nanocrystal Synthesis," *Nature*, Vol. 437, 2005, pp. 121–124.

[73] Tirosh, E., G. Shemer and G. Markovich, "Optimizing Cobalt Ferrite Nanocrystal Synthesis Using a Magneto-optical Probe," *Chem. Mater.*, Vol. 18, 2006, pp. 465–470.

CHAPTER 3

Peptide-Functionalized Quantum Dots for Live Diagnostic Imaging and Therapeutic Applications

Laurent A. Bentolila, Sören Doose, Yuval Ebenstein, Gopal Iyer, J. Jack Li, Xavier Michalet, Fabien Pinaud, James Tsay, and Shimon Weiss

3.1 Introduction

Since their first appearance as optical probes in biological imaging [1, 2], qdots have been applied in most biotechnological applications using fluorescence, including DNA array technology, immunofluorescence assays (reviewed in [3]), and cell and animal biology (reviewed in [4, 5]. Qdots have gained wide acceptance by the scientific community and the biotechnology industry as new fluorescent, nonisotopic labels of unmatched potentials. Most appealing to the biosciences are the high brightness, high resistance to photobleaching, and the ability to size-tune fluorescent emission of these inorganic-biological hybrid nanostructures. Qdots have also proved to be excellent probes for two-photon confocal microscopy and deep-tissue imaging given their large two-photon absorption cross-section [6–9]. But it is when combined with ultrasensitive microscopy techniques that qdots have shown their true potential by allowing visualization of cellular processes down to the molecular scale [10–13]. The enhanced photophysical properties of qdots can fulfill the stringent requirements needed to provide spatial, temporal, and structural information at all length scales: from the whole body down to the nanometer resolution with a single probe.

Fluorescent nanocrystals of semiconductor material, which are generally synthesized in solutions of nonpolar organic solvents using colloidal chemistry [14], require additional chemical modifications to be solubilized in aqueous buffers and functionalized for biological applications (see Chapter 1, "Colloidal Quantum Dots: Synthesis, Photophysical Properties, and Biofunctionalization Strategies," by Susumu et al. for an in-depth discussion). This can be achieved by either surfactant exchange, a process primarily driven by mass-action in which the native TOP/TOPO hydrophobic surface ligands are substituted with bifunctional amphiphilic ones, or by insulation of the original hydrophobic qdot within a heterofunctional amphiphilic coating [4, 5]. These various qdot solubilization strategies have included the following: (1) ligand exchange with small thiol-containing molecules [2, 15] or more complex ones such as oligomeric phosphines [16], dendrons [17], and peptides [18, 19]; (2) encapsulation by a layer of amphiphilic diblock [20], or triblock copolymers [21], in silica shells [1, 22], phospholipid micelles [23], polymer beads [24], polymer shells [25], or amphiphilic polysaccharides [26]; and (3) combination of layers of different molecules conferring the required colloidal stability to qdots [27, 28]. Once the qdots have been solubilized with hydrophilic ligands, those can serve as anchoring points for the chemical attachment of biomolecules to functionalize the qdot's surface. Qdot's ligands containing either an amine or a carboxyl group offer the possibility to crosslink molecules containing a thiol group [18, 23, 29] or an N-hydroxysuccinimyl-ester moiety [1, 19] using standard bioconjugation reactions.

Another approach uses electrostatic interactions between qdots and charged molecules, or proteins modified to incorporate charged domains [30]. These functionalization steps can be repeated to add or change functionality. For instance, streptavidin-coated qdots can be used in combination with biotinylated proteins, antibodies, or nucleic acids [10, 19, 20, 31–34]. By extension, a generic three-layer approach using (1) an antibody against a specific target, (2) a biotinylated secondary antibody against the first, and (3) a streptavidin-coated qdot allows qdot labeling of most types of targets [10, 20]. However, the "sandwich" approach results in large structures that may impede further use of qdots in some applications. This issue can be minimized by using small peptide derivatives for qdot solubilization and/or functionalization. The utility of peptides in qdot chemistry stems from several characteristics. Thiol-containing peptide sequences (i.e., Cysteine) have the capacity to coordinate with the nanocrystal shell surface after ligand exchange of the TOPO coating. This leads to a direct attachment of the peptide to the qdot. While small, peptides still maintain excellent molecular recognition properties that allow them to participate in ligand-receptor and protein-protein molecular interaction with high affinity. For example, it has been shown that a ~30 amino acids peptide hairpin against Texas Red has a dissociation constant K_d of ~25 pM [35]. Peptides provide selective anchor points for independent chemical modifications. They offer flexible platforms to screen vast combinatorial libraries with the aim of mutating the peptide sequences to optimize the colloidal and photo-physical properties of nano-materials [36, 37]. Finally, peptides are usually easy to synthesize or mass produce in recombinant hosts.

Our laboratory and others have harnessed these properties to develop unique peptide-based solubilization, functionalization, and targeting approaches that maintain the overall size of the qdot bioconjugate as relatively small while yielding monodisperse water-soluble qdots that remain bright and photostable. In the "conventional" two-step approach, solubilization and functionalization are usually uncoupled. Qdots are first solubilized through one of the many approaches described previously before a functional peptide sequence could be attached to the qdots' surface through covalent conjugations or self-assembly. (For a review, see [38].) We will refer to these probes as "peptide-conjugated" qdots. On the other hand, our laboratory has developed a single-step solubilization/functionalization approach based on exchanging the qdots' surface ligands with bi-functional amphiphilic peptides [19]. In the rest of this chapter, we will refer to this approach as *peptide coating*. The peptide-coating approach has been successful on several types of core and core-shell qdots encompassing the visible to the near-infrared (NIR) spectral range. In this chapter, we first describe the peptide-coating approach and briefly assess the colloidal and photophysical properties of the resulting peptide-coated particles when tested by fluorescence correlation spectroscopy (FCS) and single-molecule spectroscopy (SMS). We then continue with several examples of biological applications in which peptide-coated qdots have been used. Those include single-particle tracking of membrane receptor in live cells and combined fluorescence and micro-positron emission tomography (μPET) imaging of targeted delivery in live animals. Beyond diagnostic imaging, they also have shown utility in other sensing and therapeutic applications including the development of novel protease assays and the use of photo-induced cellular targeted killing. We finally conclude with a brief overview of future developments.

3.2 Phytochelatin Peptides: The All-in-One Solubilization/ Functionalization Approach

The use of semiconductor qdots for biological applications requires that they are water soluble and offer reactive chemical groups on their surface for the subsequent conjugation of molecules and compounds of biological interest. In contrast to the more conventional multiligand/multilayer approaches mentioned previously, our group has developed a new peptide-based family of ligands that replaces the shell surface TOPO coating and fulfills all the stringent requirements of a biocompatible imaging probe at the same time. These engineered peptides maintain most of the original qdot photophysical properties, solubilize qdots in aqueous buffers, provide a biological interface to the qdot, and allow multiple functions to be easily incorporated all in a single easy step. This surface chemistry was designed to be simple, robust, amenable to high-throughput molecular evolution, and flexible enough to suit the different needs of the experimentalists. This is achieved by exchanging the surfactants with synthetic phytochelatin-like α-peptides [19].

Phytochelatins are glutathione-related, cysteine-rich isopeptides synthesized by some plants, yeast, and bacteria strains to detoxify their environment from heavy metal ion contaminants (i.e., Cd^{2+} [39]) by inducing their nucleation into semiconductor qdot particles (i.e., CdS [40, 41]). These peptides of general structure (Glu-Cys)$_n$Gly (designed (γ-EC)$_n$G or (α-EC)$_n$G depending on the peptide linkage between the glutamate and cysteine residues) follow a strict periodicity (with n being the number of di-peptide repeats typically ranging from 2 to 4), which acts as a template for the nucleation and intracellular growth of the qdots (Figure 3.1). Interestingly, the resulting peptide-coated qdots grown in vivo show similar photo-luminescent properties when compared to the chemically synthesized ones, with the only notable exception of being less stable and more prone to degradation upon photo-excitation [41]. One possible reason is their lower crystalline quality, but it also may be due to the absence of higher band gap shell material grown on top of the semiconductor cores. For this reason, qdots grown from natural peptide templates have found very little use as probes for biological imaging.

The phytochelatin-like α-peptides developed in our laboratory have been inspired by these naturally occurring processes. Such synthetic sequences efficiently

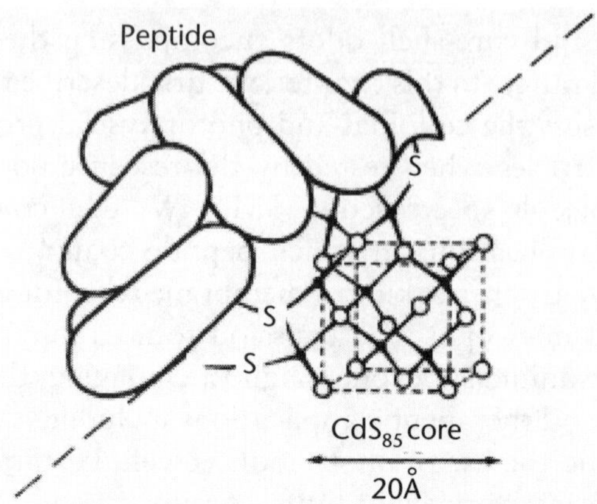

Figure 3.1 Hypothetical model structure of a natural phytochelatin peptide-coated CdS crystallite from yeast. The cysteinyl thiolates of approximately 30 $(\gamma\text{–EC})_n$G peptides are surface ligands to the core of about 85 CdS units. The yeast qdots are monodisperse with an average diameter of 20Å. Adapted from [41] with permission from Elsevier.

bind to the surface of ZnS capped CdSe qdots synthesized in vitro in the presence of TOPO surfactant. A typical amphiphilic peptide is about 20 amino acids long (Figure 3.2(a) and Table 3.1). It is composed of two distinct domains: a metal-chelating adhesive domain containing multiple cysteines (Cys) and unnatural hydrophobic amino acids 3-cyclohexylalanines (Cha), and a negatively charged hydrophilic tail domain. The hydrophobic domain is primarily responsible for the recognition and attachment to the qdot shell surface, while the hydrophilic one ensures solubilization and stability in buffers. The sequence composition of the metal-binding domain is fixed, and the spacing of the cysteinyl thiolates ensures proper anchorage on CdS and ZnS qdot's surfaces [41–43]. We have found that substituting the Cys residues by alanine (Ala) resulted in water insoluble particles, thus confirming the essential role of the Cys in binding of the peptides onto the qdot's surface. We also observed that a single adhesive domain repeat resulted in unstable qdots. We thus opted for multiple tandem repeats of Cys, which enhanced the stability of the peptide on the qdots most likely by providing better surface coverage. A similar length-dependent stability was previously reported for CdS qdots coated with phytochelatin peptides of various lengths [41]. The presence of the Cha residues around the Cys in the adhesive domain helps the solubilization of the peptides in a 9:1 (v:v) pyridine:dimethylsulfoxide (DMSO) cosolvent mixture where TOPO-coated qdots are stable, therefore limiting the formation of aggregate during the reaction. The large cyclohexyl moieties were also chosen to limit the cross-reactivity between the Cys of the adhesive domain and to compete with the hydrophobic TOPO on the qdot's surface. When the Cha residues were replaced by Ala, the peptide-coated qdots we obtained were unstable in buffers. However, we have been recently successful in replacing the unnatural amino-acid Cha by a natural one, phenylalanine (Phe), in the metal-binding domain that still preserves the stability and photophysical properties of the peptide-coated qdots [44]. One direct advantage of this substitution is that an "all natural" peptide (peptide 8 in Table 3.1) can be mass-produced in bacteria. This represents a cost-effective alternative to

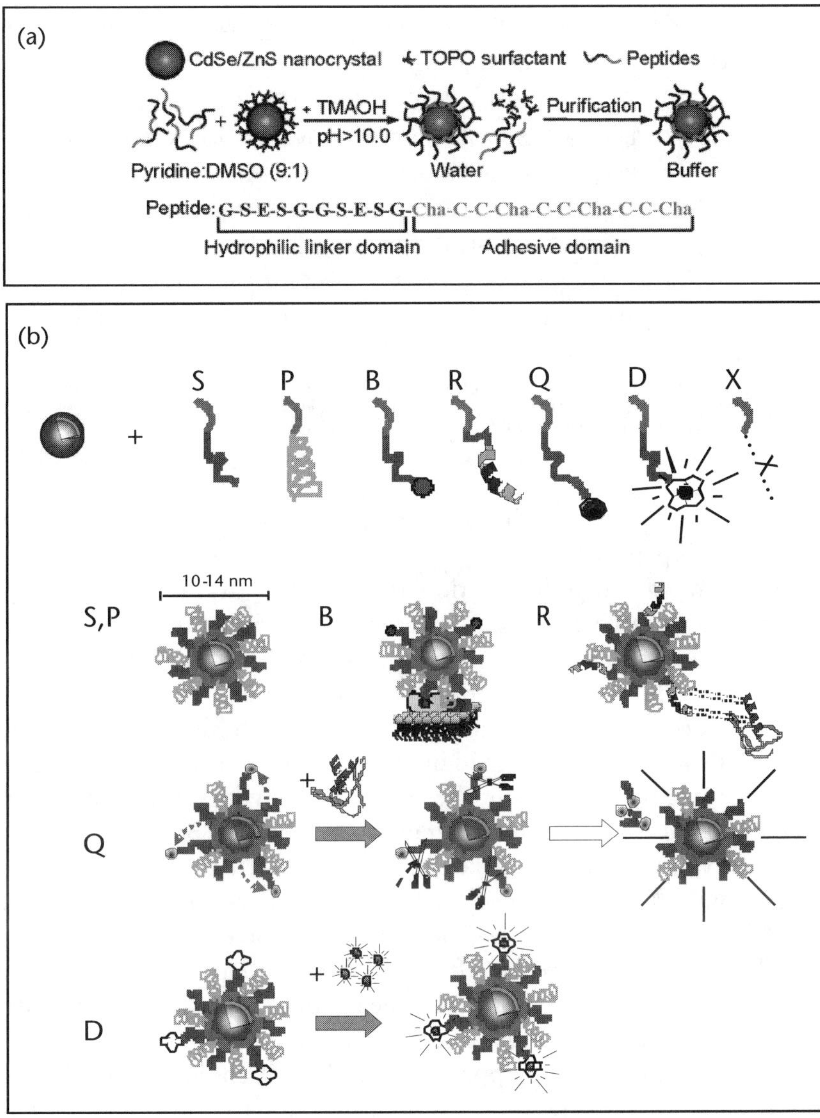

Figure 3.2 The phytochelatin peptide-coating approach: (a) Schematic representation of the surface coating chemistry of CdSe/ZnS nanocrystals with phytochelatin-related-peptides. The peptide C-terminal adhesive domain binds to the ZnS shell of CdSe/ZnS nanocrystals after exchange with the trioctylphosphine oxide (TOPO) surfactant. A polar and negatively charged hydrophilic linker domain in the peptide sequence provides aqueous buffer solubility to the nanocrystals. TMAOH: Tetramethyl ammonium hydroxide; Cha: 3-cyclohexylalanine. Adapted from [19] with permission from American Chemical Society. (b) Schematic representation of the peptide toolbox. The light blue segment contains cysteines and hydrophobic amino acids ensuring binding to the nanocrystal (adhesive domain of Figure 3.2(a)) and is common to all peptides. S: solubilization sequence (hydrophilic linker domain of Figure 3.2(a)), P: PEG, B: biotin, R: recognition sequence, Q: quencher, D: DOTA (1,4,7,10-tetraazacyclododecane-1,4,7,10-tetraacetic acid) for radionuclide and nuclear spin label chelation, X: any unspecified peptide-encoded function. Qdots solubilization is obtained by a mixture of S and P. Qdots can be targeted with biotin (B), a peptide recognition sequences (R), or other chemical moieties. Qdots fluorescence can be turned on or off by attaching a quencher (Q) via a cleavable peptide link. In the presence of the appropriate enzyme, the quencher is separated from the qdot, restoring the photoluminescence and reporting on the enzyme activity (as described in Section 3.6). For simultaneous PET (or MRI) and fluorescence imaging, qdots can be rendered radioactive by chelation of radionuclides (or nuclear spin labels respectively) using (D) DOTA (as described in Section 3.5). Adapted from [5] with permission from American Association for the Advancement of Science. (See Color Plate 3.)

Table 3.1 Phytochelatin-Related α-Peptides Used for Solubilization/Functionalization of Qdots

Nomenclature	*Peptide Sequences**	*References*
1	KGSESGGSESG(*Cha*)CC(*Cha*)CC(*Cha*)CC(*Cha*)-Cmd	[19]
2	Biotin-GSESGGSESG(*Cha*)CC(*Cha*)CC(*Cha*)CC(*Cha*)-Cmd	Ibid
3	PEG-(*Cha*)CC(*Cha*)CC(*Cha*)CC(*Cha*)-Cmd	Ibid
4	GSESGGSESG(*Cha*)CC(*Cha*)CC(*Cha*)CC(*Cha*)-Cmd	Ibid
5	Ac-GSESGGSESG(*Cha*)CC(*Cha*)CC(*Cha*)CC(*Cha*)-Cmd	Ibid
6	Suc-GSSSGGSSSG(*Cha*)CC(*Cha*)CC(*Cha*)CC(*Cha*)-Cmd	Ibid
7	FITC-GSESGGSESG(*Cha*)CC(*Cha*)CC(*Cha*)CC(*Cha*)-Cmd	[44]
8	GSESGGSESGFCCFCCFCCF-HS[b]	Ibid

*All sequences are written from N- to C-terminus. Cmd: carboxamide; Ac: N-terminal acetylation; Suc: N-terminal succinylation; *Cha*: 3-cyclohexylalanine (unnatural amino acid), PEG: hexaethyleneglycol. [b]HS: homoserine residue obtained after CNBr cleavage of methionine residue.

solid-phase peptide synthesis, which can also be technically challenging for cysteine-rich peptides.

Contrary to the adhesive domain sequence that is fixed, the hydrophobic tail sequence is variable and can be altered at will to dial in desirable intracellular homing sequences and/or functional groups for bioconjugation (Figure 3.2(b)). The inherent flexibility of this approach provides endless functionalities (in the form of a "peptide toolbox") that can be subsequently combined to create multimodal qdot imaging probes (later described in Section 3.5). But perhaps the main advantage for the experimentalist resides in the simplicity by which the peptide surface chemistry exchange is accomplished in a single reaction step (Figure 3.2(a)). The addition of tetramethylammonium hydroxide (TMAOH) base to a mixture of peptides:qdots in DMSO:pyridine (1:9) triggers the formation of cysteine thiolate anions, which initiates binding of the peptides onto the ZnS layer. The resulting peptide-coated nanoparticles precipitate out of the cosolvent and are collected by centrifugation. At this point, the qdots are readily soluble in aqueous buffers. Gel filtration and dialysis are then used to remove the excess of unbound peptides and to transfer the peptide-coated qdot into the appropriate buffer of choice. Table 3.1 lists some of the phytochelatin-related α-peptide sequences used. Recently, Zheng et al. have successfully mimicked the use of a natural phytochelatin peptide by describing a facile one-pot aqueous synthesis of glutathione-coated CdTe qdots [45].

3.3 Colloidal and Photophysical Properties of Peptide-Coated Qdots

The peptide-coating approach overcomes some of the known limitations of other capping strategies that lead to particles that either lack long-term stability [2, 15], result in large particles [20, 21], have broader size distributions [1], or do not work well with all particle sizes [23]. Because of the organic nature of the peptide coat, which provides biocompatibility in aqueous buffer, conventional analytical techniques can be used to systematically monitor the ligand-exchange reaction's efficiency. For example, we routinely use size exclusion liquid chromatography (SE-HPLC) and agarose gel electrophoresis as stringent criteria to test for batch quality and consistency. Such analysis is also instrumental in determining the size distribution of the resulting peptide-coated qdots. Figure 3.3(a) illustrates how narrow the size distribution of a typical peptide-coated qdot batch can be. For example, the tight, smearless band in the agarose gel is indicative of the deposition of a uniform peptide layer of a constant thickness, independent of the original size of the nanoparticle's core-shell structure. Figure 3.3(b) shows also how subtle variations of the hydrophilic peptide sequence can result in changes of the overall particle charge that can be easily resolved by the electrophoretic process. SE-HPLC and FCS provide an estimate of the hydrodynamic radius of the coated nanoparticles. All together, the peptide-coating approach maintains the overall size of the qdots as relatively small (8 to 13 nm, Figure 3.3(c)) compared to ~18 nm for phospholipid-coated qdots and up to 30 nm for commercial nanocrystals protected by a polymer coat as shown by FCS analysis [46]. This is definitely an advantage for cell biology applications in which interference with biological interactions and target inaccessibility due to steric hindrance need to be kept to a minimum.

Finally, peptide-coated qdots have long shelf lives and show minimum aggregation in physiological buffer over several months when kept at 4 degrees C. On the other hand, we observed that the quantum yield (QY) of the peptide-coated qdots in buffer is somewhat influenced by the composition and structure of the shell, ranging from 8–16 percent for CdSe/ZnS to 20–35 percent for CdSe/CdS/ZnS with graded shells [5]. A graded shell composition also seems to induce a slight change of emission spectra (red shift) upon peptide coating. This is suggestive of cross-talks

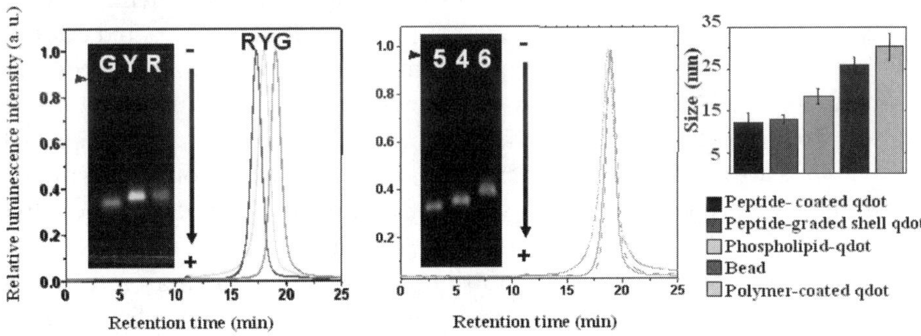

(a) (b) (c)

Figure 3.3 Characterization of peptide-coated qdots: (a) Effect of qdot size as measured by SE-HPLC and gel electrophoresis. The nomenclature of the peptides refers to the numbering in Table 3.1. Green, yellow, and red qdots emitting at 530, 565, and 617 nm, respectively, and coated with peptide 5 were separated on a size exclusion column against a 0.1M PBS mobile phase. The diameter of the peptide-coated qdots was evaluated from the elution times as 129.4Å (±15 percent), 150.3Å (±16 percent), and 164.8Å (±14 percent), respectively. Inset: 0.5 percent agarose gel electrophoresis of the same three peptide-coated qdot samples in TBE buffer pH 8.3. (b) Effect of peptide charge. Qdots coated with peptide 5 (dash), peptide 4 (dot), or peptides 6 (solid) have similar retention times on a SE-HPLC column. Inset: the same peptide-coated qdots migrate at different positions on a 0.5 percent agarose gel, in good agreement with the theoretical charge of each peptide. –►: position of the loading wells. →: direction of the applied electric field. (b) Effect of peptide charge on peptide-coated qdots. Qdots coated with peptide 5 (dash), peptide 4 (dot), or peptides 6 (solid) have similar retention times on a SE-HPLC column (same size) while having different charges as accessed by gel electrophoresis. Adapted from [19] with permission from American Chemical Society. (c) Hydrodynamic diameter of various qdot preparations deducted from FCS analysis. Adapted from [46] with permission from American Chemical Society. (See Color Plate 4.)

between the excitonic wavefunction and the peptide molecular orbitals [5]. One can envision that these sorts of interactions can be harnessed to improve the photo-physical properties of the peptide-coated qdots (e.g., as to enhance quantum yield or to reduce fluorescence intermittency by screening large libraries of peptides). Such strategies have been extremely powerful for the recognition, synthesis, and self-assembly of nanocrystals and other metallic materials in bio-engineered phage [36, 37, 47] or in bacteria [48].

3.4 Live Cell Dynamic Imaging

3.4.1 Single-Particle Tracking of Cell-Surface Membrane Receptors

As discussed previously, one of the advantages of the peptide-coating approach relies on those qdot surface properties that are easily controlled and tuned with various peptide combinations (Figure 3.2(b)). The peptide exchange chemistry can be modified to produce a large variety of functional groups that are exposed at the particle surface, allowing a number of covalent modification techniques for conjugation. In general, the presence of amines and/or thiols on the qdot surface enables the most common conjugation strategies [49, 50] and sidesteps the need to chemically prepare specialized linker molecules. For example, one can easily activate peptide-coated qdots with biotin. The qdots can also be directly coated with synthetic biotinylated peptides (peptide 2 in Table 3.1 and peptide B in Figure 3.2(b)) or via the conjugation of amine reactive biotinylation reagents (such as succinimidyl ester biotin) on a terminal lysine amino acid residue of peptide-coated qdots (peptide 1 in Table 3.1 and [51]). These biotin-terminated peptide-coated qdots show excellent reactivity with avidin, neutravidin, or streptavidin [19].

Importantly, this bioactivation approach maintains a small particle diameter, which is a valuable asset for targeting, detecting, and monitoring the trajectories of individual proteins in the plasma membrane of living cells. Their hydrodynamic radius (< 12 nm, Figure 3.3(c)) is significantly smaller than the commonly used 40-nm gold nanoparticles or 500-nm latex beads that may interfere with protein dynamics [10, 52]. Qdots also outperform the rapid photobleaching of small (1- to 4-nm) fluorescent organic labels [10, 53]. For example, we have used biotin-terminated peptide-coated qdots to target avidin fusion to glycosylphosphatidyl-inositol CD14 cell surface receptor (CD14-Av) in cultured HeLa cells (Figure 3.4 and [19]). This approach not only demonstrated specific recognition of the CD14-Av proteins on the cell membrane, but also that qdot fluorescence can be used to track the movement of single receptors in live cells over extended periods of time. Indeed, by working at subnanomolar concentration of biotin-peptide-coated-qdots to ensure that individual qdots could be distinguished optically, we were able to observe binding events and the subsequent membrane diffusion of individually labeled CD14-Av receptors, as illustrated in Figure 3.4.

The brightness and photostability of peptide-coated qdots [46, 54] allow the use of a standard CCD camera (CoolSnap *cf*, Princeton Instruments, Trenton, NJ) and rather short exposure times (~100 ms). Other experiments performed with an electron multiplying camera (Cascade 512B, Princeton Instruments) and total internal reflection (TIR) microscopy allowed the use of much shorter exposure time (20 ms

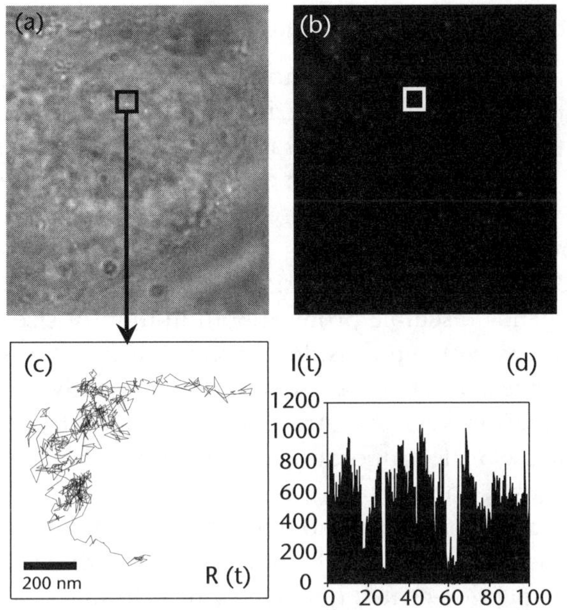

Figure 3.4 Single-particle tracking in a live-cell: (a) DIC and (b) epifluorescence images of live HeLa cells expressing the CD14-Av receptors (see main text for details). Single qdots were observed to diffuse at characteristically different rates in different regions of the membrane or inside the cytosol (data not shown). (c) The 1,000 steps (100 ms/step) trajectory, R(t), of the qdot localized in the region marked in panel (a, b), with (d) the corresponding qdot intensity, I(t). The blinking pattern (succession of on and off emission) demonstrates that a single qdot was observed. Adapted from [5] with permission from American Association for the Advancement of Science.

or less). It is worth mentioning that the trajectory of an individual receptor cannot necessarily be tracked continuously due to the intermittence in qdot's fluorescence emission (Figure 3.4(d)). Instead, we use this blinking behavior as a proof of singleness. The advantages of using qdots in these experiments become evident. Qdots' photostability can allow the observation of individual receptor trajectories for 10 to 20 min compared to ~5s with Cy3-labelled antibodies [10]. The brightness of the qdots also allows the spots to be detected with a high signal-to-noise ratio (SNR ~50), while short integration time allows the capture of the dynamics of the process. The high SNR allows better positioning accuracy (~5–10 nm) of the tracked particle and its receptor. Similar experiments by Dahan et al. [10] tracking extra-synaptic receptors also revealed that these cell-surface proteins were far more mobile than previously considered by single-particle tracking using micrometer-sized beads [55], further confirming that the size of larger load does influence diffusion properties. Long trajectory observations give access to a wealth of information on the local spatio-temporal environment of each particle, which would be accessible only through statistical analysis of hundreds of trajectories using standard fluorescent dyes [56].

3.4.2 Peptide-Mediated Intracellular Delivery and Targeting of Qdots

The delivery of biological and/or inorganic cargos across the membrane lipid bilayer of living cells toward the cell interior has many potential applications that range from the development of novel therapeutic agents to the basic understanding of gene and protein functions. Mammalian cells have evolved strategies to selectively import and export vital compounds like hydrated ions and small polar molecules. But the plasma membrane still represents a formidable barrier to the passage of larger biomolecules. Colloidal qdots consisting of an inorganic core surrounded by a layer of organic ligands resemble proteins both in term of size (in the nanometer range) and charge (negative) and thus do not freely diffuse across the lipid bilayer of live cells. For these reasons, the use of qdots has principally focused on targeting cell surface membrane markers that are easily accessible from the surrounding culture medium. The use of electroporation or transfection reagents [57] that capitalize on a receptor-mediated endocytotic translocation routes results in qdots being sequestrated and accumulated in lysosomal and endosomal vesicles that appear scattered in the cytoplasm [58, 59]. On the other hand, the direct microinjection of peptide-conjugated or peptide-coated qdots in living cells [51, 57] has allowed the targeting of qdots to subcellular compartments such as mitochondria [57] or the nucleus [60]. All of these physical approaches have, however, limited in vivo applications since they are serial, time consuming, or technically challenging, and they do not allow high-throughput screening. Thus, there is still a need to systematically explore various strategies for delivering qdots into live cells, especially those that can facilitate cell entry without the requirement for endocytosis.

To date, the use of short arginine-rich peptide sequences constitutes one of the most promising classes of ligands for the intracellular delivery of a variety of macromolecules into live cells [61] including qdots [58, 60, 62–69]. These sequences, referred to as *cell permeable peptides/peptide transduction domains* (CPP/PTD), include short segments first isolated from the human immunodeficiency virus 1 (HIV-1) transcriptional activator Tat protein, the *drosophila* homeotic transcription protein antennapedia (Antp), and the herpes simplex virus structural protein VP22 [70]. Other sequences have been identified, including homopolymers of arginine [71]. Most, if not all, PTDs carry a net positive charge (highly rich in basic residues), are less than 20–30 amino acids long, and have the ability to rapidly translocate large molecules into cells. PTDs that have been used for intracellular delivery of qdots are shown in Table 3.2.

While the mechanism responsible for uptake of PTDs and their cargos remains unclear, if not controversial, PTDs can be used to accelerate the intracellular delivery of qdots into a variety of cell types by coupling PTDs to qdots via a streptavidin-biotin link [21, 58, 60], covalently [72], by electrostatic adsorption of PTDs containing free cysteine residues [57] or not [73]. Once mono-disperse qdots are given access to the cytosol, they can be delivered to specific cellular compartments or organelles by means of different homing peptide sequences (residue R in Figure 3.2(b)). This has been elegantly demonstrated for targeting peptide-qdot conjugates to the mitochondria [57] and the nucleus [57, 60].

Table 3.2 Protein Transduction Domains Used for Intracellular Delivery and Targeting of Qdots

Localization	*Peptide Sequences**	*References*
Cytoplasmic	RRRRRRRRR	[58, 59]
	$(His)_8$-WGLA(A_{ib})SG$(R)_8$	[67]
	RKKRRYRRR	[21]
	KETWWETWWTEWSQPKKKRKV	[73]
Nuclear	PPKKKRKVPPKKKRKV	[60]
	CSSDDEATADSQHSTPPKKKRKV	[57]
	RRRRRRRRRRRKC	[72]
	APSGAQRLYGFGL	[74]
Mitochondrial	MSVLTPLLLRGLTGSARRLPVPRAKIHC	[57]
	MSVLTPLLLRGLTGSARRLPVPRAKIHWLC	[72]

*All sequences are written from N- to C-terminus. $(His)_8$: polyhistidine, A_{ib}: alpha-amino isobutyric acid.

3.5 Live Animal Imaging

The visual analysis of molecules and cellular processes in living subjects (i.e., molecular imaging) has the potential to markedly enhance earlier diagnosis of disease. Radionuclide tracers and 3-D imaging systems such as positron emission tomography (PET) and single photon emission computed tomography (SPECT) are now helping to characterize the molecular status of tumors in patients [75]. While effective, the use of radiopharmaceuticals is limited by their complex fabrication, the short half-life of the isotopes as well as other issues related to patient/provider safety, and radioactive waste disposal. The use of radioactivity-based methods is further impaired by the inability to multiplex simultaneous signals and by the lack of detection sensitivity toward small tumor burdens. (For a review, see [76].) The other alternative in deep tissue imaging relies on multiphoton fluorescence microscopy, which can capture high-resolution, 3-D images of living tissues tagged with highly specific fluorophores [77]. However, tissue absorption and scattering, in addition to limiting the light coming out of the subject, also limits the amount of incident excitation light that reaches the fluorophore. As a result, only a very limited amount of excitation light becomes available at deeper regions of the animal tissue.

Finally, conventional dye molecules suffer major limitations that include poor photostability and phototoxicity. In this section, we review how qdots provide highly sensitive alternatives to both radioactivity- and fluorophore-based methods. First, we demonstrate how the peptide-coating approach allows the tens to hundreds of nm^2 of qdots' surface area to be functionalized with a combinatorial assortment of different peptide sequences to make radiolabeled qdots for dual-modality imaging (both fluorescence and PET in a single probe). Then we show how small peptides are paving the way for the first successful targeted deliveries of qdot conjugates in live animals. This growing trend is confirming their unmatched potential as novel intravascular probes for deep-tissue imaging in various optical modalities, including two-photon confocal microscopy [6], PET [5, 78, 79], and SPECT/CT [80].

3.5.1 Near-Infrared Deep-Tissue Dual-Modality Imaging

The complex nature of mammalian tissues, through which photons are absorbed and scattered, generally limits the depth at which light-emitting probes can be imaged in vivo [81, 82]. One partial remedy is to rely on near infrared (NIR) wavelengths for excitation and/or emission. At 700 nm to 900 nm, the absorbance of all biomolecules reaches a minimum while maximizing photon penetration efficiency into and out of tissues. This provides a clear window with minimal autofluorescence for in vivo optical imaging [83]. In the past five years, the contribution of NIR qdots to this biologically relevant "therapeutic window" [84, 85], where no good fluorescent dyes exist, has been quite remarkable. For example, Kim et al. have demonstrated in pigs and mice the superiority of NIR qdots in sentinel lymph node (SLN) mapping, a major procedure in breast cancer surgery. Qdots allowed real-time image guidance throughout the procedure, virtually free of any background, 1 cm deep into the tissues [86]. These and other studies have established the great potential of qdot optical imaging as a surrogate to radioactive techniques [6, 21].

On the other hand, only radioactive tracers have the unique ability to provide both quantitative in vivo biodistribution and deeper imaging data. Based on these considerations, our laboratory created the first dual-mode qdot probe combining optical and radioactive imaging capabilities [5]. For simultaneous PET and fluorescence imaging, qdots were radiolabeled by chelation of a radionucltide (Cu64) to a DOTA (1,4,7,10-tetraazacyclododecane-1,4,7,10-tetraacetic acid) functionalized peptide (peptide D in Figure 3.2(b)). Polyethylene glycol moieties of various lengths (PEG, peptide 3 in Table 3.1 and peptide P in Figure 3.2(b)) were also added in a single-step reaction in an attempt to reduce nonspecific binding and increase blood circulation time [87]. These radiolabeled qdots were injected (~80 μCi per animal) via tail-vein into anesthetized nude mice and then dynamically imaged in a small animal mPET scanner (Concorde Microsystems Inc., Knoxville, TN). Biodistribution and mPET analysis showed rapid and marked hepatic and splenic uptake of the qdots without evidence of body clearance (Figure 3.5(a)). This known tendency is caused by specialized particle-scavenging Kupffer cells residing en masse in the reticulo-endothelial system (RES) of the liver and spleen [87]. We also observed that PEGylation beneficially increased the blood circulation half-life and somewhat slowed down liver and spleen uptake of qdots [78]. Here, one clear advantage of the

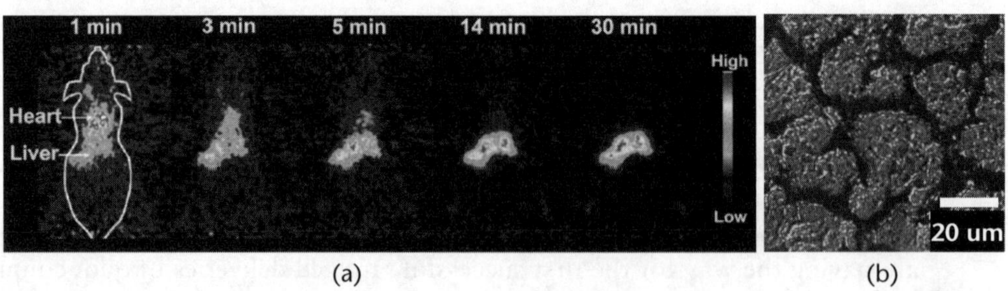

Figure 3.5 Dual-mode imaging in live animals: (a) μPET imaging of nude mice injected with radiolabeled qdots through a DOTA-functionalized peptide (see Section 3.5 for details). (b) Overlay of DIC and fluorescence images of hepatocytes from a mouse showing the accumulation of qdots within liver cells. Scale bar indicates 20 μm. Adapted from [5] with permission from the American Association for the Advancement of Science.

peptide-coating approach is that it gives us considerable latitude to modulate parameters such as peptide density and thus the overall number of functional groups (i.e., PEG moieties) or the overall charge (as shown in Figure 3.3(b)). Separate studies where free copper chloride (~78 μCi) is injected via tail-vein show that the maximum signal in the liver is only 7.8 percent of that observed when injecting mice with Cu64 radiolabeled peptide-qdots (~80 μCi). This demonstrates that even if all of the copper/peptide dissociates from the qdots, it can only lead to a small component of the overall liver signal. Moreover, biopsies of the liver observed by fluorescence light microscopy confirm this accumulation of qdots within the liver (Figure 3.5(b)).

It is important to realize that fluorescence alone cannot be measured in a fully quantitative way due to the scattering and absorption properties of living tissues as mentioned previously. There are multiple benefits to having dual-mode radioactive and optical peptide-coated qdots. First, this combination allows fluorescence imaging of qdots for tracking together with quantitative biodistribution studies of the radiotracer to access accurately their pharmaco-kinetics and targeting efficacy in living animals. Second, the dual-modality approach requires a much smaller amount of qdots (in our studies: ~25 pmol or 0.8–1.25 nmol/kg depending on the weight of the animal [78]) to yield enough contrast for PET imaging than optical imaging alone (about 10 to 100 times more qdots needed). This can significantly lower the potential cyto-toxicity risk posed by Cd^{2+} and other heavy metals leakage from the qdot inner core structure [88, 89]. Nuclear spin labels for MRI imaging could also be incorporated into qdots peptide coating using the same type of chelating group. A further step could involve TEM imaging of their precise localization within cells and tissues [10, 90]. It should therefore be possible to image targeted qdots at all scales, from the level of whole body down to the nanometer resolution using a single probe with exquisite spatio-temporal sensitivity.

3.5.2 In Vivo Targeting of Tumor Vasculature

To date, the successful targeted delivery of peptide qdots in living mice has been limited to tissue-specific vascular markers. Akerman et al. have used lung- and tumor-specific homing peptides (Table 3.3) to direct qdots to their appropriate targets. After intravenous injection in the mice, targeting was demonstrated by ex vivo fluorescence microscopy of histological sections [18]. However, no in vivo imaging was achieved. More recently, arginine-glycine-aspartic acid (RGD) peptide-conjugated qdots have been used to specifically target integrin $\alpha_v\beta_3$ in vitro [91, 92] and in living mice [63, 79]. The RGD peptide motif (Table 3.3) found in vitronectin, fibronectin, and thrombospondin [93] binds selectively to integrin $\alpha_v\beta_3$. Taking advantage of the fact that integrin $\alpha_v\beta_3$ is significantly upregulated in tumor but not in normal tissues [94, 95], Cai et al. reported the first in vivo targeting and imaging of tumor vasculature in a murine xenograph model in live animals using RGD-qdot conjugates [63, 79]. Subcutaneous tumor imaging was observed six hours post-injection (Figure 3.6(a)) and was further demonstrated by harvesting the tumor followed by ex vivo imaging using a sensitive CCD camera (IVIS200, Xenogen Corp., Alameda, CA). Qdot fluorescence signal was clearly detected in the tumor of the mouse injected with the RGD qdots, while no signal was seen in the

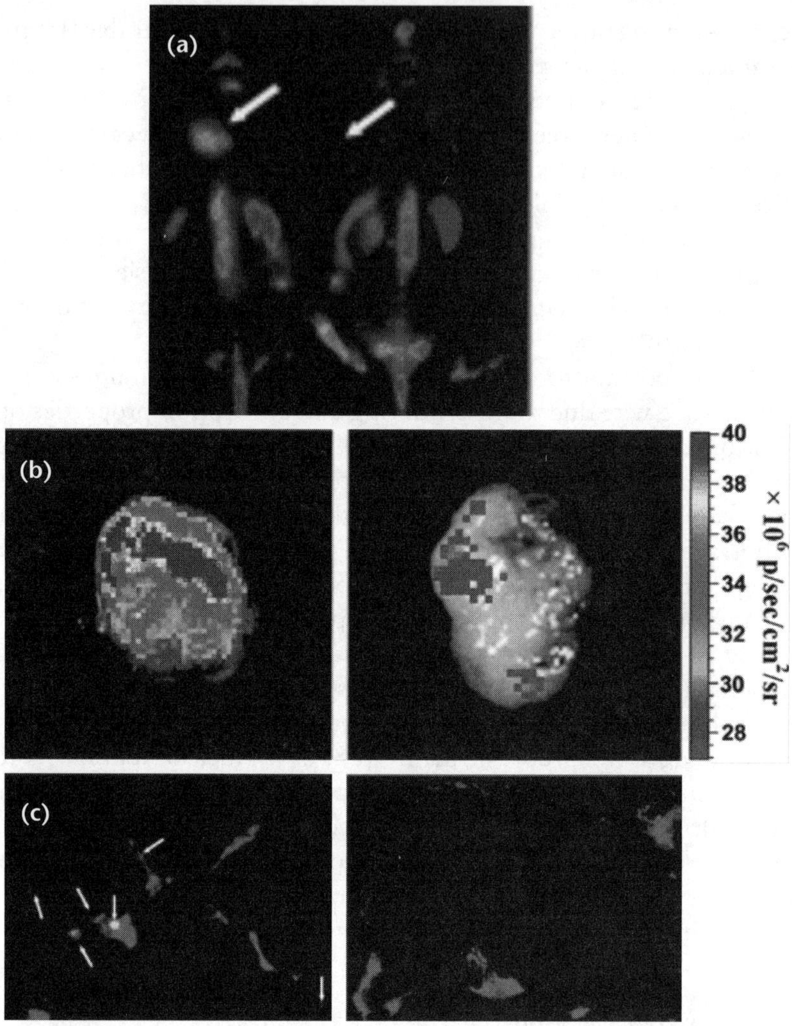

Figure 3.6 Targeting of tumor vasculature with RGD peptide-conjugated qdots: (a) In vivo NIR fluorescence imaging of U87MG tumor-bearing mice (left shoulder, pointed at with white arrows) injected with 200 pmol of RGD-qdots (left mouse) and control qdots (right mouse) six hours after injection. (b) Ex vivo fluorescence images of the same tumors, surgically removed from RGD qdots (left) and control qdots (right) injected mice. (c) Fluorescent microscope images of frozen tumor slices stained for CD31 (green) to allow visualizing of the tumor vasculature. Qdot signal is shown in red and pointed at with white arrows. Adapted from [63] with permission from the American Chemical Society. (See Color Plate 5.)

Table 3.3 Sequences of Homing Peptides Used for In Vivo Targeting

Vasculatures	*Peptide Sequences**	*References*
Lung	CGFECVRQCPERC	[18]
Tumor, blood	KDEPQRRSARLSAKPAPPKPEPKPKKAPAKK	Ibid
Tumor, lymphatic	CGNKRTRGC	Ibid
Integrin $\alpha_v\beta_3$ tumor	RGD	[63, 79]

*All sequences are written from N- to C-terminus.

tumor of the control mouse injected with qdots alone (Figure 3.6(b)). Interestingly, further fluorescence microscopy analysis of frozen sections indicated that the RGD qdots did not extravasate but stayed confined to the tumor vasculature (Figure 3.6(c)) as previously reported [18]. Overall, the advantages for using peptide qdots for tumor targeting in vivo are multiple. Compared to their peptide-dye conjugate counterparts (RGD-Cy5.5, [96]) RGD qdots showed more photostability and much stronger signal-to-background ratio. In conjunction with other specific integrin binding peptides (RGDS, LDV, DGEA, KGD, PECAM, and FYFDLR), qdots offer the unique possibility of multiplexing [91]. Peptides might also potentially be better targeting ligands than mono-clonal antibodies conjugated to qdots. Gao et al. estimated that the number of antibodies per qdots is limited to 5–6 [21], while the number of peptides can easily be optimized to provide stronger binding avidity [19]. Peptides might also be rendered multimeric to improve targeting efficiency because of the polyvalency effect [97–99]. The next step remains to improve tumor-targeting efficacy, which requires extravasation of the peptide-qdot probe as opposed to targeting the tumor vasculature where no extravasation is needed. Reducing the size of the qdot probes will lower uptake by the reticulo-endothelial system (RES), which holds the key to achieving better tissue penetration and tumor targeting.

3.6 Beyond Diagnostic Imaging: Sensing and Therapeutic Applications

Optical sensing (i.e., detection of electromagnetic radiation) is the most widely used format for detecting biological binding events and enzymatic reactions or performing quantitative immunoassays in biological systems. The goals of using qdots are ultimately to enable single-molecule detection in vivo, parallel integration of multiple signals (i.e., multiplexing), signal amplification, and resistance to photobleaching in a high-throughput format. In the following section, we review some of the most significant progress in the application of peptide qdots in biological detection.

3.6.1 Cleavable Peptides for Proteases Activity

Proteases are enzymes that regulate many essential biological processes by catalyzing the cleavage of specific peptide bonds in other proteins. They are also well known to be aberrantly regulated and activated in various diseases including cancer, stroke, and infection [100]. Hence, proteases constitute a prominent class of pharmaceutical targets for assay and drug development. For example, because protease activity is key to tumor progression and evasion (metastasis), monitoring their expression and bioactivity in vivo provide information about the metastatic potential of a tumor. Many of the sensors designed to monitor proteolytic activity exploit the low background of FRET quenched fluorophores and the high fluorescent signal resulting from unquenching after proteolysis [101]. In such FRET geometry, two fluorophores are usually held in close proximity by a short peptide linker that becomes the target of a specific protease. The main limitations of these fluorophore-based probes reside in their lack of general tunability in wavelength, which is imposed by the donor-acceptor pair. In addition, the optical properties of conventional organic fluorophores or genetically encoded fluorescent proteins are susceptible to their local environment (pH sensitivity and so on) and prone to photobleaching. In order to overcome some of these shortcomings, qdot-peptide conjugates have emerged as promising new FRET-based protease sensors. The use of qdots as energy donors capitalizes on their well-known spectroscopic benefits. Specifically relevant here is their broadband absorption and fluorescence emission spectra that can be tuned to best overlap with the acceptor absorption. With this in mind, Chang et al. designed the first qdot-peptide-gold conjugates to target collagenase. In this bioassay, collagenase cleaves between alanine and glycine of a GGLGPAGGCG target peptide to release the functionalized gold nanoparticles that quenches the qdot fluorescence [102]. This approach was however limited by steric hindrance from the gold nanoparticles, which impaired the accessibility of the collagenase to the peptide.

As an improvement of this approach, Medintz et al. have developed qdot-peptide-dye conjugates for the enzyme recognition of four different target enzymes (Table 3.4); caspase 1, thrombin, collagenase, and chymotrypsin [103]. Replacing gold with a much smaller dye molecule (Cy3 or QXL-520) possibly increased the substrate accessibility to the protease since the authors succeeded in measuring kinetic values similar to those obtained with dye-only peptides in solution. Steric constraints were also minimized by titrating the peptide-qdot ratio to be less than 5. Moreover, the low peptide number ensures that the proteolytic assays were carried out under rate-limiting substrate conditions, which means that all peptides on the qdots are likely to participate in the protease activity measurement. The net result is an increase in the sensitivity of the QD-peptide-dye probes. Finally, these QD-peptide sensors can also measure protease activity in vivo. Shi et al. used qdots directly coated with a small RGDC tetrapeptide labeled with rhodamine to quantitatively study the aberrant collagenase activity of HTB 126 cancer cell lines [104]. The kinetic rate constants of FRET signal changes of the qdot-based protease sensors were significantly higher within the cancer cells as compared to the normal HTB 125 cells. Interestingly, the qdot FRET-based probes could discriminate between normal and cancerous cells within 10 min. By extension, changing the peptide sequence would enable high throughput screening of the activity of specific proteolytic enzymes in real-time in an array/multiplex format. This could provide a unique protease signature for each cancer patient to personalize ongoing therapeutic strategies.

Table 3.4 Sequences of Cleavable Peptides Used for Measuring Protease Activity

Target Enzymes	*Peptide Sequences**	*References*
Collagenase	GGLGPAGGCG	[102]
	RGDC	[104]
	$(His)_6$-AL(A_{ib})AAGGPAC	[103]
Caspase-1	$(His)_6$-GL(A_{ib})AAGGWEHDSGC	Ibid
Thrombin	$(His)_6$-GLA(A_{ib})SGFPRGRC	Ibid
Chymotrypsin	$(His)_6$-GL(A_{ib})AAGGWGC	Ibid

*All sequences are written from N- to C-terminus. $(His)_6$: polyhistidine, A_{ib}: alpha-amino isobutyric acid.

3.6.2 Photodynamic Therapy

Photodynamic therapy (PDT) refers to a kind of cancer treatment based on three synergistic components: a photosensitizer (PS), light, and oxygen molecules present in tissues [105, 106]. Photosensitizers are nontoxic chromophores that generate reactive oxygen species (ROS) such as free radicals (hydroxyl radical: •OH and superoxide: $\bullet O_2^-$) and single oxygen ($^1O_2$) upon light irradiation. These compounds act locally to cause irreversible oxidative damages to enzymes, proteins, nucleic acids, mitochondria, and membranes with the result of inducing apoptosis, necrosis, and cell death. In the clinic, the effectiveness of a PDT treatment relies on the retention and accumulation of the PS into tumor tissues followed by its selective destruction by ROS generated through laser irradiation of specific wavelength and directed to the sensitized local area. Compared with conventional surgery, this approach is minimally invasive. However, current FDA-approved PSs (such as Photofrin) are far from being ideal. They are poorly soluble, unstable, have low targeting selectivity, and show some spontaneous skin phototoxicity triggered by regular daylight (which goes with the fact that their excitation wavelengths are not optimal for deep tissue penetration). Given these major drawbacks, qdots have garnered much attention as potentially novel PSs or, at least, as cofactors of conventional PSs [107, 108]. Qdots main benefits relate to their resistance to photobleaching, emission, and absorption tunability in the NIR for deep tissue excitation, large absorption coefficients, continuous absorption bands that can be used to extend the range of excitation of conventional PSs through Förster (fluorescence) resonance energy transfer (FRET), and the availability of active-targeting approaches to introduce a degree of selectivity in PDT treatments. Qdots as PS carriers could boost singlet oxygen yield (through FRET) for better PDT efficacy over PSs alone. They also have the potential to act as imaging and therapeutic agents simultaneously.

Early attempts to harness the full capabilities of qdots in PDT have been limited due to the poor solubility and/or instability of the qdot-PS conjugates in the aqueous environment [109–111]. We recently developed novel qdot-PS bioconjugates based on our unique phytochelatin peptide-coating technology that preserved both the photophysical properties of the qdots and of the PSs [112]. Figure 3.7 describes the conjugation schemes used to covalently attach two PSs, rose bengal and chlorin e6, to phytochelatin peptides (peptide 1 in Table 3.1). The versatility of our mix-and-match peptide approach allowed us to carefully control the number of PSs conjugated to the qdots by simply changing the stoichiometry of PS-conjugated peptides to peptides of other functionalities (PEG, biotin, and so on; see Figure 3.2(b)) during the mass exchange process. Typically, 1 to 30 PSs could be grafted per qdots. It is worth mentioning that the number of PSs directly correlated with the size (i.e., surface area) of the qdots; the bigger the qdots, the more PSs could be added [112]. FRET was evident between the qdots (acting as donors) and PSs (acting as acceptors). Figure 3.7(c) shows the dramatic increase of fluorescence of both rose bengal (attached to green qdots) and chlorin e6 (attached to red qdots) as a result of FRET (red curve) in comparison with the fluorescence of PSs alone at the same concentration (black curves). An important conclusion is that the peptide coating layer is thin enough to allow easy energy transfer between qdots and the PSs. Finally, we found that the qdot-PS conjugates produced singlet oxygen either by exciting the PS

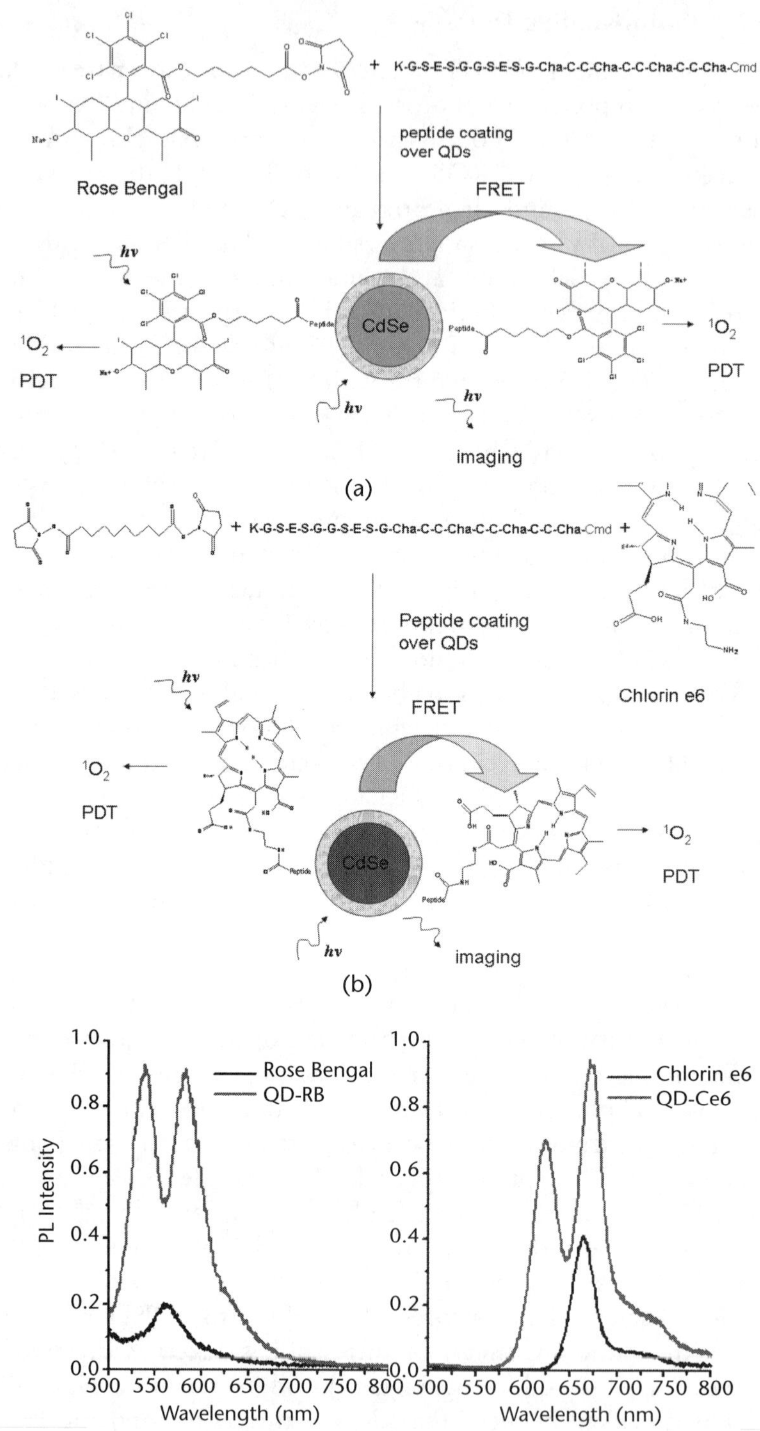

(c)

Figure 3.7 Production of singlet oxygen with peptide-coated qdot-photosensitizer probes: (a) Scheme of conjugations of rose bengal and (b) chlorin to phytochelatin peptides. (c) Photoluminescence spectra of the conjugates. (left) rose bengal peptide-coated qdots (gray curve) and rose bengal alone (black curve). (right) Chlorin e6-conjugated QDs (gray curve) and chlorin e6 alone (black curve). The same concentration of each photosensitizer was excited at 450 nm. Adapted from [112] with permission from the American Chemical Society.

directly or indirectly through the FRET process. We are currently testing these qdot-PS conjugates for their ability to kill cells in culture. The next step would be to customize multifunctional qdot-PS probes able to specifically target cancer cells, absorb large quantities of light, and destroy tumors through singlet oxygen generation deep into tissue using NIR qdots and conjugation to NIR-absorbing photosensitizers.

3.7 Conclusion and Perspectives

Several key features make the peptide-coating approach advantageous for biological applications of qdots. First and foremost is its simplicity, since a single, simple reaction step can achieve both solubility in aqueous environment and bioactivation of the nanoparticles. Second, this approach is highly versatile and allows the testing of various peptide sequences simultaneously to encode multifunctional and multimodal capabilities in a single probe. Finally, the peptide-based approach maintains the overall size of the qdot probe as relatively small. For example, it has recently been demonstrated that a small (< 5 nm) hydrodynamic radius is crucial for renal clearance of qdots intravenously injected into mice [113]. Without a way to excrete or biodegrade qdots into inert components, toxicity becomes an issue and imaging is impaired. Fortunately, the "peptide toolbox" gives us considerable latitude to modulate parameters such as peptide density, overall charge, hydrophilicity/hydrophobicity, and incorporation of moieties like high molecular weight PEG. In particular, PEG helps to increase biocompatibility, to neutralize nonspecific adsorption of serum proteins, and to increase circulation time in vivo. Therefore, peptide engineering might provide a rational path to the optimization of the pharmacokinetic parameters of IV-administrated functionalized qdots, while maintaining the final size of the functionalized probes as small as possible. Future research utilizing smaller, NIR-emitting qdots such as InAs-based qdots [114] may further promote extravasations of the qdots from the blood vasculature to target solid tumors. Active targeting strategies using peptides could also be combined with cytotoxic agents in the form of photodynamic therapy treatments.

At the cellular level, peptides offer wide potentials for novel applications. New affinity pairs will certainly emerge from in vitro directed molecular evolution to enable multiplexing studies [115]. New peptide sequences will facilitate crossing the cell membrane to go beyond the study of cell surface membrane markers to intracellular processes such as trafficking and signal transduction. Interestingly, recent studies are making use of extracellular proteases to modulate the cellular uptake of peptide-conjugated qdots [116]. Modulating the uptake of nanoparticles into cells with tumor-specific proteases may lead to their selective accumulation in tumor cells for further targeted destruction. Finally, new peptide qdot–based systems will be capable of sensing at the single-molecule level. Capitalizing on the advantages of both peptides and qdots may bring us closer to the ultimate goal of probing biological systems at all length scales: from the whole-body down to the cellular and molecular level with a single probe.

Acknowledgments

We would like to thank our valuable colleagues in the field and ask for their forgiveness if some of their studies could not be cited within the space limits of this review. The development of the peptide-coated qdots was made possible thanks to the contribution of past and present members of our laboratory. Finally, we would like to express our appreciation to Tal Paley for her editorial assistance. Fluorescent microscopy images in Figure 3.5 were obtained at the California NanoSystems Institute Advanced Light Microscopy/Spectroscopy Shared Facility at UCLA. This work was supported by funds from the National Institute of Health, Grant No. 2 R01 EB000312-06A2.

References

[1] Bruchez, M.P., et al., "Semiconductor nanocrystals as fluorescent biological labels," *Science,* 1998. 281: 2013–2015.

[2] Chan, W.C.W. and S.M. Nie, "Quantum dot bioconjugates for ultrasensitive nonisotopic detection," *Science,* 1998. 281(5385): 2016–2018.

[3] Alivisatos, P., "The use of nanocrystals in biological detection," *Nat. Biotechnol.,* 2004. 22(1): 47–52.

[4] Medintz, I.L., et al., "Quantum dot bioconjugates for imaging, labelling and sensing," *Nat. Mater,* 2005. 4(6): 435–46.

[5] Michalet, X., et al., "Quantum dots for live cells, in vivo imaging, and diagnostics," *Science,* 2005. 307(5709): 538–44.

[6] Larson, D., et al., "Water-soluble quantum dots for multiphoton fluorescence imaging in vivo," *Science,* 2003. 300: 1434–1436.

[7] Bharali, D.J., et al., "Folate-Receptor-Mediated Delivery of InP Quantum Dots for Bioimaging Using Confocal and Two-Photon Microscopy," *Journal of the American Chemical Society,* 2005. 127(32): 11364–11371.

[8] Ferrara, D.E., et al., "Quantitative 3D fluorescence technique for the analysis of en face preparations of arterial walls using quantum dot nanocrystals and two-photon excitation laser scanning microscopy," *American Journal of Physiology,* 2006. 290(1, Pt. 2): R114–R123.

[9] Serrano, E.E. and V.B. Knight, "Multiphoton imaging of quantum dot bioconjugates in cultured cells following Nd: YLF laser excitation," *Proceedings of SPIE-The International Society for Optical Engineering,* 2005. 5705(Nanobiophotonics and Biomedical Applications II): 225–234.

[10] Dahan, M., et al., "Diffusion dynamics of glycine receptors revealed by single-quantum dot tracking," *Science,* 2003. 302(5644): 442–445.

[11] Lidke, D.S., et al., "Reaching out for signals: filopodia sense EGF and respond by directed retrograde transport of activated receptors," *J. Cell Biol.,* 2005. 170(4): 619–626.

[12] Warshaw, D.M., et al., "Differential labeling of myosin V heads with quantum dots allows direct visualization of hand-over-hand processivity," *Biophys. J.,* 2005. 88(5): L30–L32.

[13] Bentolila, L.A., X. Michalet, and S. Weiss, "Quantum optics: colloidal fluorescent semiconductor nanocrystals (quantum dots) in single-molecule detection and imaging.," *Single-Molecules and Nanotechnology,* R. Rigler and H. Vogel, Editors. 2008, Springer-Verlag: Heidelberg, pp. 53–81.

[14] Yin, Y. and A.P. Alivisatos, "Colloidal nanocrystal synthesis and the organic-inorganic interface," *Nature,* 2005. 437(7059): 664–670.

[15] Pathak, S., et al., "Hydroxylated quantum dots as luminescent probes for in situ hybridization," *J. Am. Chem. Soc.,* 2001. 123(17): 4103–4104.

[16] Kim, S. and M.G. Bawendi, "Oligomeric Ligands for luminescent and stable nanocrystal quantum dots," *J. Am. Chem. Soc.,* 2003. 125(48): 14652–14653.

[17] Guo, W., et al., "Conjugation chemistry and bioapplications of semiconductor box nanocrystals prepared via dendrimer bridging," *Chem. Mater.,* 2003. 15(16): 312–3133.

[18] Akerman, M.E., et al., "Nanocrystal targeting in vivo," *Proc. Natl. Acad. Sci,* USA, 2002. 99(20): 12617–12621.

[19] Pinaud, F., et al., "Bioactivation and Cell Targeting of Semiconductor CdSe/ZnS Nanocrystals with Phytochelatin-Related Peptides," *J. Am. Chem. Soc.,* 2004. 126: 6115–6123.

[20] Wu, X.Y., et al., "Immunofluorescent labeling of cancer marker Her2 and other cellular targets with semiconductor quantum dots," *Nature Biotechnol.,* 2003. 21(1): 41–46.

[21] Gao, X., et al., "In vivo cancer targeting and imaging with semiconductor quantum dots," *Nature Biotechnol.,* 2004. 22: 969.

[22] Gerion, D., et al., "Synthesis and properties of biocompatible water-soluble silica-coated CdSe/ZnS semiconductor quantum dots," *J. Phys. Chem. B,* 2001. 105(37): 8861–8871.

[23] Dubertret, B., et al., "In vivo imaging of quantum dots encapsulated in phospholipid micelles," *Science,* 2002. 298(5599): 1759–1762.

[24] Gao, X., W.C.W. Chan, and S. Nie, "Quantum-dot nanocrystals for ultrasensitive biological labeling and multicolor optical encoding," *J. Biomed. Opt.,* 2002. 7(4): 532–537.

[25] Pellegrino, T., et al., "Hydrophobic nanocrystals coated with an amphiphilic polymer shell: A general route to water soluble nanocrystals," *Nano Lett.,* 2004. 4(4): 703–707.

[26] Osaki, F., et al., "A Quantum Dot Conjugated Sugar Ball and Its Cellular Uptake. On the Size Effects of Endocytosis in the Subviral Region," *J. Am. Chem. Soc.,* 2004. 126: 6520–6521.

[27] Mattoussi, H., et al., "Self-assembly of CdSe-ZnS quantum dot bioconjugates using an engineered recombinant protein," *J. Am. Chem. Soc.,* 2000. 122(49): 12142–12150.

[28] Sukhanova, A., et al., "Biocompatible fluorescent nanocrystals for immunolabeling of membrane proteins and cells," *Anal. Biochem.,* 2004. 324(1): 60–67.

[29] Mitchell, G.P., C.A. Mirkin, and R.L. Letsinger, "Programmed assembly of DNA functionalized quantum dots," *J. Am. Chem. Soc.,* 1999. 121(35): 8122-8123.

[30] Goldman, E.R., et al., "Conjugation of luminescent quantum dots with antibodies using an engineered adaptor protein to provide new reagents for fluoroimmunoassays," *Anal. Chem.,* 2002. 74(4): 841–847.

[31] Bentolila, L.A. and S. Weiss, "Single-step multicolor fluorescent in situ hybridization analysis using semiconductor quantum dot-DNA conjugates," *Cell Biochemistry and Biophysics,* 2006. 45(1): 59–70.

[32] Chan, P., et al., "Method for multiplex cellular detection of mRNAs using quantum dot fluorescent in situ hybridization," *Nucleic Acids Res,* 2005. 33(18): e161.

[33] Jaiswal, J.K., et al., "Long-term multiple color imaging of live cells using quantum dot bioconjugates," *Nature Biotechnol.,* 2003. 21(1): 47–51.

[34] Mansson, A., et al., "In vitro sliding of actin filaments labelled with single quantum dots," *Biochem. Biophys. Res. Commun.,* 2004. 314(2): 529–34.

[35] Marks, K.M., M. Rosinov, and G.P. Nolan, "In Vivo Targeting of Organic Calcium Sensors via Genetically Selected Peptides," *Chem. Biol.,* 2004. 11: 347–356.

[36] Whaley, S.R., et al., "Selection of peptides with semiconductor binding specificity for directed nanocrystal assembly," *Nature,* 2000. 405(6787): 665–668.

[37] Lee, S.-W., et al., "Ordering of Quantum Dots Using Genetically Engineered Viruses," *Sciences,* 2002. 296: 892–895.

[38] Zhou, M. and I. Ghosh, "Quantum dots and peptides: a bright future together," *Peptide Science,* 2007. 88(3): 325–339.

[39] Cobbett, C.S., "Heavy metal detoxification in plants: Phytochelatin biosynthesis and function," *Iubmb Life,* 2001. 51(3): 183–188.

[40] Dameron, C.T., et al., "Biosynthesis of cadmium sulphide quantum semiconductor crystallites," *Nature,* 1989. 338: 596–597.

[41] Dameron, C.T. and D.R. Winge, "Peptide-Mediated Formation of Quantum Semiconductors," *Trends in Biotechnology,* 1990. 8(1): 3–6.

[42] Sukhanova, A., et al., "Highly Stable Fluorescent Nanocrystals as a Novel Class of Labels for Immunohistochemical Analysis of Paraffin-Embedded Tissue Sections," *Laboratory Investigation,* 2002. 82(9): 1259.

[43] Bae, W. and R.K. Mehra, "Cysteine-capped ZnS nanocrystallites: Preparation and characterization," *Journal of Inorganic Biochemistry,* 1998. 70(2): 125–135.

[44] Iyer, G., et al., "Solubilization of quantum dots with a recombinant peptide from Escherichia coli," *Small,* 2007. 3(5): 793–798.

[45] Zheng, Y., S. Gao, and J.Y. Ying, "Synthesis and cell-imaging applications of glutathione-capped CdTe quantum dots," *Advanced Materials,* 2007. 19: 376–380.

[46] Doose, S., et al., "Comparison of Photophysical and Colloidal Properties of Biocompatible Semiconductor Nanocrystals Using Fluorescence Correlation Spectroscopy," *Anal Chem.,* 2005, 77(7): 2235–42.

[47] Mao, C., et al., "Virus-based toolkit for the directed synthesis of magnetic and semiconducting nanowires," *Science,* 2004. 303(5655): 213–217.

[48] Brown, S., "Engineered iron oxide-adhesion mutants of the Escherichia coli phage λ receptor. Proc Natl Acad Sci USA, 1992. 89: 8651–8655.

[49] Waggoner, A., "Covalent labeling of proteins and nucleic acids with fluorophores," *Methods in Enzymology,* 1995. 246(5): 362–73.

[50] Hermanson, G., *Bioconjugate Techniques,* 1996, San Diego, CA: Academic Press, Inc.

[51] Pinaud, F., et al., "Advances in fluorescence imaging with quantum dot bio-probes," *Biomaterials,* 2005. 27(9): 1679–1687.

[52] Saxton, M.J. and K. Jacobson, "Single-particle tracking: applications to membrane dynamics," *Annu. Rev. Biophys. Biomol. Struct.,* 1997. 26: 373–399.

[53] Ueda, M., et al., "Single-molecule analysis of chemotactic signaling in Dictyostelium cells," *Science,* 2001. 294(5543): 864–867.

[54] Tsay, J.M., et al., "Enhancing the photoluminescence of peptide-coated CdSe nanocrystals with shell composition and UV irradiation," *Journal of Physical Chemistry,* 2005.

[55] Meier, J., et al., "Fast and reversible trapping of surface glycine receptors by gephyrin," *Nat. Neurosci.,* 2001. 4(3): 253–60.

[56] Schmidt, T., et al., "Imaging of single molecule diffusion," *Proceedings of the National Academy of Sciences USA,* 1996. 93: 2926–2929.

[57] Derfus, A.M., W.C.W. Chan, and S.N. Bhatia, "Intracellular delivery of quantum dots for live cell labeling and organelle tracking," *Adv. Mater.,* 2004. 16(12): 961–966.

[58] Lagerholm, B.C., et al., "Multicolor Coding of Cells with Cationic Peptide Coated Quantum Dots," *Nano Letters,* 2004. 4(10): 2019–2022.

[59] Silver, J. and W. Ou, "Photoactivation of quantum dot fluorescence following endocytosis," *Nano Lett,* 2005. 5(7): 1445–1449.

[60] Chen, F. and D. Gerion, "Fluorescent CdSe/ZnS Nanocrystal-Peptide Conjugates for Long-term, Nontoxic Imaging and Nuclear Targeting in Living Cells," *Nano Letters,* 2004. 4(10): 1827–1832.

[61] Wadia, J.S. and S.F. Dowdy, "Protein transduction technology," *Curr Opin Biotechnol,* 2002. 13(1): 52–56.

[62] Anikeeva, N., et al., "Quantum dot/peptide-MHC biosensors reveal strong CD8-dependent cooperation between self and viral antigens that augment the T cell response," *Proc. Natl. Acad. Sci. USA,* 2006. 103(45): 16846–16851.

[63] Cai, W., et al., "Peptide-Labeled Near-Infrared Quantum Dots for Imaging Tumor Vasculature in Living Subjects," *Nano Lett.*, 2006. 6(4): 669–676.

[64] Kim, Y., et al., "Targeting Heat Shock Proteins on Cancer Cells: Selection, Characterization, and Cell-Penetrating Properties of a Peptidic GRP78 Ligand," *Biochemistry*, 2006. 45(31): 9434–9444.

[65] Xue, F., et al., "Enhancement of intracellular delivery of CdTe quantum dots (QDs) to living cells by Tat conjugation," *Journal of Fluorescence*, 2007. 17(2): 149–154.

[66] Zhou, M., et al., "Peptide-Labeled Quantum Dots for Imaging GPCRs in Whole Cells and as Single Molecules," *Bioconjugate Chem.*, 2007. 18(2): 323–332.

[67] Delehanty, J.B., et al., "Self-Assembled Quantum Dot-Peptide Bioconjugates for Selective Intracellular Delivery," *Bioconjugate Chem.*, 2006. 17(4): 920–927.

[68] Medintz, I.L., et al., "Designer Variable Repeat Length Polypeptides as Scaffolds for Surface Immobilization of Quantum Dots," *J. Phys. Chem. B*, 2006. 110(22): 10683–10690.

[69] Vu, T.Q., et al., "Peptide-Conjugated Quantum Dots Activate Neuronal Receptors and Initiate Downstream Signaling of Neurite Growth," *Nano Lett.*, 2005. 5(4): 603–607.

[70] Prochiantz, A., "Protein and peptide transduction, twenty years later a happy birthday," *Advanced Drug Delivery Reviews*, 2008. 60(4-5): 448–451.

[71] Wender, P.A., et al., "The design, synthesis, and evaluation of molecules that enable or enhance cellular uptake: peptoid molecular transporters," *Proc. Natl. Acad. Sci. USA*, 2000. 97(24): 13003–13008.

[72] Hoshino, A., et al., "Quantum dots targeted to the assigned organelle in living cells," *Microbiology and Immunology*, 2004. 48(12): 985–994.

[73] Mattheakis, L.C., et al., "Optical coding of mammalian cells using semiconductor quantum dots," *Anal. Biochem.*, 2004. 327(2): 200–208.

[74] Biju, V., et al., "Quantum dot-insect neuropeptide conjugates for fluorescence imaging, transfection, and nucleus targeting of living cells," *Langmuir*, 2007. 23(20): 10254–10261.

[75] Gambhir, S.S., "Molecular imaging of cancer with positron emission tomography," *Nat. Rev. Cancer*, 2002. 2(9): 683–693.

[76] Massoud, T.F. and S.S. Gambhir, "Molecular imaging in living subjects: seeing fundamental biological processes in a new light," *Genes Dev*, 2003. 17(5): 545–580.

[77] Helmchen, F. and W. Denk, "Deep tissue two-photon microscopy," *Nature Methods*, 2005. 2(12): 932–940.

[78] Schipper, M.L., et al., "microPET-based biodistribution of quantum dots in living mice," *J. Nucl. Med.*, 2007. 48(9): 1511–1518.

[79] Cai, W., et al., "Dual-function probe for PET and near-infrared fluorescence imaging of tumor vasculature," *J. Nucl. Med.*, 2007. 48(11): 1862–1870.

[80] Woodward, J.D., et al., "In vivo SPECT/CT imaging and biodistribution using radioactive Cd[125m]Te/ZnS nanoparticles," *Nanotechnology*, 2007. 18(17): 175103.1–175103.5.

[81] Tromberg, B.J., et al., "Non-invasive in vivo characterization of breast tumors using photon migration spectroscopy," *Neoplasia*, 2000. 2(1-2): 26–40.

[82] Rice, B.W., M.D. Cable, and M.B. Nelson, "In vivo imaging of light-emitting probes," *J. Biomed. Opt.*, 2001. 6(4): 432–440.

[83] Weissleder, R., et al., "In vivo imaging of tumors with protease-activated near-infrared fluorescent probes," *Nat. Biotechnol.*, 1999. 17(4): 375–378.

[84] Weissleder, R., "A clearer vision for in vivo imaging," *Nat. Biotechnol.*, 2001. 19(4): 316–317.

[85] Frangioni, J.V., "In vivo near-infrared fluorescence imaging," *Curr. Opin. Chem. Biol.*, 2003. 7(5): 626–34.

[86] Kim, S., et al., "Near-infrared fluorescent type II quantum dots for sentinel lymph node mapping," *Nature Biotechnol.*, 2004. 22(1): 93–97.

[87] Ballou, B., et al., "Noninvasive imaging of quantum dots in mice," *Bioconjug. Chem.*, 2004. 15(1): 79–86.

[88] Kirchner, C., et al., "Cytotoxicity of Colloidal CdSe and CdSe/ZnS Nanoparticles," *Nano Lett.*, 2005. 5(2): 331–338.

[89] Derfus, A.M., W.C.W. Chan, and S.N. Bhatia, "Probing the Cytotoxicity of Semiconductor Quantum Dots," *Nano. Lett.*, 2004. 4(1): 11–18.

[90] Giepmans, B.N., et al., "Correlated light and electron microscopic imaging of multiple endogenous proteins using Quantum dots," *Nature Methods*, 2005. 2(10): 743–749.

[91] Shi, P., et al., "Peptide-Directed Binding of Quantum Dots to Integrins in Human Fibroblast," *IEEE Transactions on Nanobioscience*, 2006. 5(1): 15–19.

[92] Lieleg, O., et al., "Specific integrin labeling in living cells using functionalized nanocrystals," *Small*, 2007. 3(9): 1560–1565.

[93] Xiong, J.P., et al., "Crystal structure of the extracellular segment of integrin alpha Vbeta3 in complex with an Arg-Gly-Asp ligand," *Science*, 2002. 296(5565): 151–155.

[94] Hood, J.D. and D.A. Cheresh, "Role of integrins in cell invasion and migration," *Nat. Rev. Cancer*, 2002. 2(2): 91–100.

[95] Jin, H. and J. Varner, "Integrins: roles in cancer development and as treatment targets," *Br. J. Cancer*, 2004. 90(3): 561–565.

[96] Chen, X., P.S. Conti, and R.A. Moats, "In vivo near-infrared fluorescence imaging of integrin alphavbeta3 in brain tumor xenografts," *Cancer Res.*, 2004. 64(21): 8009–8014.

[97] Mammen, M., S.-K. Choi, and G.M. Whitesides, "Polyvalent Interactions in Biological Systems: Implications for Design and Use of Multivalent Ligands and Inhibitors," *Angew. Chem. Int. Ed.*, 1998. 37: 2754–2794.

[98] Chen, X., et al., "Micro-PET imaging of alphavbeta3-integrin expression with 18F-labeled dimeric RGD peptide," *Mol. Imaging*, 2004. 3(2): 96–104.

[99] Wu, Y., et al., "microPET imaging of glioma integrin {alpha}v{beta}3 expression using (64)Cu-labeled tetrameric RGD peptide," *J. Nucl. Med.*, 2005. 46(10): 1707–1718.

[100] Richard, I., "The genetic and molecular bases of monogenic disorders affecting proteolytic systems," *J. Med. Genet.*, 2005. 42(7): 529–539.

[101] Funovics, M., R. Weissleder, and C.H. Tung, "Protease sensors for bioimaging," *Anal. Bioanal. Chem.*, 2003. 377(6): 956–963.

[102] Chang, E., et al., "Protease-activated quantum dot probes," *Biochem. Biophys. Res. Commun.*, 2005. 9(334): 1317–1321.

[103] Medintz, I.L., et al., "Proteolytic activity monitored by fluorescence resonance energy transfer through quantum-dot-peptide conjugates," *Nature Material*, 2006. 5(7): 581–589.

[104] Shi, L., et al., "Synthesis and application of quantum dots FRET-based protease sensors," *J. Am. Chem. Soc.*, 2006. 128(32): 10378–10379.

[105] Dougherty, T.J., "Photosensitizers: therapy and detection of malignant tumors," *Photochemistry and Photobiology*, 1987. 45(6): 879–889.

[106] Ochsner, M., "Photophysical and photobiological processes in the photodynamic therapy of tumours," *Journal of Photochemistry and Photobiology Biology*, 1997. 39(1): 1–18.

[107] Bakalova, R., et al., "Quantum dots as photosensitizers?" *Nature Biotechnology*, 2004. 22(11): 1360–1361.

[108] Samia, A.C., S. Dayal, and C. Burda, "Quantum dot-based energy transfer: perspectives and potential for applications in photodynamic therapy," *Photochemistry and Photobiology*, 2006. 82(3): 617–625.

[109] Samia, A.C., X. Chen, and C. Burda, "Semiconductor quantum dots for photodynamic therapy," *Journal of the American Chemical Society*, 2003. 125(51): 15736–15737.

[110] Hsieh, J.M., et al., "Iridium-complex modified CdSe/ZnS quantum dots; a conceptual design for bifunctionality toward imaging and photosensitization," *Chemical Communications*, 2006. 6: 615–617.

[111] Shi, L., B. Hernandez, and M. Selke, "Singlet oxygen generation from water-soluble quantum dot organic dye nanocomposites," *Journal of the American Chemical Society*, 2006. 128(19): 6278–6279.

[112] Tsay, J.M., et al., "Singlet Oxygen Production by Peptide-Coated Quantum Dot-Photosensitizer Conjugates," *J. Am. Chem. Soc.*, 2007. 129(21): 6865–6871.

[113] Choi, H.S., et al., "Renal clearance of quantum dots," *Nature Biotechnology*, 2007. 25(10): 1165–1170.

[114] Aharoni, A., et al., "Synthesis of InAs/CdSe/ZnSe core/shell1/shell2 structures with bright and stable near-infrared fluorescence," *J. Am. Chem. Soc.*, 2006. 128(1): 257–264.

[115] Boder, E.T., K.S. Midelfort, and K.D. Wittrup, "Directed evolution of antibody fragments with monovalent femtomolar antigen-binding affinity," *Proc. Natl. Acad. Sci. USA*, 2000. 97(20): 10701–10705.

[116] Zhang, Y., M.K. So, and J. Rao, "Protease-modulated cellular uptake of quantum dots," *Nano Letters*, 2006. 6(9): 1988–1992.

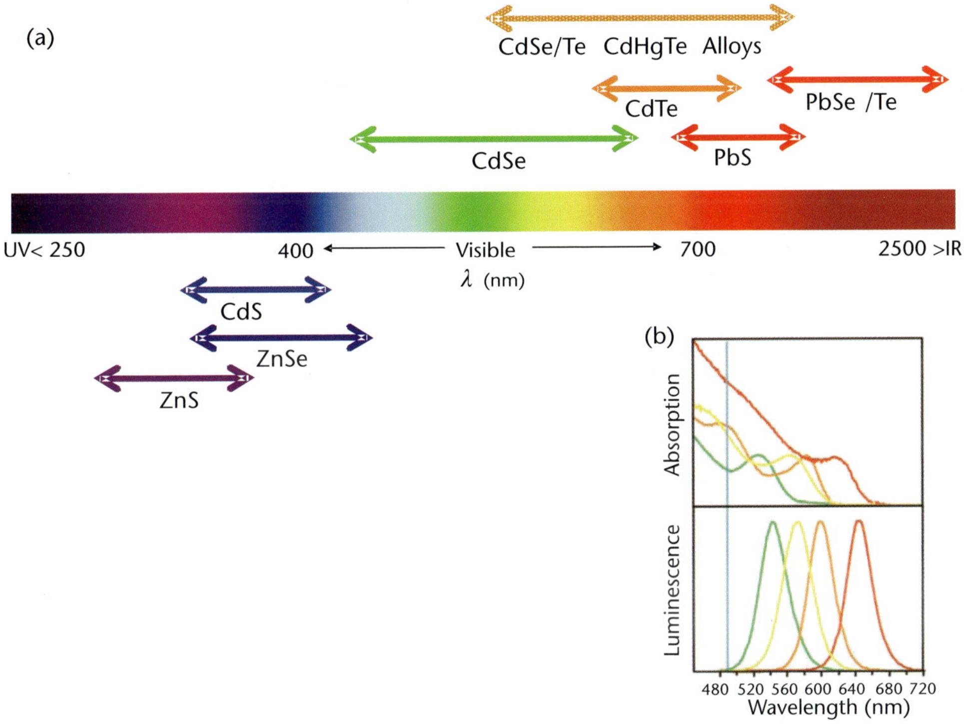

Color Plate 1 (a) Representative set of emission spectral windows for several types of QD materials. Core materials of II–VI, III–V and hybrid "III–VI" are shown. Partially reproduced from [5], with permission from NPG. (b) A representative example of absorption and normalized emission spectra collected for solutions of CdSe-ZnS QDs. Partially reproduced from [4], with permission from AAS. Other materials not represented here include InP and InAs QDs.

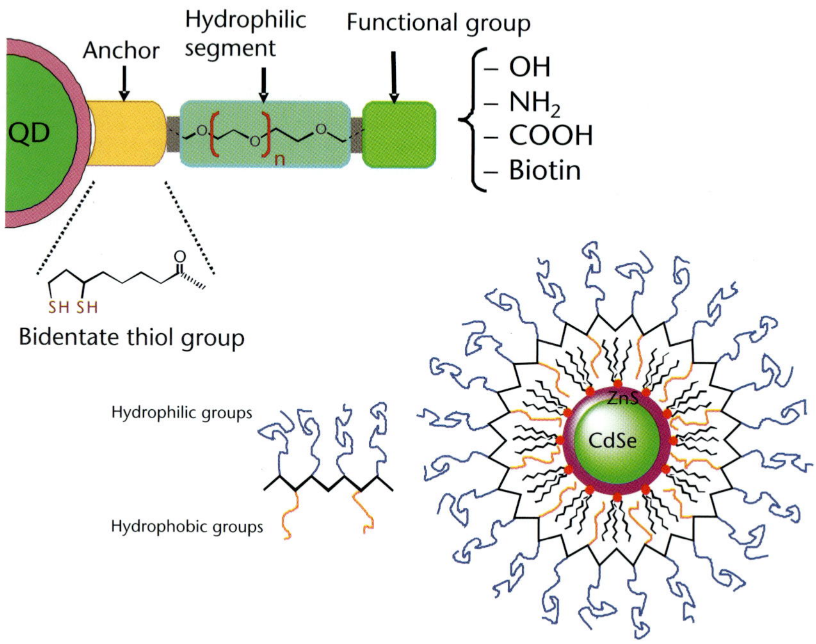

Color Plate 2 (top) Schematic representation of a QD capped with modular hydrophilic ligands based on the DHLA motif. Each ligand molecule has a central tunable length PEG segment, an anchoring dithiol head, and a terminal functional group that can be chemically modified. Reproduced from [92], with permission from the American Chemical Society. (bottom) Schematic representation of the strategy based on encapsulation of QDs with di-block copolymer shell. The polymer chain contains hydrophobic and hydrophilic blocks. The hydrophobic block is expected to strongly interact with the TOP/TOPO cap while the hydrophilic block promotes compatibility with aqueous environments.

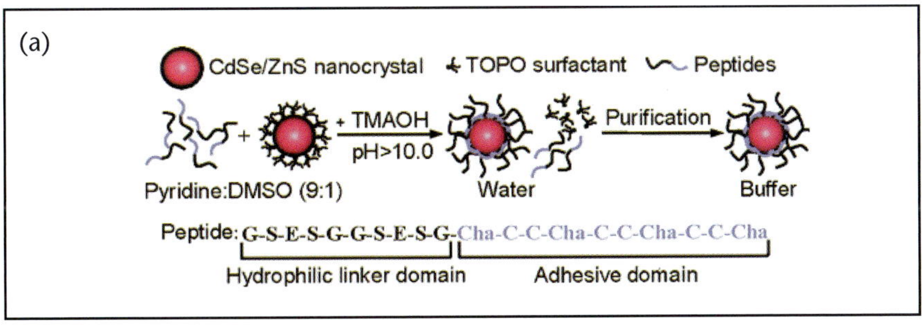

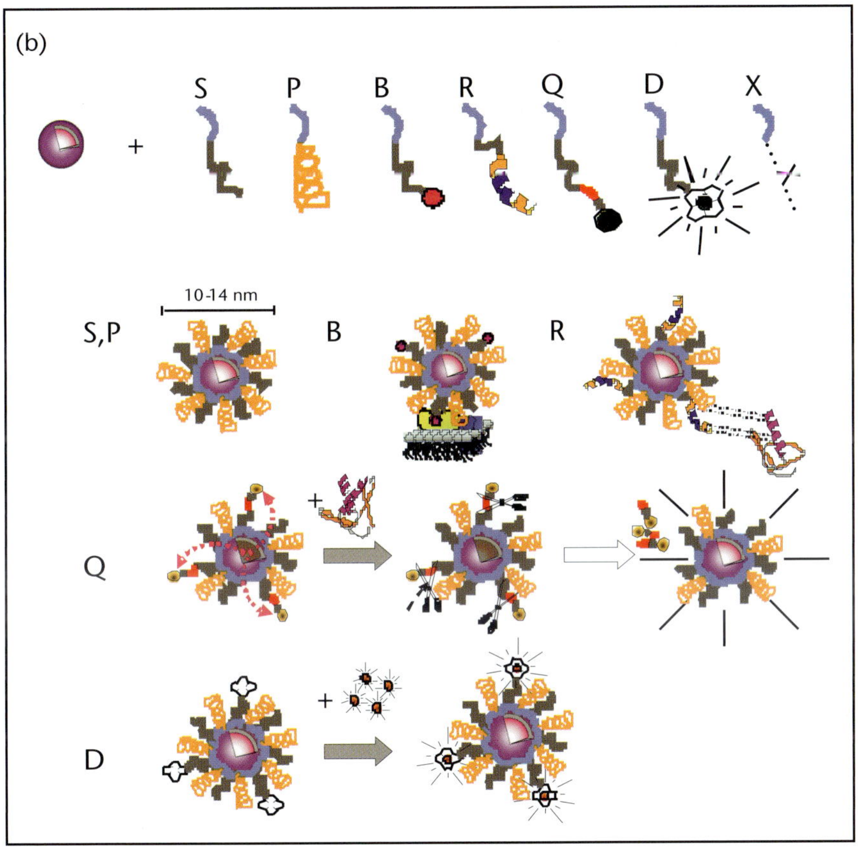

Color Plate 3 The phytochelatin peptide-coating approach: (a) Schematic representation of the surface coating chemistry of CdSe/ZnS nanocrystals with phytochelatin-related-peptides. The peptide C-terminal adhesive domain binds to the ZnS shell of CdSe/ZnS nanocrystals after exchange with the trioctylphosphine oxide (TOPO) surfactant. A polar and negatively charged hydrophilic linker domain in the peptide sequence provides aqueous buffer solubility to the nanocrystals. TMAOH: Tetramethyl ammonium hydroxide; Cha: 3-cyclohexylalanine. Adapted from [19] with permission from American Chemical Society. (b) Schematic representation of the peptide toolbox. The light blue segment contains cysteines and hydrophobic amino acids ensuring binding to the nanocrystal (adhesive domain of Figure 3.2(a)) and is common to all peptides. S: solubilization sequence (hydrophilic linker domain of Figure 3.2(a)), P: PEG, B: biotin, R: recognition sequence, Q: quencher, D: DOTA (1,4,7,10-tetraazacyclododecane-1,4,7,10-tetraacetic acid) for radionuclide and nuclear spin label chelation, X: any unspecified peptide-encoded function. Qdots solubilization is obtained by a mixture of S and P. Qdots can be targeted with biotin (B), a peptide recognition sequences (R), or other chemical moieties. Qdots fluorescence can be turned on or off by attaching a quencher (Q) via a cleavable peptide link. In the presence of the appropriate enzyme, the quencher is separated from the qdot, restoring the photoluminescence and reporting on the enzyme activity (as described in Section 3.6). For simultaneous PET (or MRI) and fluorescence imaging, qdots can be rendered radioactive by chelation of radionuclides (or nuclear spin labels respectively) using (D) DOTA (as described in Section 3.5). Adapted from [5] with permission from American Association for the Advancement of Science.

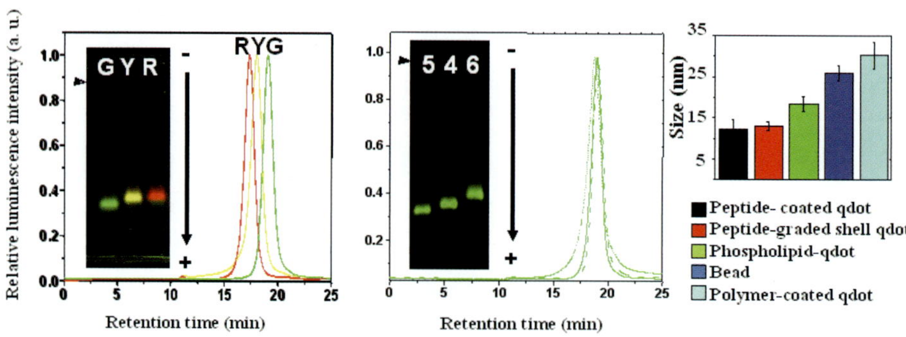

(a) (b) (c)

Color Plate 4 Characterization of peptide-coated qdots: (a) Effect of qdot size as measured by SE-HPLC and gel electrophoresis. The nomenclature of the peptides refers to the numbering in Table 3.1. Green, yellow, and red qdots emitting at 530, 565, and 617 nm, respectively, and coated with peptide 5 were separated on a size exclusion column against a 0.1M PBS mobile phase. The diameter of the peptide-coated qdots was evaluated from the elution times as 129.4Å (±15 percent), 150.3Å (±16 percent), and 164.8Å (±14 percent), respectively. Inset: 0.5 percent agarose gel electrophoresis of the same three peptide-coated qdot samples in TBE buffer pH 8.3. (b) Effect of peptide charge. Qdots coated with peptide 5 (dash), peptide 4 (dot), or peptides 6 (solid) have similar retention times on a SE-HPLC column. Inset: the same peptide-coated qdots migrate at different positions on a 0.5 percent agarose gel, in good agreement with the theoretical charge of each peptide. –►: position of the loading wells. →: direction of the applied electric field. (b) Effect of peptide charge on peptide-coated qdots. Qdots coated with peptide 5 (dash), peptide 4 (dot), or peptides 6 (solid) have similar retention times on a SE-HPLC column (same size) while having different charges as accessed by gel electrophoresis. Adapted from [19] with permission from American Chemical Society. (c) Hydrodynamic diameter of various qdot preparations deducted from FCS analysis. Adapted from [46] with permission from American Chemical Society.

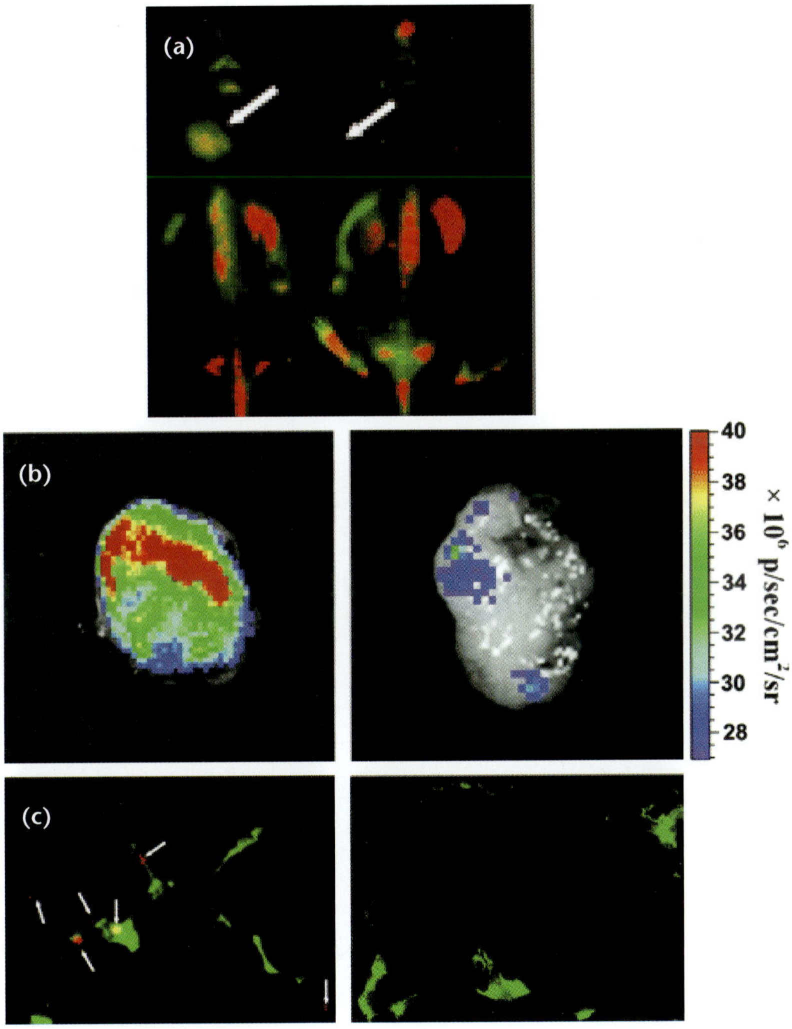

Color Plate 5 Targeting of tumor vasculature with RGD peptide-conjugated qdots: (a) In vivo NIR fluorescence imaging of U87MG tumor-bearing mice (left shoulder, pointed at with white arrows) injected with 200 pmol of RGD-qdots (left mouse) and control qdots (right mouse) six hours after injection. (b) Ex vivo fluorescence images of the same tumors, surgically removed from RGD qdots (left) and control qdots (right) injected mice. (c) Fluorescent microscope images of frozen tumor slices stained for CD31 (green) to allow visualizing of the tumor vasculature. Qdot signal is shown in red and pointed at with white arrows. Adapted from [63] with permission from the American Chemical Society.

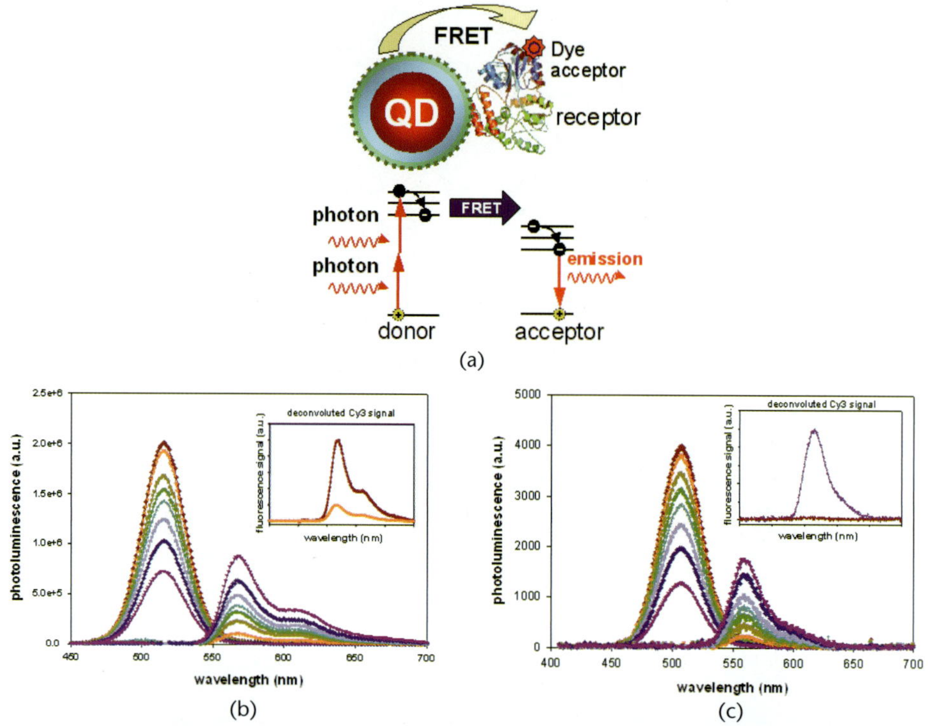

Color Plate 6 (a) Schematic of two-photon excitation and FRET with a QD-protein-dye conjugate. Deconvoluted PL spectra of QDs and Cy3 as a function of an increasing number of MBP-Cy3 per 510-nm QD using both (b) conventional and (c) two-photon excitation. The inset in each shows a comparison between FRET-induced Cy3 PL and the contribution due to direct conventional or two-photon excitation collected for a control MBP-Cy3 sample. Figure adapted from [27] and reproduced with permission. © Wiley-VCH Verlag GmbH & Co. KGaA.

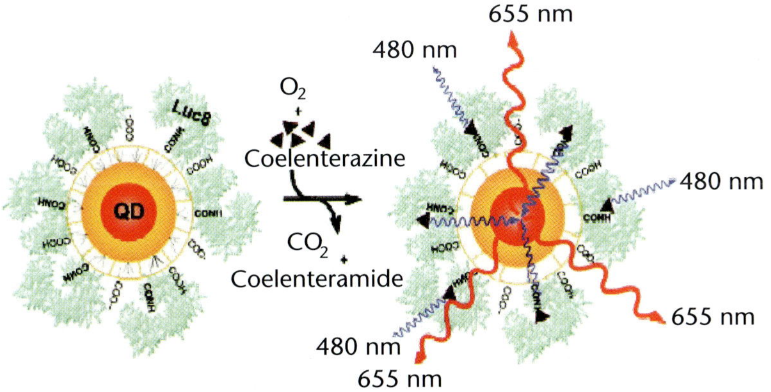

(a)

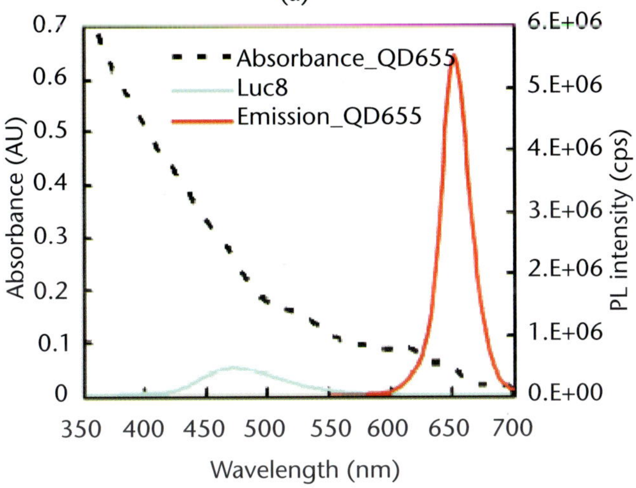

(b)

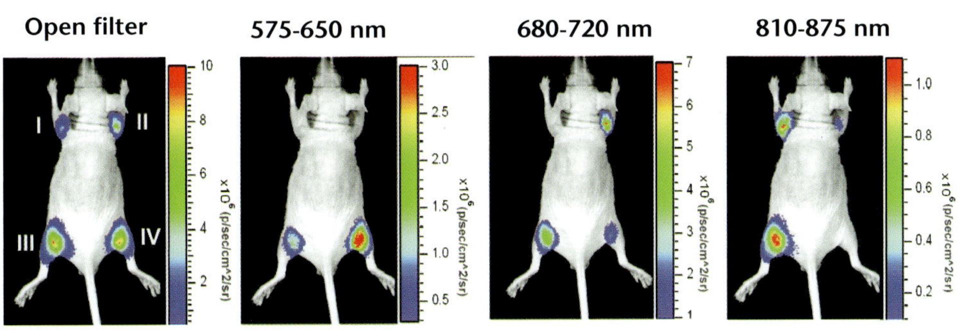

(c) (d) (e) (f)

Color Plate 7 (a) Schematic of QD-Luc8 BRET assemblies. The bioluminescent energy from Luc8-catalyzed oxidation of coelenterazine is transferred to the QDs resulting in their emission. (b) Absorption and emission spectra of QD655 (ex = 480 nm) and spectrum of the bioluminescent light emitted in the oxidation of coelenterazine substrate by Luc8. (c) Multiplexed in vivo bioluminescence imaging of the following conjugates intramuscularly injected at the indicated sites in a mouse: (I) QD800-Luc8 15 pmol (II) QD705-Luc8 15 pmol (III) mixture of QD665-Luc8, QD705-Luc8 and QD800-Luc8 (IV) QD665-Luc8 5 pmol. Images (c–f) were collected with the indicated filters. Figures provided by J. Rao, Stanford University, reprinted with permission of the NPG [64].

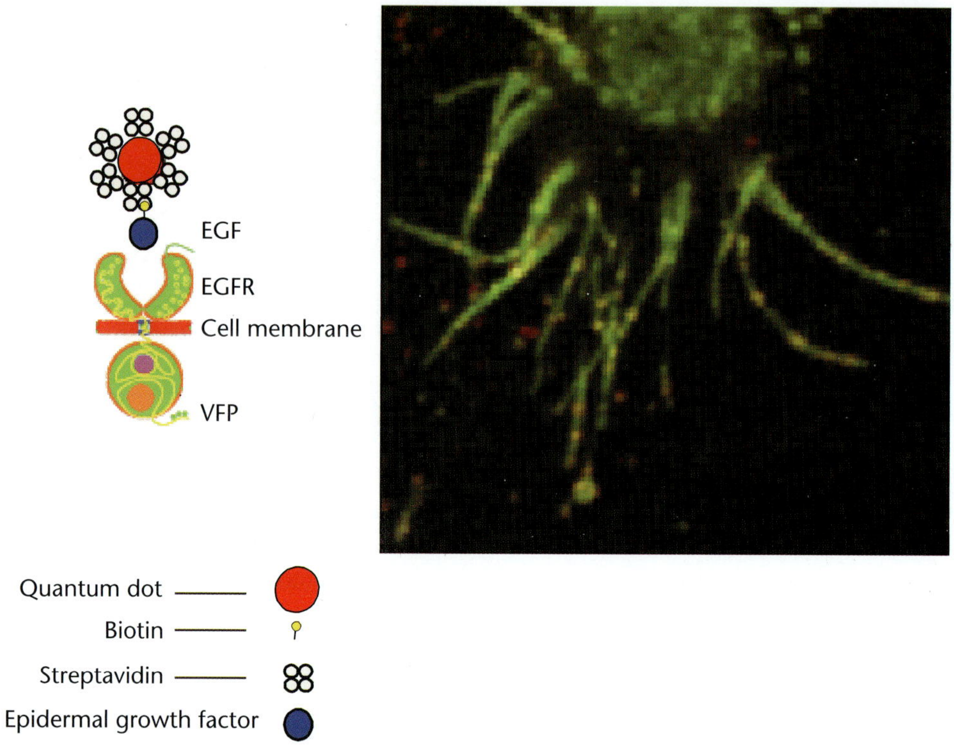

Color Plate 8 Strategy to study the binding of QD-EGF to the EGF receptor (EGFR), and the resultant activation and endocytosis of the receptor into living cells. The image displays A431 cells expressing ERB1-EGFP 20 min after addition of biotinylated EGF bound to Streptavidin QD-605. For further details, see [20].

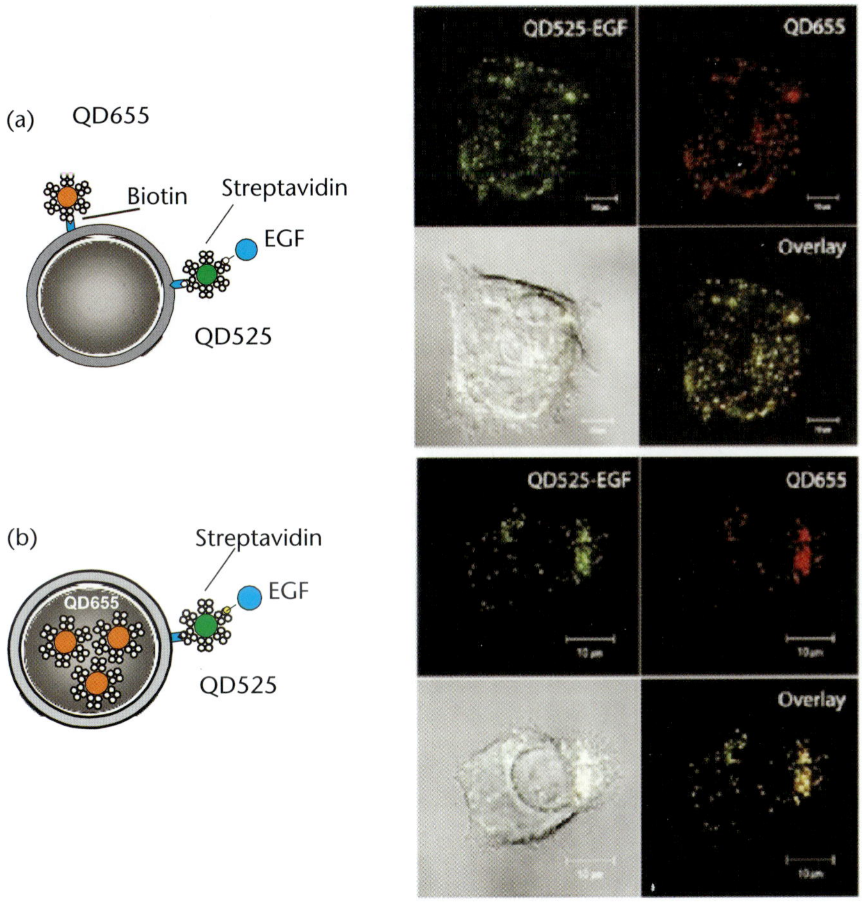

Color Plate 9 Preparation of liposomes attached to and/or containing QDs: (a) Surface labeling of lipid particles with QD525-EGF and untargeted QD655. (b) Lipid particles with encapsulated QD655 and surface labeled with QD525-EGF. QD-655 are either encapsulated or decorate the liposome surface. In a second conjugation step, preformed QD525-EGF complexes in 1:2 molar ratio target the liposomes for specific cell delivery. The images depict the cellular uptake of dual QD-labeled liposomes by live A431 cells, detected as colocalized dots in endosomal vesicles after 2h incubation at 37 degrees C according to strategies (a) and (b).

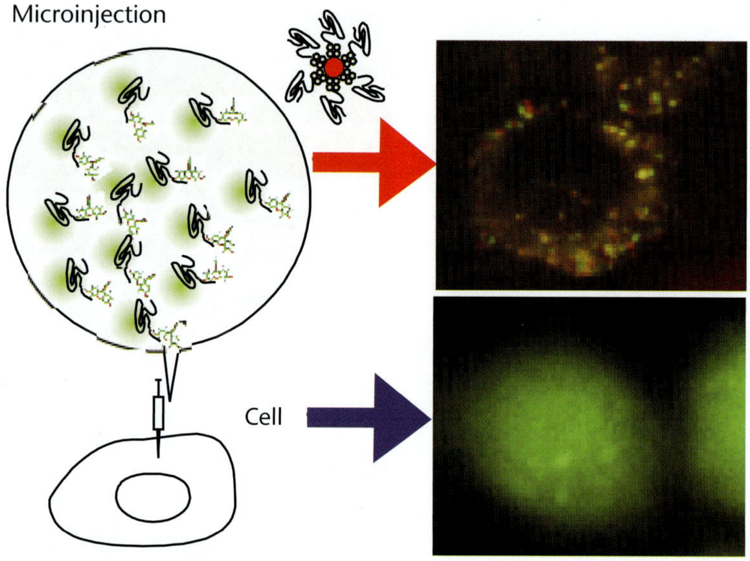

Color Plate 10 QDs acting as specific nucleation sites for ∝-synuclein (AS) in living cells. Cells were microinjected with AS in the presence or absence of AS-QDs-605 (40:1 protein:QD ratio) and observed after 24h of incubation. A mixture 2 nM AS-QDs-605 and 100 mM of AS-TC labeled with FlAsH was microinjected into HeLa cells (upper panel, red arrow). QDs were detected, colocalizing to a pronounced degree with AS aggregates. Lower panel, blue arrow, microinjection of 100 mM of AS-TC labeled with FlAsH in the absence of QDs; little or no aggregation was observed.

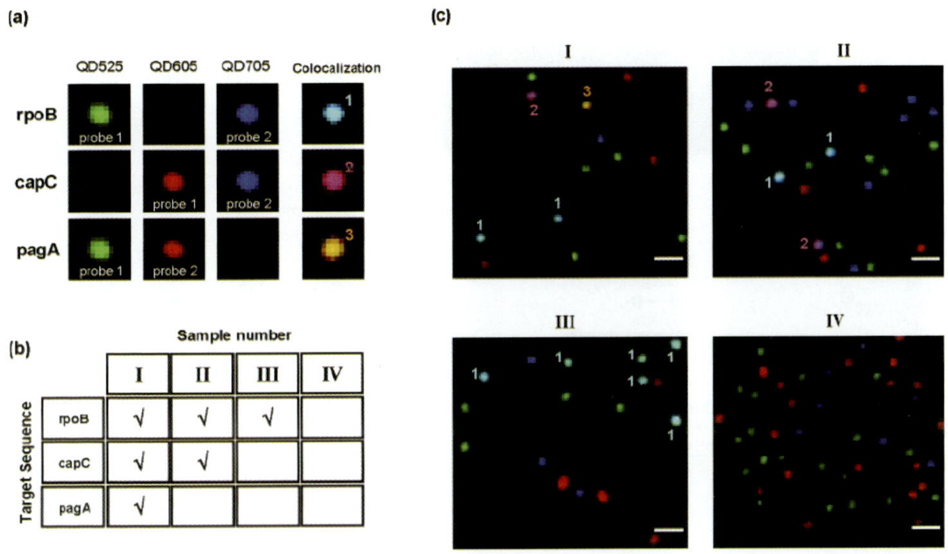

Color Plate 11 Simulated multiplexed analysis of anthrax-related genetic targets: (a) color pallet for the three pairs of target-specific QD nanoprobes and their resulting colocalized fluorescent images upon sandwich hybridization; (b) four samples containing different combinations of the three targets, rpoB, capC, and pagA. Checks represent the existence of certain target sequences. Sample IV does not contain any target and is used as a negative control. (c) Fluorescent images I, II, III, and IV correlate with samples I, II, III, and IV, respectively. (Bar dimension is 1 μm.). Reprinted by permission from the American Chemical Society [9], © 2003.

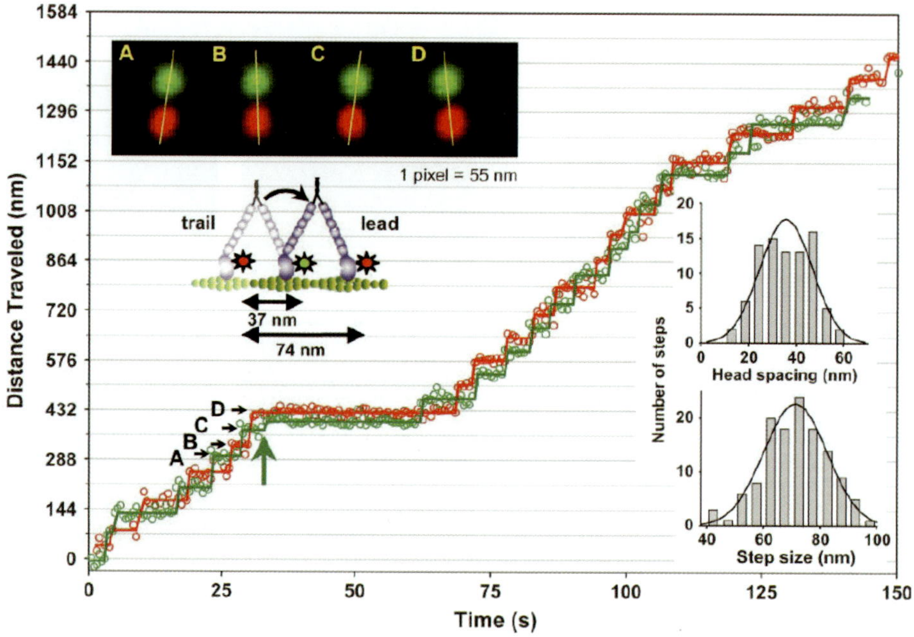

Color Plate 12 Myosin V processive runs with heads labeled with different color QDs. Green and red open circles are the two different QD positions determined by Gaussian fits. Solid lines are the average QD positions between steps, with the onset of steps determined by eye. Upper left are averaged QD images for steps labeled A–D. The yellow lines connect QD centers emphasizing alternating relative head positions. The green arrow identifies the substep. Lower right are histograms of interhead spacing and step size. Reprinted by permission from the Biophysical Society [33], © 2005.

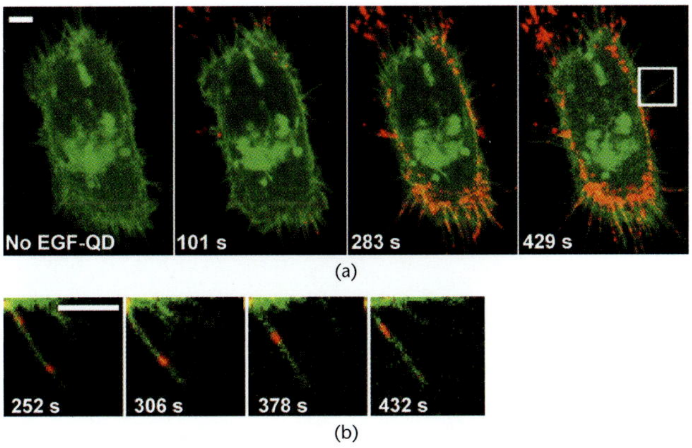

Color Plate 13 Retrograde transport of EGF-QDs (red) on filipodia. (a) A431 cell expressing receptor erbB3-mCitrine (green); maximum intensity projection of four 0.5-μm confocal sections as a function of time. (b) Magnified image of filipodium indicated in the last panel of (a), showing the uniform migration of the EGF-QDs toward the cell body with a velocity of ~ 10 nm/s. All scale bars, 5 μm. Reprinted by permission from Macmillan Publishers Ltd: *Nature Biotechnology* [42], © 2004.

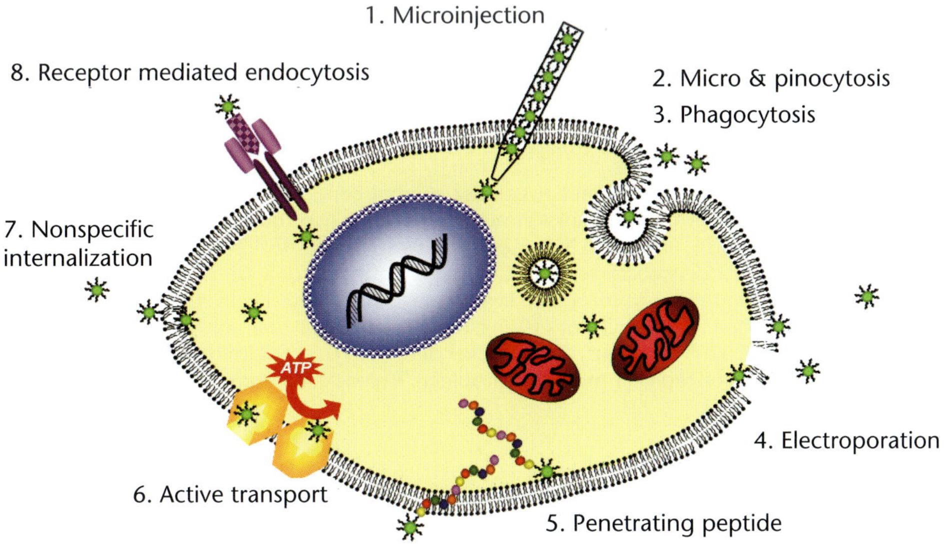

Color Plate 14 Cellular uptake mechanisms available for the internalization of quantum dots.

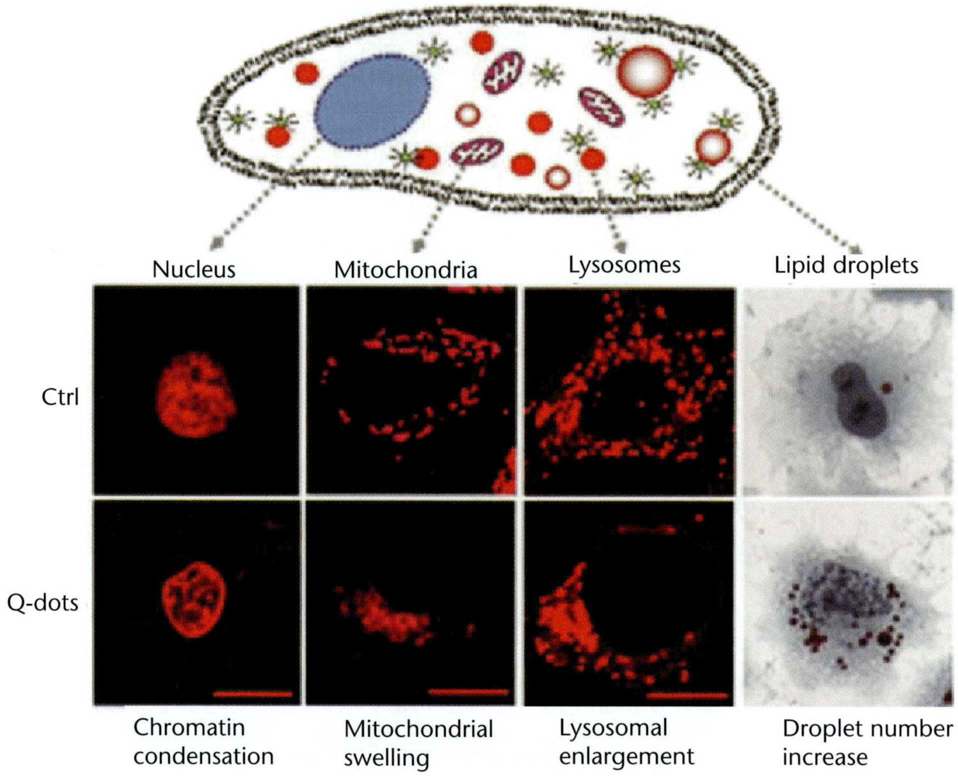

Color Plate 15 Organelle states and functions under normal conditions and under oxidative stress; Top: schematic representation of the cellular compartments observed. Top row: organelles under normal conditions. Bottom row: changes in organelles exposed to quantum dots for 24 hours. Column 1: nuclei are deformed and often have condensed chromatin. Column 2: mitochondria are swollen and often localized in the perinuclear region. Column 3: lysosomes are swollen in Q-dot treated cells. Column 4: lipid droplets are more abundant and enlarged in CdTe Q-dot (10 mg mL^{-1}) treated cells than in the untreated controls. Cells were stained with Draq5 (0.5 mM, nucleus), MitoTracker deep red (0.5 mM, mitochondria); LysoTracker DND 99 (0.5 mM, lysosomes) and oil red O (1 mM, lipid droplets). Reproduced from [83] by permission of the Royal Society of Chemistry.

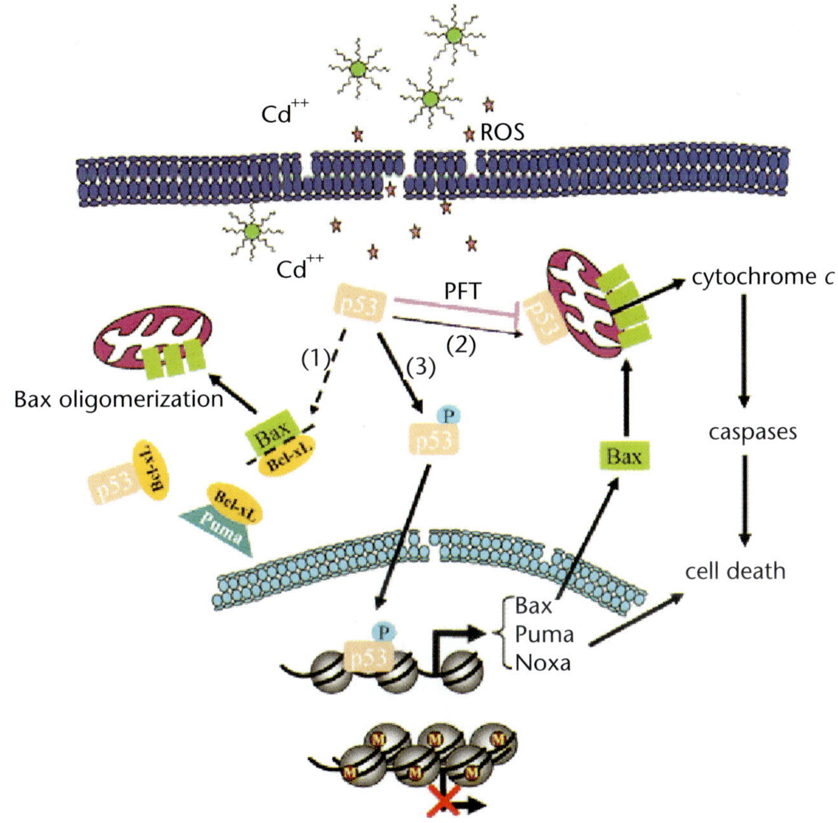

Color Plate 16 Schematic representation of the changes induced by QDs at the cellular epigenic and genomic levels. QDs release reactive oxygen species (ROS)and free cadmium ions extra- and intracellularly, triggering changes in the epigenome through chromatin condensation and histone hypoacetylation. QDs induce increased protein levels and activation of the transcription factor p53 resulting in: 1 cytosolic p53 directly activating Bax by freeing it from its binding proteins and facilitating the mitochondrial accumulation of Bax; 2. p53 proteins can mistranslocate to the mitochondria, leading to membrane permeabilization and consequential cell death. Pifithrin-á (PFT), a specific inhibitor of p53, can prevent this mistranslocation, and thereby can partially prevent QD-induced cell death; 3 activated (phosphorylated) p53 induces the transcription of proapoptotic genes, including Bax, Puma, and Noxa. Bax proteins accumulate and oligomerize at the mitochondrial membrane, forming pores and releasing cytochrome c, leading to cell death. Puma facilitates Bax mitochondrial accumulation by occupying Bax-binding proteins (i.e., Bcl-xL), freeing cytosolic Ba. Reproduced from [97] with permission from Springer Science and Business Media.

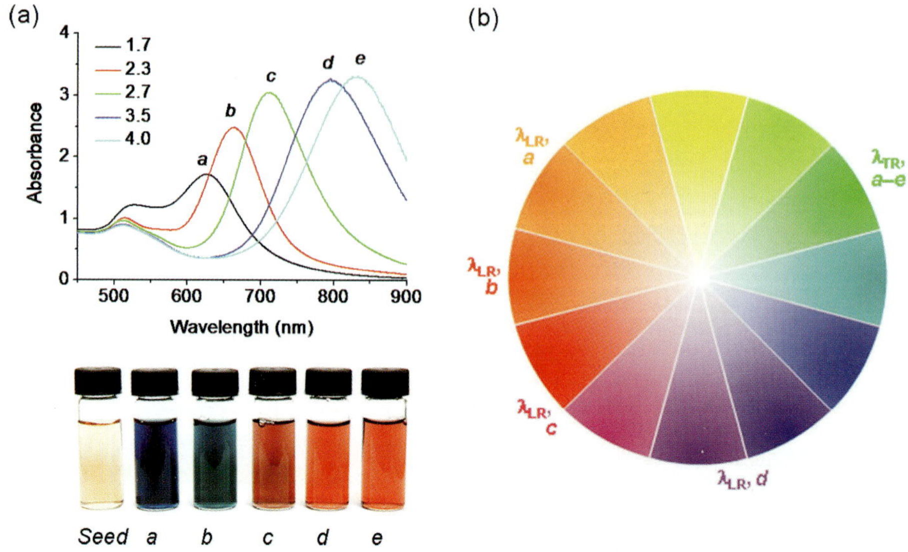

Color Plate 17 (a) Optical absorption spectra of GNRs with different aspect ratios; (b) color wheel with reference to λ_{LR} (and λ_{TR}) for GNR samples *a–e*.

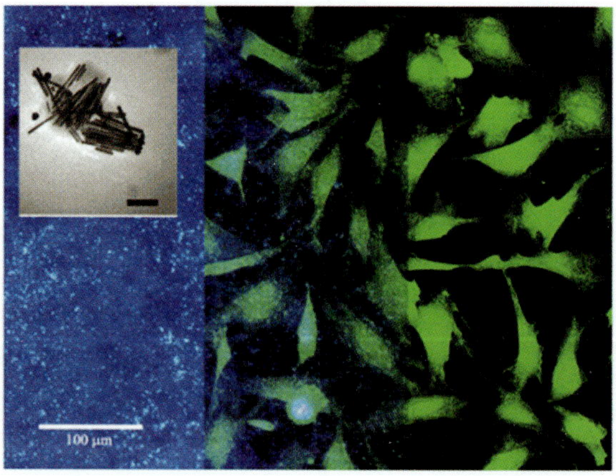

Color Plate 18 Partially overlapping dark-field and fluorescence images of GNRs incubated with cardiac fibroblasts [242]. TEM image of GNRs shown in upper-left inset. Reprinted with permission from the American Chemical Society.

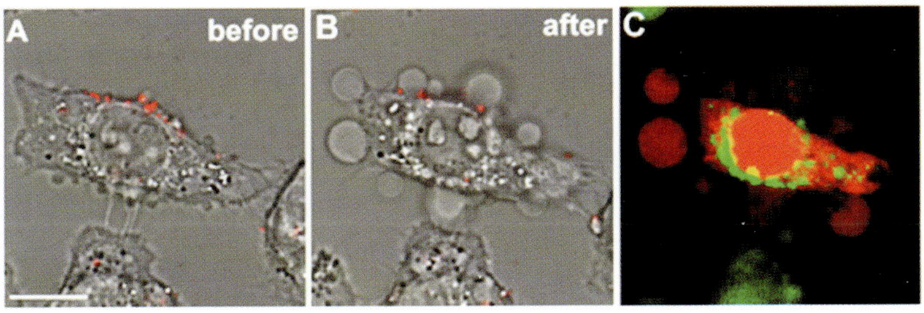

Color Plate 19 (a, b) Folate-conjugated GNRs (red) targeted to the membranes of KB cells, before and after a 1-min exposure to a scanning NIR laser (12 J/cm^2). (c) Evidence for "optoporation" was obtained by using ethidium bromide (red) and a fluorescent dye indicating high levels of intracellular Ca^{2+} (green) [279]. Reprinted with permission from Wiley-VCH Publishing.

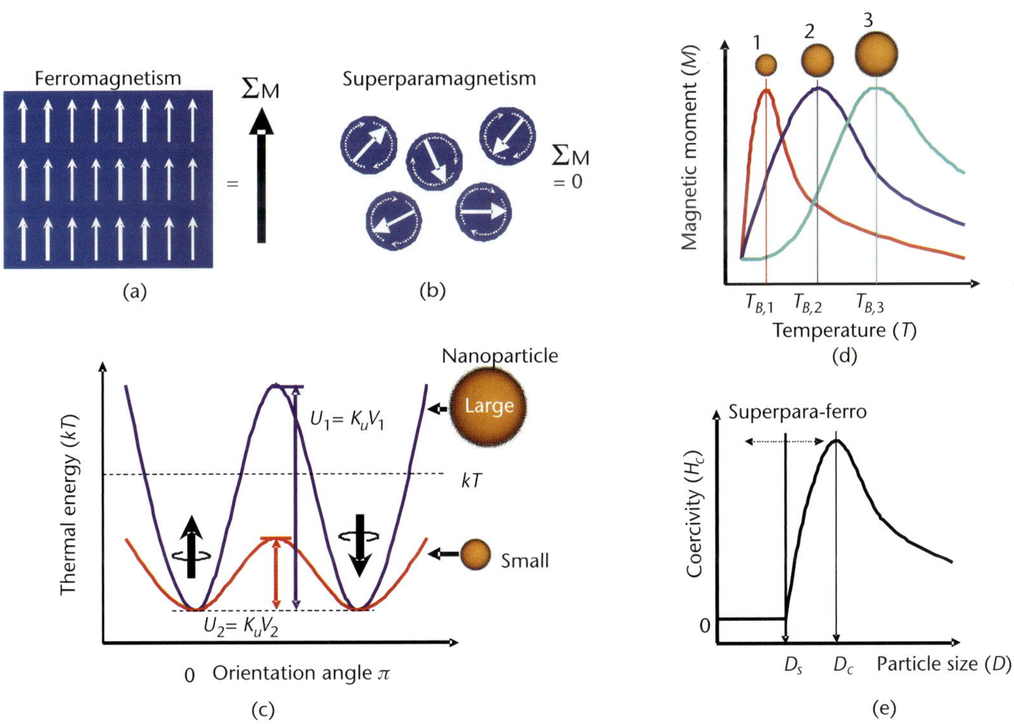

Color Plate 20 The main characteristics of nanoscale magnetism. Magnetic spin structures of (a) ferromagnetism which has a significant amount of net magnetization (M) after the external magnetic field (B_0) has disappeared and (b) superparamagnetism in which the net magnetization (M) becomes zero. (c) Energy diagram of magnetic nanoparticles of different particle sizes. In large particle, anisotropy energy (U_1) is higher than thermal energy (kT) which results in ferromagnetism (top), and in a small particle, anisotropy energy (U_2) is lower than kT which results in superparamagnetism (bottom). (d) Size-dependent zero-field cooling curves indicating changes in the blocking temperature (T_B). (e) Size-dependent coercivity (H_c) curve, in which magnetic domain structures changes from multidomain ferromagnetism to single-domain and superparamagnetism.

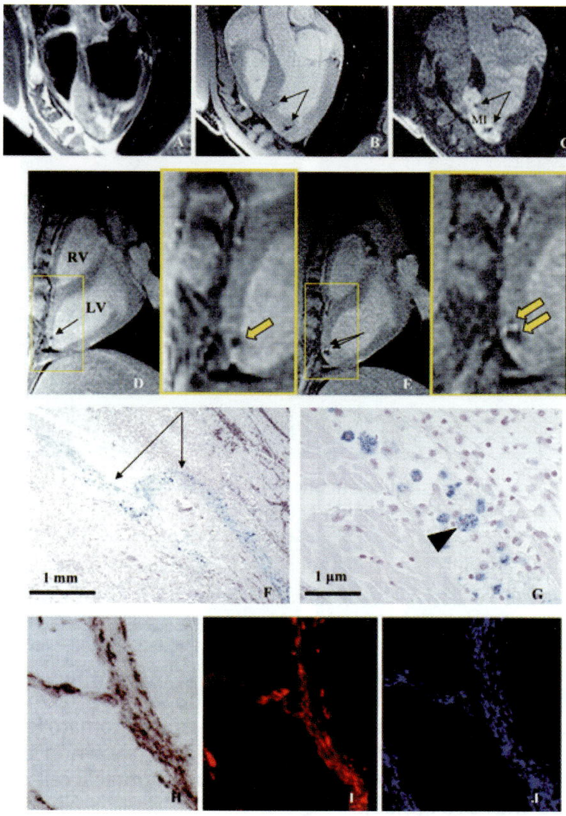

Color Plate 23 Representative hypointense lesions in FSE (A), FGRE (B), and DE-MRI (C) of MR-MSC injection sites (arrows) within 24 hr of injection. MR-MSCs were injected in the infarct (MI, hyperintense region in C). Long-axis MRIs showing hypointense lesions (arrows) caused by MR-MSCs acquired within 24 hr (D) and one week (E) of injection, with inset at right demonstrating expansion of lesion over one week. Needle tract (arrow) of MR-MSCs is demonstrated in the histological section at one week after injection with Prussian blue staining (F) as cells with blue iron inclusions (arrowhead) that are excluded from nucleus (G). Iron inclusion from DAB-enhanced Prussian blue staining (H) matches colabeling with DiI (I) and DAPI fluorescent dyes (J) on adjacent histological sections at ×20 magnification at 24 hr after MSC injection in another animal, indicating Feridex is still contained within original MSCs. LV indicates left ventricle; RV, right ventricle. (Used with the permission of *Circulation.*)

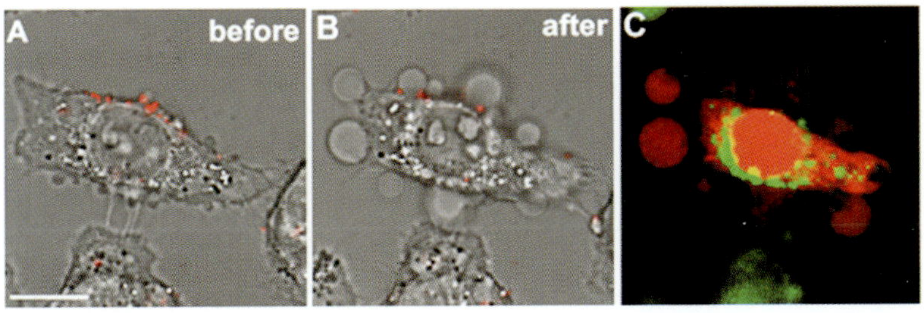

Color Plate 19 (a, b) Folate-conjugated GNRs (red) targeted to the membranes of KB cells, before and after a 1-min exposure to a scanning NIR laser (12 J/cm^2). (c) Evidence for "optoporation" was obtained by using ethidium bromide (red) and a fluorescent dye indicating high levels of intracellular Ca^{2+} (green) [279]. Reprinted with permission from Wiley-VCH Publishing.

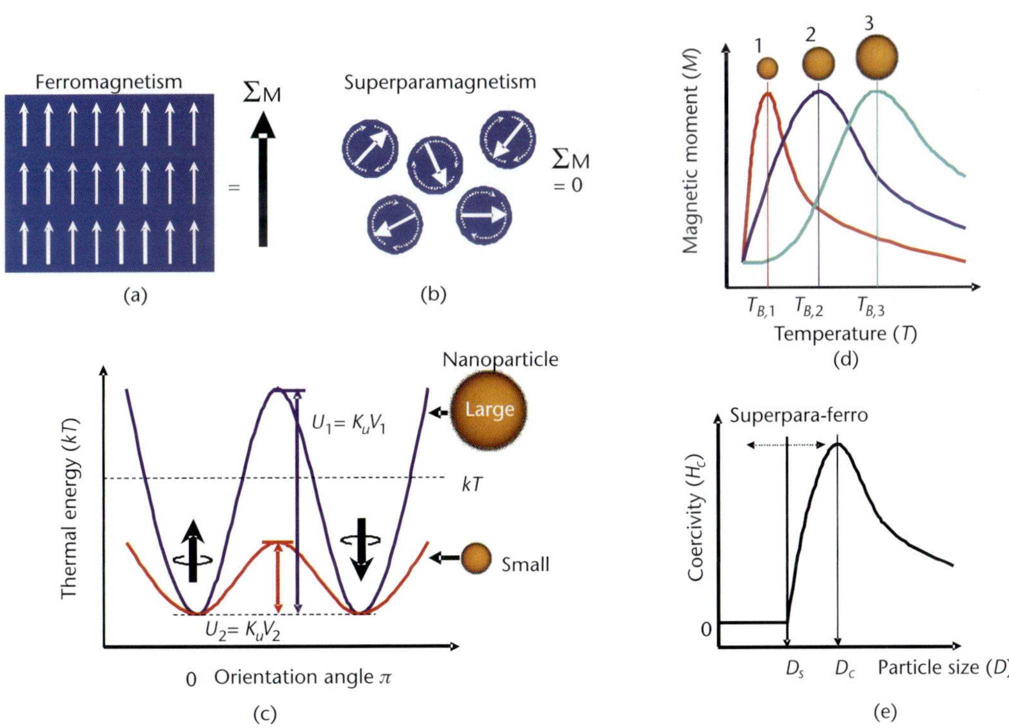

Color Plate 20 The main characteristics of nanoscale magnetism. Magnetic spin structures of (a) ferromagnetism which has a significant amount of net magnetization (M) after the external magnetic field (B_0) has disappeared and (b) superparamagnetism in which the net magnetization (M) becomes zero. (c) Energy diagram of magnetic nanoparticles of different particle sizes. In large particle, anisotropy energy (U_1) is higher than thermal energy (kT) which results in ferromagnetism (top), and in a small particle, anisotropy energy (U_2) is lower than kT which results in superparamagnetism (bottom). (d) Size-dependent zero-field cooling curves indicating changes in the blocking temperature (T_B). (e) Size-dependent coercivity (H_c) curve, in which magnetic domain structures changes from multidomain ferromagnetism to single-domain and superparamagnetism.

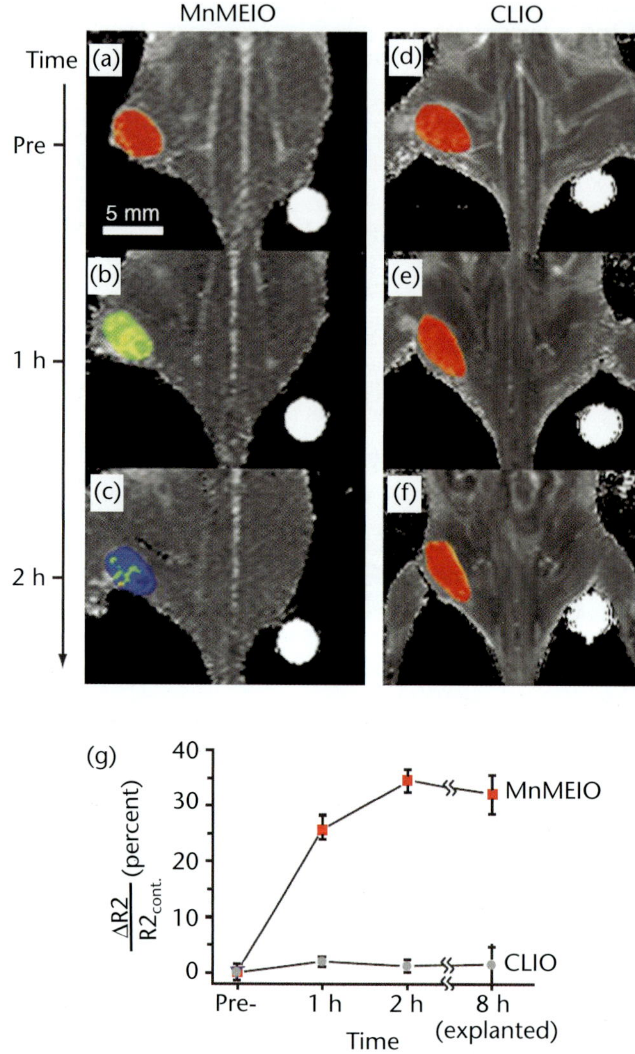

Color Plate 21 Highly sensitive in vivo cancer detection by utilization of MnMEIO-Herceptin nanoparticles. (a–c) Color mapped MRI of the tumor-bearing mouse at different temporal points following injection of MnMEIO-Herceptin nanoparticles, and (d–f) CLIO-Herceptin nanoparticles. (g) Time-dependent $\Delta R2/R2_{control}$ changes at the tumor site after injection of MnMEIO-Herceptin probes (blue square) and CLIO-Herceptin probes (red circle). (Reproduced with permission from [17]. © 2007 Nature Publishing Group.)

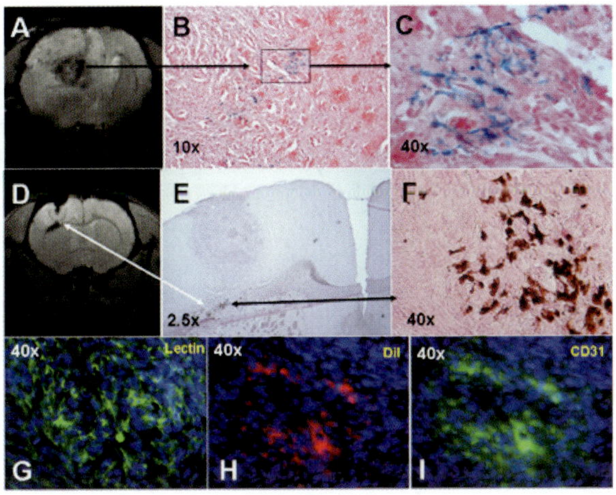

Color Plate 22 Representative cases of magnetically labeled endothelial progenitor cells' (EPCs) tracking in an implanted brain tumor in a rat model by 7 Tesla MR system. Tumors were created in nude rats by implanting U251 glioma cell line. Double-labeled (iron plus dye DiI) EPCs were administered on day seven after tumor implantation, and MRI was obtained on day 14 (seven days after intravenous administration of magnetically labeled EPCs). Panels A to C: T2*-weighted MRI image shows low signal intensity areas surrounding the tumor, indicating accumulation of magnetically labeled cells (A), which are confirmed by Prussian blue staining in the corresponding histological section (10x, B) and (40x, C). Note the blue cells within the box in the B and in C panels. Panels D to F: T2*W images show hypointense voxels around and in the tumor extension in the corpus callosum (white arrows in D and E). DAB-enhanced Prussian blue staining shows iron positive cells (E and F). Panels G to I: The section stained for endothelial lining (G, FITC-labeled tomato lectin) shows extensive formation of new vessels within the tumor, and the corresponding area (shown in the consecutive section) also shows DiI positive cells (H, red cells), which are also positive for endothelial cell marker CD31 (I, green cells). Nuclei of the cells are stained with DAPI (blue).

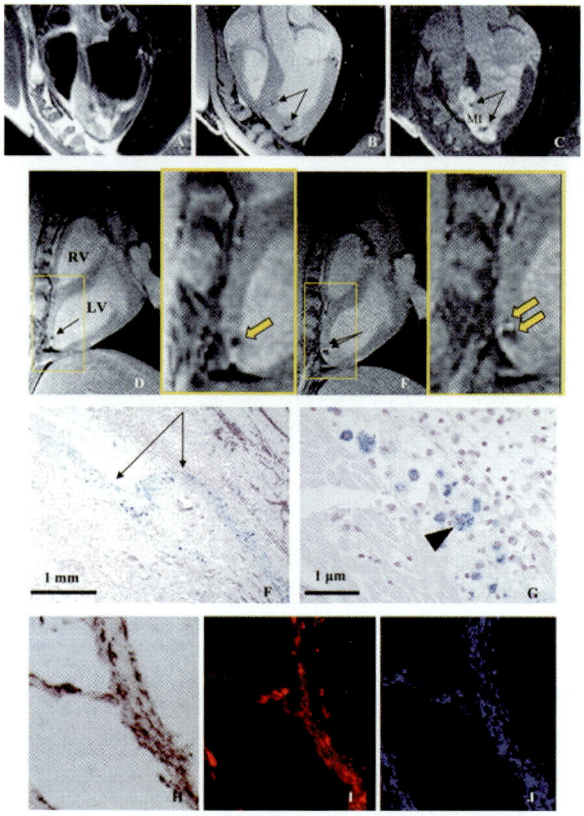

Color Plate 23 Representative hypointense lesions in FSE (A), FGRE (B), and DE-MRI (C) of MR-MSC injection sites (arrows) within 24 hr of injection. MR-MSCs were injected in the infarct (MI, hyperintense region in C). Long-axis MRIs showing hypointense lesions (arrows) caused by MR-MSCs acquired within 24 hr (D) and one week (E) of injection, with inset at right demonstrating expansion of lesion over one week. Needle tract (arrow) of MR-MSCs is demonstrated in the histological section at one week after injection with Prussian blue staining (F) as cells with blue iron inclusions (arrowhead) that are excluded from nucleus (G). Iron inclusion from DAB-enhanced Prussian blue staining (H) matches colabeling with DiI (I) and DAPI fluorescent dyes (J) on adjacent histological sections at ×20 magnification at 24 hr after MSC injection in another animal, indicating Feridex is still contained within original MSCs. LV indicates left ventricle; RV, right ventricle. (Used with the permission of *Circulation.*)

CHAPTER 4

Resonance Energy Transfer-Based Sensing Using Quantum Dot Bioconjugates

Igor L. Medintz and Hedi Mattoussi

4.1 Introduction and Background

One of the most common activities in all of biological research is monitoring of protein-protein interactions and protein tracking. This can provide information on a broad range of processes including cellular signaling pathways, drug interactions, pathogen detection, molecular structure/function, and genetic expression. Although simple in concept, the complexity arises from difficulties in implementation and data analysis. Förster or fluorescence resonance energy transfer (FRET) provides a powerful spectroscopic tool to probe these complex biological phenomena. Its use has steadily expanded in the past three decades, facilitated by progress in both developing sophisticated detection systems and the ever-growing range of available fluorophores.

FRET is a photophysical process that involves the nonradiative transfer of excitation energy from an excited state donor molecule (D) to a proximal ground-state acceptor molecule (A) [1]. Efficient FRET requires that two key criteria are satisfied: (1) proximity between donor and acceptor, because the process is driven by dipole-dipole interactions, and (2) the donor emission must have a sizable overlap with the acceptor absorption profile (i.e., they share spectral overlap) [1]. Although an in-depth review of the FRET formalism is not warranted here, we will provide a few expressions that are important to the current discussion. The rate of energy transfer between a donor and an acceptor separated by a center-to-center distance, r, can be expressed as:

$$k_{D-A} = \frac{B \times Q_D I}{\tau_D r^6} = \left(\frac{1}{\tau_D}\right) \times \left(\frac{R_0}{r}\right)^6 \tag{4.1}$$

where Q_D and τ_D designate the donor photoluminescence (PL) quantum yield and its exciton radiative lifetime, respectively. The constant B is a function of the refractive index of the medium n_D, Avogadro's number N_A, and the dipole orientation parameter, κ_p:

$$B = \frac{[9{,}000 \times (\ln 10)]\kappa_p^2}{128\pi^5 n_D^4 N_A} \tag{4.2}$$

The Förster radius R_0 designates the separation distance corresponding to 50 percent FRET efficiency and is given by:

$$R_0 = (BQ_D I)^{1/6} = \left(9.78 \times 10^3 n_D^{-4} \kappa_p^2 Q_D I\right)^{1/6} \left(\text{in Å}\right) \tag{4.3}$$

where I is the integral of the spectral overlap between donor PL and acceptor absorption, $J(\lambda)$. The orientation factor κ_p^2 varies from 0 (for perpendicular alignment of the donor and acceptor dipoles) to 4 (for parallel orientation) [1]. The energy transfer efficiency defined as:

$$E = \frac{k_{D-A}}{k_{D-A} + \tau_D^{-1}} = \frac{R_0^6}{R_0^6 + r^6} \tag{4.4}$$

accounts for the fraction of excitons that are transferred from the donor to the acceptor nonradiatively. Experimentally, E is determined from either steady-state or time-resolved fluorescence measurements using:

$$E = 1 - \frac{F_{DA}}{F_D} \text{(steady-state), or } E = 1 - \frac{\tau_{DA}}{\tau_D} \text{ (time-resolved)} \tag{4.5}$$

where the donor fluorescence intensity in the absence (F_D) and presence (F_{DA}) of the acceptors are used; similarly, τ_D and τ_{DA} designate the donor excited state fluorescent lifetime in the absence and presence of the acceptors [1].

The strong sixth power dependence of FRET efficiency on r makes this process ideally suited for probing nanoscale separation distances in the range of 10–100Å, which has resulted in the technical qualification of FRET as a "spectroscopic ruler." FRET is ideally suited for assessing the size of biomolecules or probing changes in protein conformation. Indeed, FRET using conventional organic or protein-based fluorophores has been applied to probe nanoscale interactions for an array of biological phenomena, which can be broadly grouped in two main areas [1]. The first area is a signal transduction modality for a myriad in vitro and in vivo biosensors of small molecule targets, such as nutrients and intracellular second messengers, or alternatively to sense specific enzymatic events, such as proteolysis [2-4]. The second area is a tool for elucidating the structure, conformation, and specific interactions of biomolecules, with applications ranging from monitoring real-time protein folding to determining the overall structure of protein-protein and DNA-protein complexes [5 , 6–9].

Effective implementation of FRET in biology hinges on the ability to meet two challenges: reproducible methods for labeling biomolecules with donor and acceptor molecules, and, more importantly, the spectroscopic properties of the fluorophores. In general, controlled labeling of the target biomolecules with fluorophores (donor/acceptor) at known and distinct sites is the most desirable format. This can allow good control over the measured FRET efficiencies and provide information on subtle changes in protein (or peptide, DNA) conformation resulting from interactions with target molecules or changes in the surrounding conditions [2]. To date, the most common donor molecules have been organic dyes or fluorescent proteins, while both emissive and nonemissive, or "dark," quenching dyes were used as acceptors [2]. Some of the inherent photophysical properties of these materials have limited further progress of FRET-based assays and sensing in biology. Limitations can arise from low quantum yields, pH sensitivity, and susceptibility to both chemical and photo-degradation, along with broad absorption and emission profiles. The latter results in substantial overlap between donor and acceptor absorption/emission spectra; it also results in significant direct excitation contribution to the acceptor emission [1, 2, 10]. Thus, effective implementation of FRET often requires complex instrumentation to provide tunable excitation and allow signal detection and sophisticated data analysis that permit careful deconvolution of complex raw PL spectra.

Luminescent semiconductor nanocrystals or quantum dots (QDs) offer unique optical and spectroscopic properties that can potentially overcome some of these limitations and improve FRET use in biological as well as nonbiological applications [10, 11]. In this chapter, we first describe the QD photophysical properties of direct relevance to FRET. We then discuss the progress made using QDs and FRET in biology by describing various biosensing configurations, and finally we provide some assessment of where QD-based FRET may be evolving in the near future.

4.2 Unique Attributes of Quantum Dots As FRET Donors

As compared to conventional organic- and protein-based fluorophores, nanocrytalline semiconductor quantum dots are characterized by several unique properties. These include broad absorption spectra extending to the UV, with very high extinction coefficients, along with tunable narrow-symmetric PL (with full width at half-maximum, FWHM, <40 nm; see Figure 4.1). Tuning of the QD emission is driven by quantum confinement effects and is primarily governed by the nanocrystal size and materials composition [12–16]. Additionally, QDs exhibit high PL yields, a strong resistance to both photo- and chemical degradation, and pronounced photobleaching thresholds. Cumulatively, these properties impart to QDs five unique attributes as FRET donors that are unavailable with conventional fluorophores [10].

4.2.1 Improving the Spectral Overlap by Tuning QD Emission

When using conventional organic dyes, the D-A pair is usually chosen to have sizable spectral overlap (e.g., fluorescein-rhodamine and Cy3-Cy5 are some of the most commonly used pairs), but the ability to tune the degree of that overlap is limited due to the relatively narrow absorption bands of conventional fluorophores [1, 2]. In comparison, for QD-dye D-A pairs, the spectral overlap with a given dye can be easily tuned by changing the QDs size/color used. As an illustrative example, Figure 4.1(a) shows the PL emission of 3 CdSe-ZnS core-shell QD dispersions with emission centered at 510, 530, and 555 nm plotted against the absorption of Cy3 acceptor, together with the corresponding overlap function, $J(\lambda)$. Plots clearly show that as Cy3 has an absorption maximum at ~555 nm, the spectral overlap improves dramatically for QDs emitting at 555 nm (R_0 varies from ~ 47Å to 57Å for these pairs). Since QD emissions can be tuned from the UV to the near IR, this would imply that with a judicious choice of core materials and nanocrystal size, a QD donor can be selected for optimized spectral overlap with essentially any potential fluorophore acceptor [10, 11].

4.2.2 Significant Reduction of Direct Excitation of the Acceptor

Organic dye and protein fluorophores are characterized by broad absorption spectra coupled with small Stoke's shifts. Experimentally, this means that the donor and acceptor absorption spectra usually exhibit considerable overlap, regardless of the excitation wavelength used, and there is always a significant direct excitation contribution to the acceptor emission. Thus, FRET analysis usually requires careful deconvolution of composite spectra to clearly isolate donor and acceptor emissions and accurately determine FRET efficiencies and sensitization of the acceptor. This contrasts with QD-dye pairs, where the ability to efficiently excite the QD at virtually any wavelength below the first absorption peak allows one to select a line corresponding to the acceptor's absorption minimum. This can substantially reduce direct excitation contribution of the acceptor emission. This feature is illustrated in Figure 4.1(b), where a 590-nm emitting QD donor is paired with a Cy5 dye acceptor. For this pair, excitation at any wavelength below 520 nm will produce little to no direct excitation contribution to Cy5 emission. Indeed, 350-nm excitation of this configuration resulted in a direct Cy5 excitation contribution ~40 times *smaller* than the FRET-sensitized emission [17].

4.2.3 Increase FRET Efficiency by Arraying Multiple Acceptors around a Single QD

QDs are significantly larger in size than organic dyes and their surfaces provide multiple sites for attaching dyes or dye-labeled biomolecules. This allows for a configuration where a single nanocrystal can simultaneously interact with multiple acceptors. Applying the Förster concepts within such a configuration translates a proportional increase in the overlap integral (or FRET cross-section) with an increasing number of acceptors per donor and a concomitant enhancement in the rate of FRET. This in turn induces a substantial enhancement in the overall FRET efficiency compared to one-to-one D-A pairs. For a simple conjugate configuration where multiple acceptors n are arrayed at a given distance r around a central QD (centro symmetric configuration with fixed separation distance), (4.4) can be developed to [18]:

$$E = \frac{nR_0^6}{nR_0^6 + r^6} \tag{4.6}$$

This assumes that a dipole-orientation κ^2 value of 2/3 (characteristic of random distribution of dipoles) provide a proper description for QD-dye pairs, which is justified by the partial random orientation of the QD dipole and the inability to control

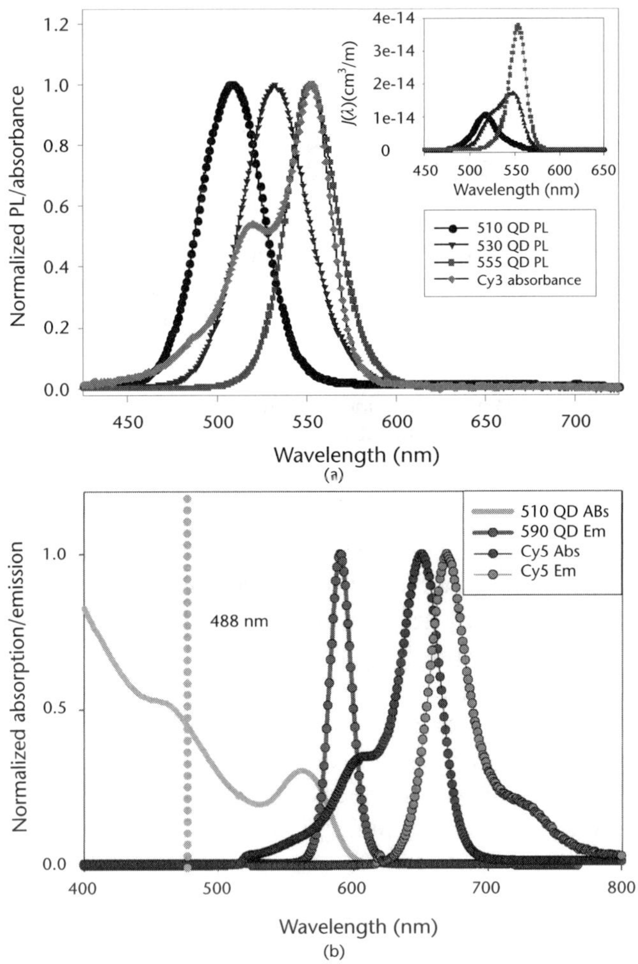

Figure 4.1 (a) Normalized absorption spectra (ε_A) of Cy3 dye and photoemission spectra of the three CdSe-ZnS core-shell QD solutions. Inset shows plots of the resulting overlap functions, $J(\lambda) = P_{LD-corr}(\lambda) \times \lambda^4 \times \varepsilon_A(\lambda)$, and highlights the effects of size-tuning the QD emission on the degree of spectral overlap for a given acceptor dye (Cy3). Adapted from [18] and reprinted with permission from the American Chemical Society (ACS). (b) Normalized absorption and emission spectra for 590-nm CdSe-ZnS core/shell donor QDs and Cy5 acceptor dye. The position of a 488-nm laser excitation line is shown in gray. Note the minimal Cy5 absorption at this wavelength.

the orientation of the dye-acceptor dipoles conjugated (such as protein dye, peptide dye, or DNA dye) to the QD surface [18]. The anticipated effect of (4.6) is schematically illustrated in Figure 4.2, where a central QD (with a nominal radius of 30Å) is interacting with protein-acceptors attached to its surface; the dye is located at a distance of 70Å from the QD center. For a nominal R_0 value of 56Å, (4.4) predicts a FRET efficiency of ~22 percent for a single QD-single dye pair ($n = 1$) [19]. In comparison, for $n = 5$ the anticipated efficiency using (4.6) increases to ~58 percent. CdSe-ZnS QDs have diameters ranging from 20–80Å depending upon emission [11, 16]. They can thus accommodate several small to medium-size dye-labeled proteins (molecular weight ~10–60 kD) and an even larger number of dye-labeled DNAs and peptides [17, 20]. This particular feature implies that dyes with lower absorptivity

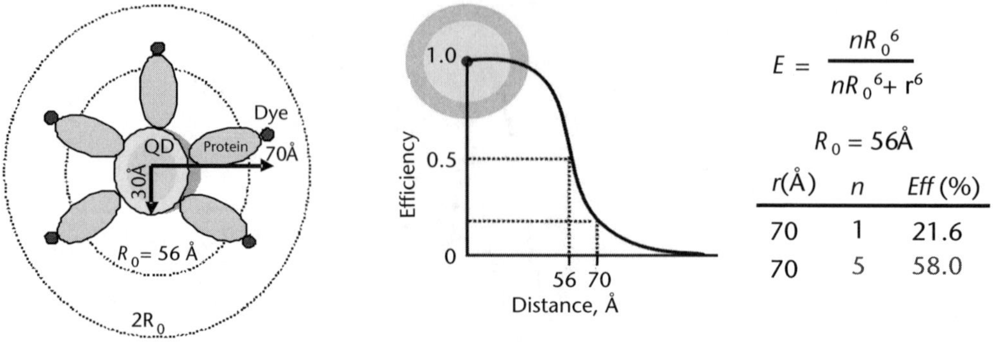

Figure 4.2 Demonstration of improved FRET efficiency E derived from arraying multiple acceptor dyes around a single QD donor acting as a protein scaffold. Figure adapted from [21] and reprinted with permission of the Nature Publishing Group (NPG).

and weaker overlap can still be used if several copies were arrayed around a QD donor. It also implies that a broad dynamic FRET range can be realized for a donor-acceptor pair by varying n. Utilization of this concept within QD-FRET–based biosensors can result in a significant increase in the range of FRET signals accessible for a sensing event [19]. In this configuration, the QD plays a dual role of a nanoscale scaffold for arraying multiple copies of dye-labeled (and unlabeled) receptor molecules and as a central exciton donor. This has in fact, both by design or default, been utilized in a number of QD-based FRET sensors to detect small molecule targets (see further discussion later) [21–24].

4.2.4 Achieving Multiplex FRET Configurations with One Excitation Source

The ability to follow two or three functions/processes simultaneously within the same cell using FRET could provide invaluable information on how a myriad of cellular events are spacio-temporally correlated. QD donors offer unique advantages for realizing multiplexed FRET. Even though the most obvious configuration to achieve this would use multiple dye-labeled receptors conjugated to the same QD donor, we have recently demonstrated that multiplex FRET with QDs is much simpler to implement using a converse configuration where multiple QD donors emitting at distinct wavelengths are paired with the same acceptor dye [25]. QDs self-assembled with maltose binding protein (MBP), site-specifically labeled with a dark-quenching acceptor, were used, as schematically represented for a *three-plex* scenario in Figure 4.3(a). As can be seen in the panels shown in Figure 4.3(b)–(e), only the PL of a particular QD conjugated to dye proteins within the mixture can be selectively quenched (or modulated) by FRET; those unconjugated are essentially unaffected. We have further expanded this configuration to a four-channel FRET system using four QD colors. This study also showed that emissive and dark (nonemissive) dyes alike can be used for effective multiplexed FRET within the same sample [25]. The study has further shown that a configuration using one QD donor and multiple color acceptors entails more complicated spectral deconvolution because of the broad emission spectra of organic dyes. In addition, nonradiative energy transfer between dyes attached to the same donor may be nonnegligible, further complicating the analysis.

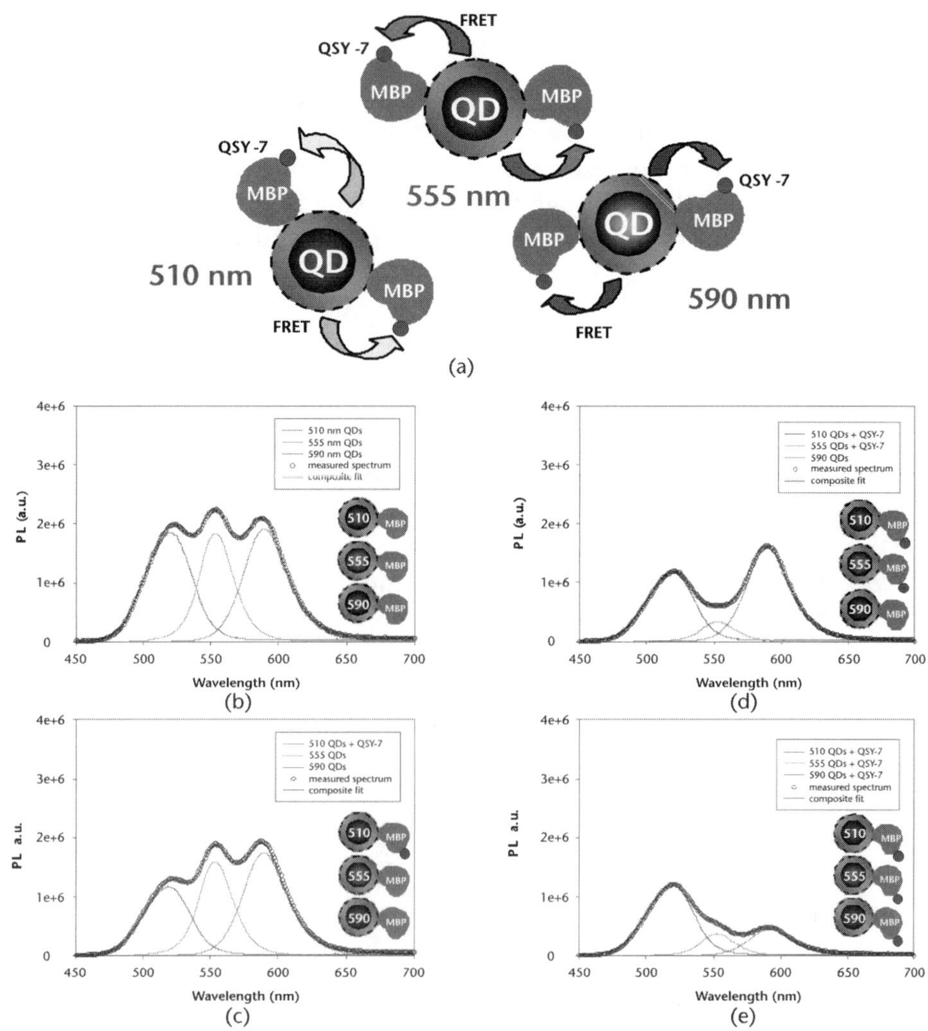

Figure 4.3 (a) Schematic representation of the FRET multiplexing configuration. Three distinct QD donors conjugated to QSY-7-labeled MBP are shown. (b–e) Deconvoluted PL spectra for the system using three QD donors interacting with QSY-7 quencher. The composite spectrum is shown as open circles (O); the fitted spectrum as a solid black line. (b) No QSY-7 dyes are present. (c) Only conjugates of the 510-nm QDs are QSY-7-labeled. (d) 510- and 555-nm QDs are conjugated to MBP-QSY-7. (e) All three QDs have dye-labeled MBP. Cartoons representing labeled and unlabeled QD conjugates are shown in the insets. Adapted from [25] and reprinted with permission from the ACS.

4.2.5 Multiphoton FRET Configurations

Fluorescence driven by multiphoton excitation utilizes IR sources that are ideally located within the tissue optical transparency window; it allows deep penetration (~1 mm) with limited overall photodamage and is thus highly desirable for deep tissue imaging [26]. FRET using conventional fluorophores driven by two-photon excitation has been extremely limited, primarily due to their low multiphoton absorption profiles [27]. In contrast QDs have very high two-photon action cross sections, ~2–3 orders of magnitude larger than the best available dyes (8–20,000 Geppert-Mayer-GM units at 800-nm excitation) [27]. It has been shown that two-photon fluorescence using luminescent QDs enabled imaging at greater depths than what was allowed with standard dye fluorophores, while using less average excitation power. For example, QDs allowed visualization of vasculature hundreds of micrometers deep through the skin of living mice [28]. The strong difference in two-photon action cross-section between dots and dyes suggest that FRET with QDs driven by two-photon excitation in the NIR could provide additional advantages to what was described for one-photon excitation earlier. Using the same QD-MBP-dye conjugates introduced previously, we demonstrated that two-photon excitation could specifically exploit the vast disparity in cross-sectional absorption efficiencies between QDs and dyes, to provide FRET sensitization with essentially negligible direct excitation contribution to the dye-acceptor signal. The steady-state data shown in Figure 4.4 indicate that there is a full equivalence between the FRET processes driven by either mode of excitation, a property also confirmed by excited-state lifetime measurements [27]. Data also show that under one-photon excitation, the direct excitation contribution to the acceptor emission though small is not negligible. In comparison, such contribution is essentially zero under

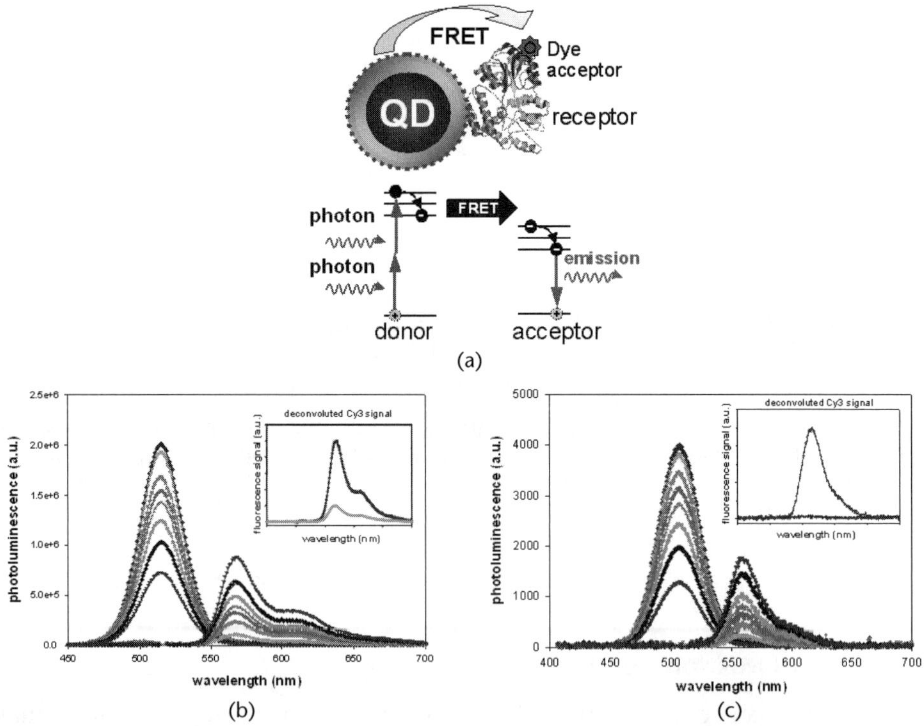

Figure 4.4 (a) Schematic of two-photon excitation and FRET with a QD-protein-dye conjugate. Deconvoluted PL spectra of QDs and Cy3 as a function of an increasing number of MBP-Cy3 per 510-nm QD using both (b) conventional and (c) two-photon excitation. The inset in each shows a comparison between FRET-induced Cy3 PL and the contribution due to direct conventional or two-photon excitation collected for a control MBP-Cy3 sample. Figure adapted from [27] and reproduced with permission. © Wiley-VCH Verlag GmbH & Co. KGaA. (See Color Plate 6.)

two-photon excitation. Multiphoton FRET with QD donors can thus remove the need to correct for background contribution and substantially increases the measured signal-to-noise ratios. This configuration may be beneficial for intracellular FRET sensing and imaging where the dye signal (due to FRET) could be easily distinguished from any background contribution [27].

4.3 FRET-Based Biosensing with Quantum Dots

Within the context of this discussion, we loosely define *biosensing* as the detection of either a biological molecule or biological process with a QD-conjugate assembly that incorporates other dye-labeled biomolecules and where signal transduction results from changes in FRET interactions. We categorize these sensors by a combination of their overall composite structure and the targeted ligand or targeted biological process. We focus on selected representative examples to highlight the sensing mechanisms and examine both their benefits and limitations.

4.3.1 Competitive Sensing Using QD-Protein Conjugates

In this format, the sensors consist of QD-protein conjugates and are primarily directed to the detection of small molecule targets. The sensor specificity is provided by the protein's ability to recognize and bind to its cognate target. The competition format uses a dye-labeled analog with known affinity to the protein receptor and is first captured by the QD-protein receptor conjugates. This is accomplished by either preassembling the protein and dye-labeled analog prior to conjugation onto the QD surface or by adding the analog dye to the sample containing the QD-protein assemblies. Formation of the QD-protein-analog-dye complex brings the dye in close proximity to the QDs and results in FRET-induced loss of the QD emission. The target molecule, when added to the solution, will compete off the analog and bind to the receptor protein, which removes the acceptor away from the nanocrystal surface, reduces FRET interactions, and produces progressive recovery of the QD emission. Analysis of the QD PL recovery also provides some insights into conjugate sensing kinetics of the target molecule. Alternatively the target and analog could be simultaneously added to the QD-protein conjugates, but in this case one monitors the reduction in FRET efficiencies measured in the presence of the competing target molecule. Three specific examples employing this sensing strategy were recently reported.

The first QD sensing assembly was demonstrated by our group and utilized MBP self-assembled on the QD surface to specifically target the nutrient sugar maltose [21]. Prior to QD-conjugate assembly, MBP was allowed to prebind a beta-cyclodextrin (BCD) analog of maltose that was covalently labeled with a QSY-9 dark quenching acceptor to form MBP-BCD-QSY9 complexes. Multiple copies of these complexes were self-assembled onto the QD surface by utilizing a pentahistidine (His_5) sequence located at the proteins C-terminus [29]. The His_5 sequence coordinates to the surface of ZnS-overcoated QDs through metal-affinity interactions. The proximity of the MBP-BCD-QSY9 complex to the nanocrystal results in efficient FRET-induced quenching of the QD emission. Subsequent addition of maltose competed for MBP binding, displaced the BCD-QSY9, and resulted in a concentration dependent increase of QD PL [21]. The maltose dissociation constant K_D of ~7 μM, extrapolated from the FRET recovery data, correlated well with the 1–10 μM values reported for solution-phase wild-type MBP. Further testing of this sensor with a variety of sugars confirmed its binding specificity only for sugars containing α1-4 glucosidic linkages such as those found in maltosides. These results indicate that MBP retains its binding characteristics after self-assembly onto the QD surface.

Modified versions of this same FRET-based sensor for the sugar maltose have also been demonstrated, employing QD-MBP conjugates in either one- or two-photon excitation modes [27] and in a reagentless configuration [30, 31]. For the reagentless configuration, MBP was labeled with Cy3 at a unique site within the proteins binding pocket and self-assembled onto the QDs surface. Addition of increasing concentrations of maltose resulted in an obligatory rearrangement of the MBP structure, and as the protein's conformation closed around the dye, it changed the dye's emission efficiency. While the system was primarily excited by the QD donor (with a given FRET efficiency), the net result was a concentration dependent change in Cy3 acceptor emission, allowing PL ratiometric monitoring of maltose presence [27, 30].

In the second example, a sensing assembly targeting the explosive trinitrotoluene (TNT) in aqueous environments was constructed and characterized; see schematics in Figure 4.5 [22]. In this case, a single chain antibody fragment specifically selected against TNT (αTNT-ScFV) and expressing a C-terminal polyhistidine sequence was conjugated to the QDs and used as the recognition protein. An explosive analog-dye complex was synthesized consisting of the dark quenching dye (BHQ-10) attached to the TNT analog trinitrobenzene via a diaminopentane linker (BHQ-10-TNB); see Figure 4.5(b) for structure. When the preassembled αTNT-ScFV-BHQ-10-TNB construct was immobilized on the QD surface via His-metal affinity, the net result was a FRET-based quenching of the QD PL, with efficiency that depended on the number of constructs attached to the nanocrystal surface and the QD-dye spectral overlap. The quenched assembly was exposed to a variety of different explosives and only TNT elicited a significant concentration-dependent increase in QD PL, see Figure 4.5(c). The QD-ScFv-BHQ-10-TNB sensing assembly was also tested against several extracts derived from explosive-contaminated soils and was able to provide accurate measures of the TNT concentrations [22].

A variation of the competitive format explored FRET-based QD immunosensing. The sensing assemblies consist of QDs conjugated to a capture antibody specific to the target-antigen and a second dye-labeled reporter antibody also having specific affinity to the target antigen; the antibodies have no affinity for each other. When the target antigen is added to the solution, it binds to the capture and reporter antibodies forming a sandwich structure immobilized on the nanocrystal. This brings the dye in proximity of the QD surface and produces a FRET-induced quenching of its photoemission. The rate of quenching depends on the target concentration. In one example, 565-nm emitting QD donors were conjugated to monoclonal antibodies specific for estrogen receptor β (ER-β) (antigen), and Alexa Fluor 633 dye was used to label a polyclonal anti-ER reporter antibody

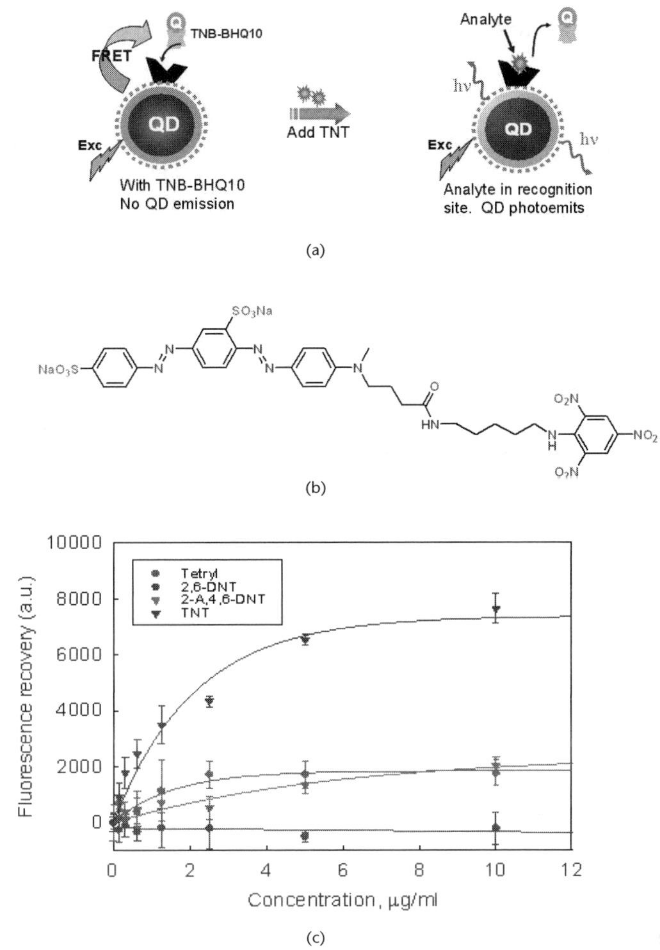

Figure 4.5 (a) Schematic of the QD-anti-TNT FRET sensor assembly. When TNB-BHQ-10 is bound to the QD-anti-TNT conjugate, QD fluorescence is quenched. As TNT is added to the assay, it competes for binding to the antibody fragment and the QD fluorescence increases following TNB-BHQ-10 release. (b) Chemical structure of the TNB-BHQ-10 quencher analogue. (c) Results from testing of the QD-anti-TNT sensor with TNT and the indicated TNT analogues. These assemblies were constructed using 530-nm emitting QDs. Adapted from [22] and reprinted with permission from the ACS.

[32]. In the presence of the target ER-β, a sandwich structure was formed on the QD surface, which brought the dyes closer to the nanocrystal surface and resulted in sizable FRET interactions and QD PL loss. A donor-acceptor separation distance of ~80–90Å was derived from the FRET data, which reflected the rather large size of the molecules (antibodies) involved. In general, QD-FRET based immunosensing can frequently be complicated by (1) the large size of antibodies and (2) the lack of unique sites on the antibodies for dye-labeling and attachment to the QD, which ultimately results in both a heterogeneous distribution of D-A separation distances and mixed antibody avidity.

4.3.2 Sensing Enzymatic Activity Using QD-Peptide and QD-Oligonucleotide Substrates

Proteases function in myriad normal and aberrant biochemical processes and play key roles in pathogenic virulence. This has made this super-family of enzymes important clinical and pharmaceutical targets [33, 34]. FRET-based sensing is perhaps the most common approach to detecting protease activity. This sensing configuration is based on cleavage of the peptide substrate, and it differs from the one based on competition for binding sites, discussed earlier for maltose and TNT. The sensing assemblies reported to date mostly consist of QDs conjugated to peptide-substrates. The peptides, as the smaller building blocks of proteins, provide a particular amino acid recognition/cleavage sequence that is integral to the sensor's overall function. Assembling multiple copies of dye-labeled peptides on a QD surface brings the acceptors in close proximity to the nanocrystal and induces a ratio-dependent quenching of the QD PL. The ratio-dependent FRET efficiencies could also be used as standard curves to which subsequent change in FRET signature are compared. Once the QD-peptide-dye assemblies are formed and the solution is equilibrated, addition of an enzyme specifically *cleaves* the protease-recognized sequence and displaces the dye away from the nanocrystal surface, resulting in progressive reduction of FRET interactions and recovery of QD emission. As the rate of peptide cleavage is a kinetic process, it will depend on the protease concentration, and this can be tracked from the PL recovery following substrate cleavage.

In a first example, Rosenzweig and coworkers used peptide substrates expressing a cysteine at one terminus and labeled with a rhodamine-dye acceptor at the other end [35, 36]. The peptide-dye were used to surface functionalize CdSe-ZnS QDs via cap exchange. The section spanning the center of the peptide sequence was designed to be recognized and cleaved by either of the peptidases trypsin or collagenase. Once fully assembled, the close proximity of the acceptor dye to the QD surface resulted in efficient FRET and loss of QD PL. Recovery of the emission was generated following incubation with either enzyme. The presence of an inhibitor was shown to substantially decrease the rate of fluorescence recovery, indicative of a reduction in protease activity. The authors also showed that the conjugate sensor could detect the presence of extra secreted proteases in media derived from cancerous cell cultures. This initial study demonstrated that proteolytic activity could be qualitatively followed over time with QD-peptide substrates both in vitro and in clinically relevant samples.

In the second example, we developed a series of tailored QD-peptide sensing assemblies capable of monitoring the proteolytic activity of several enzymes [20]. In this study, we used a modular peptide design where each peptide incorporated within its linear structure: (1) an N-terminal His_6 sequence for self-assembly onto CdSe-ZnS QDs, (2) a helix-linker spacer to provide rigidity and extension away from the QD surface, (3) an exposed protease recognition sequence, and (4) a C-terminal cysteine-thiol for specific dye-labeling; see schematic Figure 4.6(a). The advantage of the modular design resides in the fact that the specificity of the substrate toward a specific enzyme could be altered by changing the central recognition sequence, while maintaining the same overall peptide structure. The data on the loss of FRET efficiency versus increasing ratio of dye-labeled peptides self-assembled on a QD provide a "standard curve," which could be used to translate relative changes

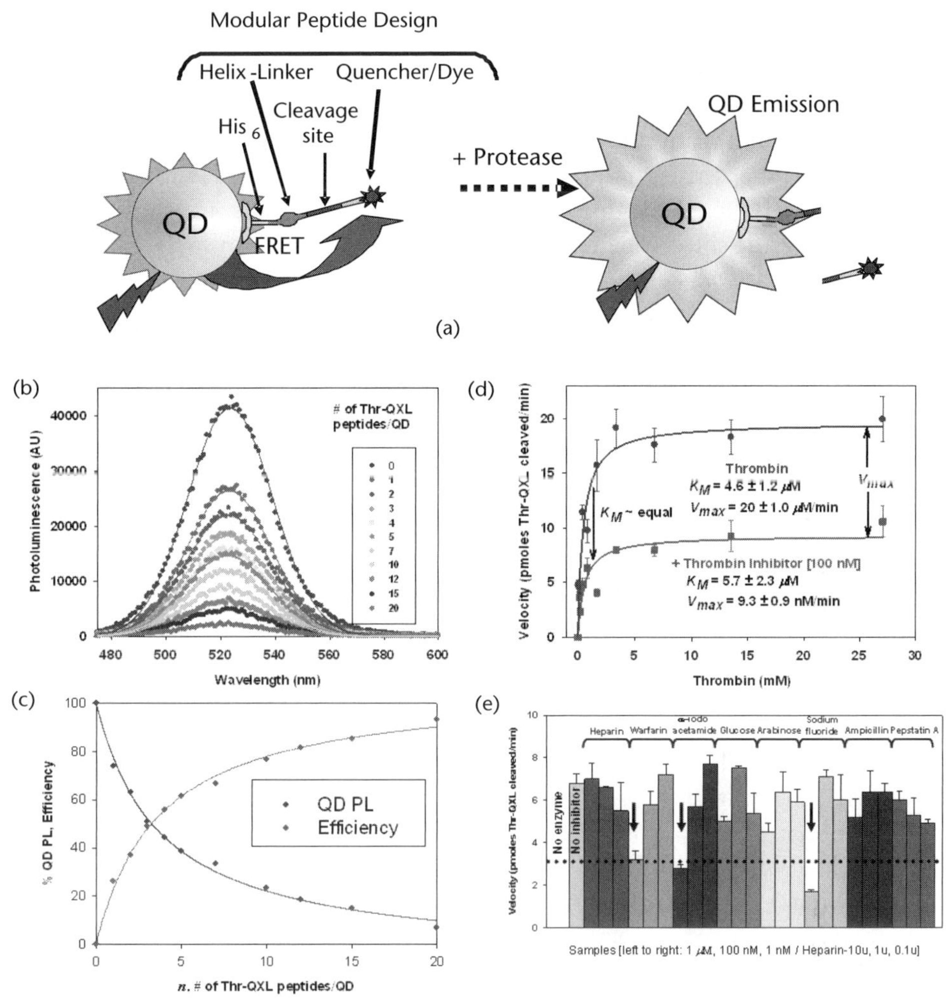

Figure 4.6 (a) Schematic diagram of the self-assembled QD-peptide protease nanosensors. Dye-labeled modular peptides containing appropriate cleavage sequences are self-assembled onto the QD. FRET from the QD to the proximal acceptors quenches the QD PL. Specific protease cleaves the peptide and alters FRET. (b) PL spectra for an increasing ratio of thrombin peptide labeled with QXL (Thr-QXL) per 522 nm QD and (c) plot of QD PL loss versus Thr-QXL:QD ratio together with corresponding FRET efficiency versus *n*. (d) Results of assaying a constant amount of QD-Thr-QXL peptide substrate versus increasing thrombin concentration in the absence and presence of 100-nM thrombin inhibitor. (e) Results of assaying the inhibitory effects of the eight indicated compounds on the thrombin nanosensor at three concentrations (1 μM, 100 μM, and 1 nM; heparin concentration in units). The no-inhibitor control yields velocity of ~7.0 picomoles peptide cleaved/min. A value of 3.5 picomoles peptide cleaved/min is designated as significant yielding three "hits" of interest (arrows). Figures adapted from [20] and reprinted with permission of the NPG.

in FRET signature/efficiency measured in the presence of a given concentration of the target enzyme into units of enzymatic activity; see Figure 4.6(b, c). This same standard curve also allows a choice of specific ratio of peptide-acceptors per QD for use in the substrate assembly that would correspond to large dynamic change in FRET following proteolytic cleavage. Using both emissive and dark-quenching acceptor dyes, four sensing assemblies targeted to the proteases caspace-1, thrombin, collagenase, and chymotrypsin were constructed and tested. Figure 4.6(b) shows a representative set of PL spectra for 520-nm emitting QD versus an increasing ratio of thrombin peptide substrate labeled with QXL-520 dark quenching acceptor; the corresponding relative QD PL decay and FRET efficiency versus number of dye-labeled peptides per QD or standard curves are shown in Figure 4.6(c). Figure 4.6(d) shows the results from the thrombin assay where QD-thrombin-peptide substrate was exposed to an increasing concentration of thrombin in the presence and absence of a specific thrombinase inhibitor. Applying the standard Michaelis-Menten kinetic analysis to the enzyme assay, the Michaelis constant K_M, maximal velocity V_{max} along with the inhibitor constant K_i (where appropriate) and turnover number k_{cat} were derived, both for this and the other systems tested. Further analysis of the data also allowed determination of the mechanism of inhibition (i.e., competitive versus noncompetitive). We further tested the ability of such QD-peptide substrates to screen for potential inhibitors against a given enzyme in a pharmaceutical-type screening assay. Figure 4.6(e) shows the results collected from screening eight potential inhibitor compounds, each at three different concentrations tested against thrombin QD-peptide substrate; the arrows indicate the compounds that showed loss of enzymatic activity exceeding 50 percent. These three "hits" correspond to compounds known to inhibit thrombin activity, which confirm the specificity of the assay format [20]. The ability to easily switch between targeted proteases by changing a small modular unit within the peptide sequences, combined with the ability to perform quantitative experiments, will be especially useful to monitoring many proteases.

The third example did not employ a peptide, but rather substituted a synthetic molecule as a substrate. Using this scheme, Rao and coworkers reported the assembly and testing of QD-substrates for sensing β-lactamase activity [37]. β-lactamases (Blas) are enzymes of bacterial origin that hydrolyze drugs such as penicillin and the cephalosporins and are responsible for bacterial antibiotic resistance [37, 38]. β-lactamases are also very effective enzymatic reporters for processes such as promoter activation and protein interactions and have been incorporated into many pharmaceutical screens where their expression and activity are directly monitored both in vivo and in vitro [37, 38]. The authors first synthesized and labeled a core Bla recognized lactam chemical substrate with a Cy5-acceptor at one terminus and a biotin at the other terminus. Biotin enabled the dye-labeled substrate to self-assemble onto 605-nm streptavidin-coated QDs (Invitrogen); see Figure 4.7. Although the assembly resulted in efficient FRET quenching of the QD, the rather small chemical substrate prevented effective interactions with the larger size enzyme, and additional modification of the substrate design by providing a longer lateral extension (a spacer) was necessary to overcome steric constraints and allow unhindered enzyme access to the Bla binding site on the QD-substrate. Addition of the lactamase enzyme to a solution of the QD-substrates resulted in time-dependent change in FRET efficiency and allowed monitoring of enzyme activity over time (see Figure 4.7).

These examples of QD-substrates suggest that they could potentially be applied to many other screening and diagnostic assays. For instance, the sensor for lactamase activity could be directly incorporated as is into pharmaceutical library screening assays for Bla inhibitors (i.e., drugs targeting bacterial antibiotic resis-

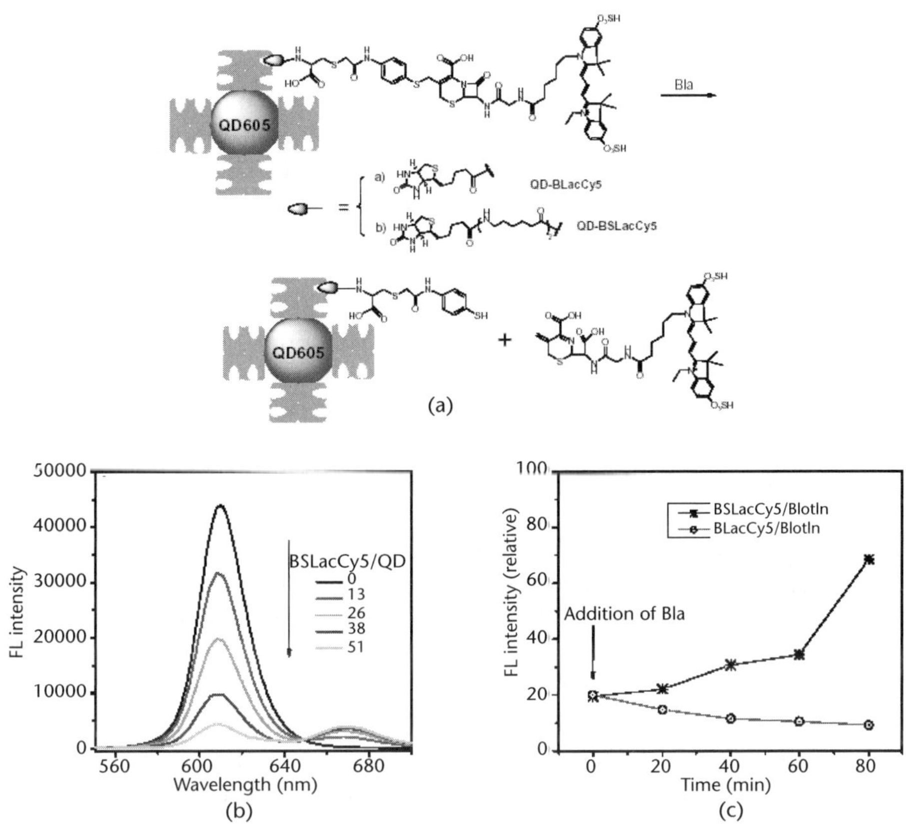

Figure 4.7 (a) Schematic of the β-lactamase sensor. The Bla substrate is labeled with Cy5 and immobilized onto QDs. Bla activity cleaves the lactam ring and releases Cy5, restoring the QD fluorescence. (b) PL from binding different ratios of extended BSLacCy5 per QD. (c) Activation of the self-assembled quantum dot probes by Bla (0.03 mg/mL) over time. The QD probes contain substrate and extended length substrate. Only cleavage with the extended substrate is noted. Figures provided by J. Rao, Stanford University, and reprinted with permission of Elsevier [37].

tance enzymes). The major challenge for all QD conjugates capable of sensing enzyme activity in vitro will be whether or not they can be extended to in vivo assays. Intracellular monitoring of the activity of caspace(s), lactamases, and a variety of other enzymatic processes inside live cells will be highly desirable, as it brings these systems closer to practical use of these QD-assemblies.

4.3.3 Detection of Hybridization Using QD-Nucleic Acid Conjugates

For this family of sensors, the nucleic acids such as DNA or RNA provide the QD assemblies with two types of recognitions. The first is a direct sequence complementarity, such as that exploited in DNA arrays and DNA molecular beacons [39, 40]. The second recognition functionality is derived from the three-dimensional structure of oligonucleotides, and it characterizes aptamers' interactions with larger nonnucleotidyl targets [41]. One representative example of sensing based on direct DNA hybridization was reported by Banin and coworkers [42]. They attached an average of six copies of thiolated DNA probe onto CdSe-ZnS QDs emitting at 580 nm, while Texas Red was used to label the complementary target DNA sequence. When QD-DNA probes and dye-labeled targets were mixed, changes in QD PL due to FRET interactions between QD and proximal dye allowed real-time monitoring of hybridization. Addition of DNase I enzyme digested the duplex DNA structures and resulted in partial QD PL recovery. The authors also observed that direct nonspecific interactions (such as electrostatic binding) between the QD surfaces and target DNAs could complicate the experimental conditions, data collection, and analysis. This issue constitutes a major hurdle to using QD-DNA as sensing assemblies, because charged groups are often used in promoting water transfer of the nanocrystals (see Chapter 1 by Susumu et al.). The same concept of QD-FRET sensing driven by hybridization was applied to the selection of highly effective small-interfering RNA (siRNA) sequences with specific affinity to the respective mRNA targets [43]. Bakalova and coworkers constructed QD-siRNA conjugates that served as hybridization probes using nanocrystals encapsulated with triblock copolymers and coupled single-stranded siRNA to the QDs via EDC (1-ethyl-3-(3-dimethylaminopropyl)carbodiimide) condensation. The target mRNA was amplified in the presence of Cy5-labeled nucleotides, providing Cy5-mRNA. FRET signature, namely the loss of QD PL coupled with an increase in the dye emission, was observed only when the QD-siRNA probes were exposed to mRNA and had both good accessibility and high affinity; any mismatch between siRNA and mRNA resulted in negligible FRET interactions [43].

Implementing QD-based FRET sensing in a multiplexed format has been rather scarce. One of the main difficulties is reducing the effects of cross-reactivity of the substrates, where often a single substrate can recognize multiple target molecules, albeit with different affinities. Algar and Krull investigated the possibility of performing a *two-plex* FRET based on direct hybridization using QD-oligonucleotide conjugates [44]. For this, two distinct color CdSe-ZnS QDs emitting at 525 nm and 605 nm were conjugated to two distinct DNA-probes. Hybridization of these conjugates with two distinct targets, one labeled with Cy3 and the other with Alex647, was investigated (see Figure 4.8). The mixture of these conjugate probes and targets was excited with a single line, and the fluorescence emission was separated in two optical channels: a green channel ($450 < \lambda < 600$ nm) isolating the FRET interactions for the 525-nm QD paired with Cy3, which allowed for detection of target one, while a red channel ($\lambda >$ 600 nm) isolated the signal from the 605-nm-QD Alexa647 pair specific to DNA target 2. This is slightly different from what was described in Section 4.2.4. The authors reported nano-molar limits of detection in a sample mixture containing both targets. Interestingly, they also found that the use of a common nucleic acid intercalating dye (ethidium bromide) as the acceptor could increase the signal-to-noise ratio by fivefold (from 2 to ~10) for the 525-nm QD substrate. This format may be expandable to 3-4 simultaneous sensors, and small improvements such as the use of an intercalating dye could potentially increase sensitivity substantially [44].

In contrast to pure sequence-driven complementarity discussed earlier, there are examples using QD-DNA conjugates to recognize larger nonnucleotidyl biomolecular targets. Ellington and coworkers adapted the three-dimensional recognition and binding properties of aptamers to detect the presence of thrombin enzyme [45]. Conjugates were formed using biotinylated aptamers specific for thrombin enzyme and commercial streptavidin-QDs. Specific partially complemen-

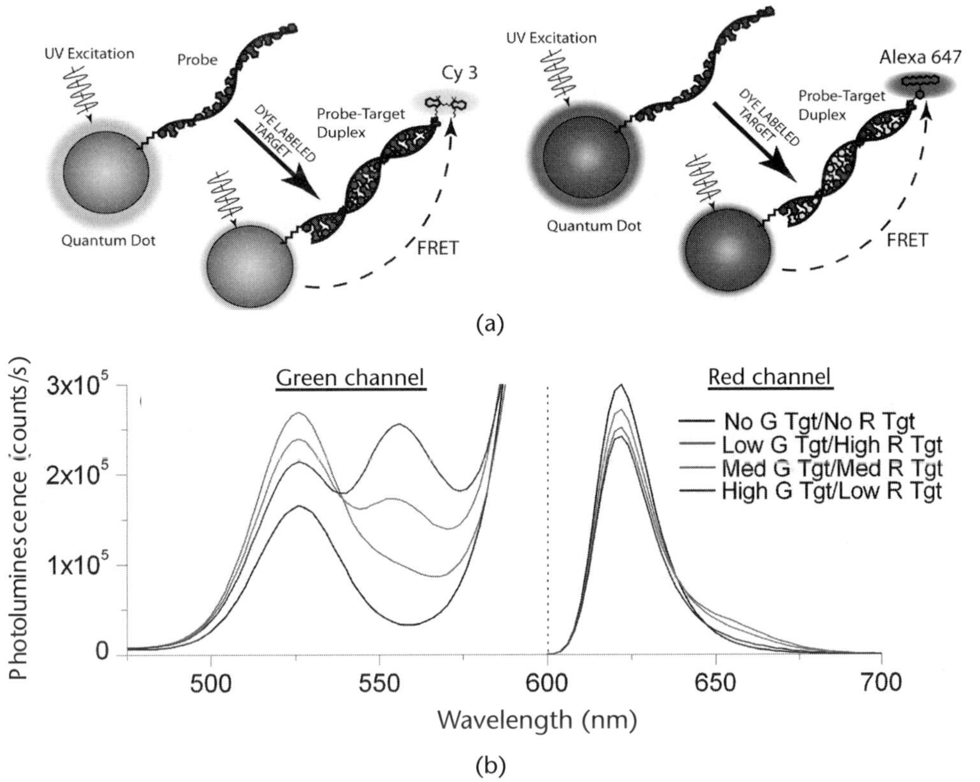

Figure 4.8 QD–FRET strategy for two-color nucleic acid detection. (a) Simultaneous excitation of QDs without significant excitation of Cy3 or Alexa647. When probe oligonucleotides were conjugated to QDs, hybridization with a Cy3 or Alexa647 labeled target oligonucleotide yielded FRET-sensitized emission from the dyes. (b) Two-color experiment demonstrating the ability to detect two different labeled oligonucleotide sequences simultaneously via FRET-sensitized emission. When different concentrations of labeled target are added, the changes in each channel are monitored for results. Figure provided by U.J. Krull, University of Toronto, and reprinted with permission of Elsevier [44].

tary acceptor-labeled DNA sequences were allowed to hybridize onto the QD-aptamer conjugates, resulting in quenching of the QDs emission. Rather high average dye-to-QD ratios were needed due to the large streptavidin-QD size. Addition of the protease thrombin displaced the quencher-DNA, resulting in a concentration dependent increase/recovery in QD PL. Effects of concentration and temperature on the enzymatic interactions were monitored, while a control experiment testing the sensor against a different target enzyme, lysozyme, did not significantly affect the QD PL; this reflects that the QD-aptamer's specificity was maintained. In this study, the presence/absence of enzyme is detected, but not its activity or viability. The sensing configuration for thrombin enzyme described here is based on a competition displacement, analogous to what was shown for the detection of maltose and TNT discussed in Section 4.3.1. The QD-aptamer-DNA-dye assembly was also tested for its ability to detect complementary and noncomplementary oligonucleotides. Two different oligonucleotides were synthesized; one perfectly complementary to the aptamer on the QD and one containing a two-base-pair internal mismatch (double mutant sequence). They found that addition of the perfectly complementary sequence resulted in a steady time-dependent increase of the QD fluorescence, due to displacement of the DNA dye away from the nanocrystal and loss of FRET. Furthermore, these changes were recorded only at temperatures near the melting point of the aptamer-DNA complex. In comparison, the presence of the second double mutant oligonucleotide had no effects. These specific changes result from displacement of the dye-labeled partially complementary sequence, which occurs only in the presence of a perfectly complementary sequence and near the melting temperature [45]. Overall, these measurements confirm that the aptamers on the nanocrystal surface maintain their biological activity.

In another example, Zhang and Johnson utilized the specificity of an RNA sequence for a peptide derived from the human immunodeficiency virus (HIV) Rev responsive element (RRE IIB RNA); see Figure 4.9 [24]. Biotinylated RRE IIB RNA was attached to streptavidin-QDs and the conjugate assembly was used to capture Cy5-labeled Rev peptide, resulting in FRET interactions with efficiencies that depended on the target concentration. The authors further assessed the inhibitory effects of neomycin B on Rev-RRE binding by exposing a solution of QD-conjugates to increasing concentration of Rev-peptide in the presence of a fixed concentration of neomycin B; for this a fixed QD-RRE conjugate concentration with a given average RRE-to-QD ratio were used in the assay. They indeed found that the dissociation constant K_d increased by ~4 in the presence of neomycin B (see Figure 4.9(b)), which suggests that this sensor could potentially function in the screening of pharmaceuticals targeting HIV-1 virus.

4.3.4 pH and Ion Sensing

Sensing of pH and local ion concentration is important to many aspects of biological research. Subcellular organelles/compartments are often kept at different pH from

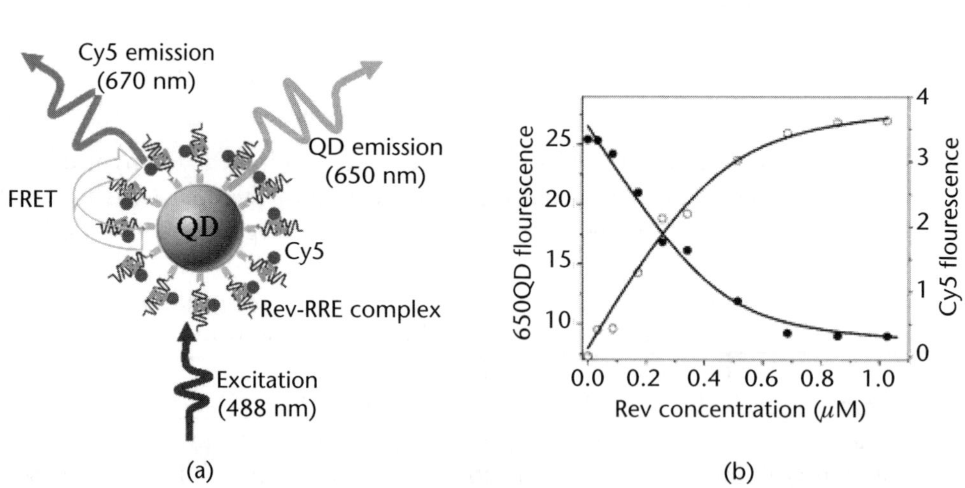

Figure 4.9 (a) Conceptual scheme of the QD-based nanosensor for Rev-RRE interaction assay based on FRET between 605QD and Cy5. FRET occurred between the 605QD and Cy5 upon illumination of the 605QD/Rev-RRE/Cy5 assemblies with 488nm excitation. (b) Titration of RRE RNA in the presence of neomycin B with increasing Rev concentration. The solid curves are fits of 605QD and Cy5 fluorescence data. Figure provided by L.W. Johnson, York College CUNY, and reprinted with permission of the ACS [24].

that of the surrounding environment, necessitating maintenance of an active proton gradient. Sodium and potassium ion channels exploit these concentration gradients to power a variety of active transmembrane transport systems and for neuronal signaling. Bursts in intracellular calcium can provide important indication of how live cells respond to external stimulations [46, 47]. Cumulatively, this has driven the need for designing sensors that monitor local changes in pH or particular ion concentration within live cells, in order to help understand the underlying processes.

Many of the commonly known pH sensors utilize fluorescent dyes whose emission and/or absorption are sensitive to the local concentration of hydrogen protons. Coupling this basic sensing process to a QD has allowed preliminary sensors to be designed and characterized. We will describe four representative examples using QD-based FRET interactions to probe changes in the pH and ionic concentration of solution samples. In the first example, Snee and coworkers coupled a pH-sensitive squaraine dye with an equilibrium response to pH to the surface of QDs [48]. The dye was conjugated via EDC coupling to QDs encapsulated by a hydrophobically modified poly(acrylic acid) layer, which promoted proximal FRET interactions between dot and dye. Because the dye's absorption profile is a function of pH, the efficiency of the FRET interactions also becomes a function of the environment pH. In particular, modulation of the FRET efficiency by variations in the solution pH produces net ratiometric dependence between the emissions of the NC and dye (as shown in Figure 4.10); pH values below and above the p*K*a of the dye (~8.5) were explored. This provided the authors with a unique tool to measure the solution pH, by simply taking the ratio of the QD and dye peak intensities or comparing them to the value at the isosbestic point. As the isosbestic point does not vary for normalized fluorescence plots, this provides for a good internal reference. Because the ratiometric measurements are potentially not sensitive to fluctuations in the overall collected signals, such an approach is potentially more accurate and more reliable than "conventional chemo" or biosensors that utilize one signal response (i.e., either brightening or darkening).

Using a slightly different rationale, Raymo and coworkers utilized a photochromic dye to realize pH sensing [49, 50]. They started by assembling an organic ligand complex that incorporates a thioctic acid group and a photochromic 4-nitrophenylazophenoxy chromophore. When the ligands are mixed with hydrophobic QDs they "associate" with the native capping shell and form QD-photochromic dye conjugates. They reported that transformations of the organic ligands in the presence of either acid or base regulate the photoluminescence intensity of the nanoparticles. This is caused by a photochromic transformation of the dye absorption, which in turn alters the rate of energy transfer between QD and dye. They then employed these QD-ligand complexes to probe the pH of aqueous solutions in biphasic systems with the assistance of a phase-transfer catalyst. Specifically, they showed that the PL of a $CHCl_3$ phase containing Bu_4NCl and QD-ligand complexes traces the pH of an overlaid aqueous phase. In particular, they found that pH change from 3.2 to 10.7 in the aqueous phase translates into a PL decrease reaching up to 29 percent of that measured originally in the organic phase. The need for a biphasic medium to realize pH sensing limits the biological relevance of this system in comparison to the first example discussed earlier.

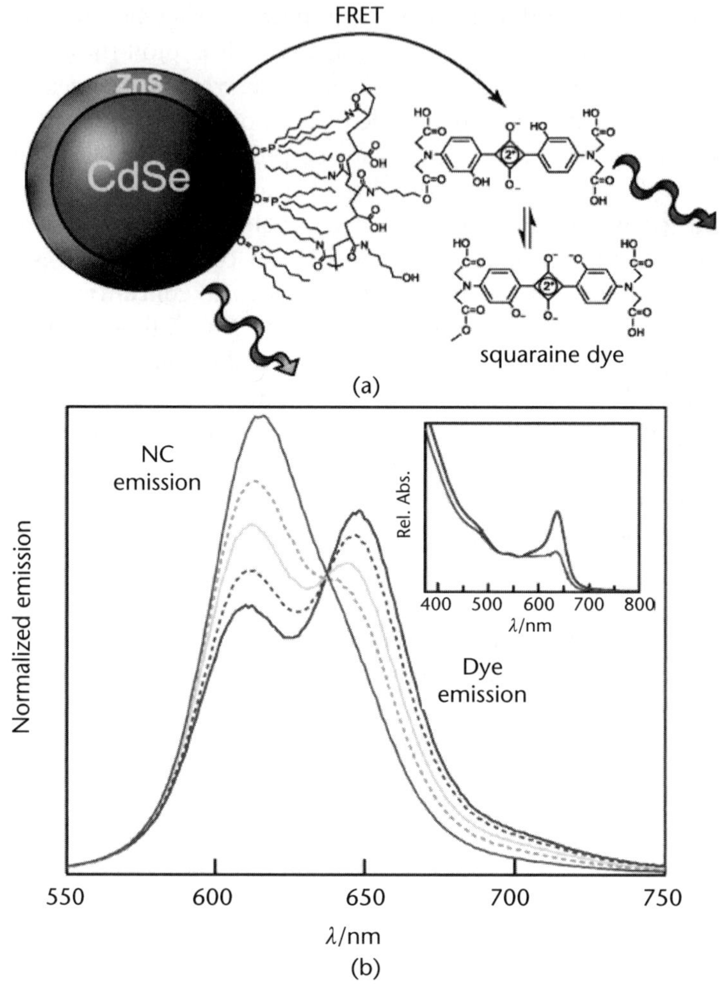

Figure 4.10 (a) pH sensor constructed from CdSe-ZnS QDs encapsulated with an amphiphilic polymer upon which a pH-sensitive squaraine dye is conjugated. FRET efficiency is modulated by the environment as the dye's absorption profile is a function of pH. (b) Emission profile of a QD-squaraine dye conjugate changes as a function of pH with ex = 380 nm. The normalized spectra show pH dependence with an isosbestic point appearing at 640 nm. The absorbance of the squaraine dye is suppressed in the conjugate at basic pHs, as shown in the inset. Figures provided by D. Nocera, MIT, and reprinted with permission of the ACS [48].

Attempts aimed at detecting specific ions such K^+ and Cl^- using QDs and FRET have also been reported recently. In one study, Ruedas-Rama and coworkers assembled 1-μm-size polyacrylic beads in which green-emitting CdSe-ZnS QDs (at 540 nm), a Cl^- sensitive lucigenin dye, and K^+-selective-valinomycin coupled to chromoionophore I acceptor (Cm I) were simultaneously embedded [51]. In this construct the K^+ sensitive chomorionophore dye (Cm I) undergoes a photochromic blue shift of its absorption and emission spectra, resulting in a significant spectral overlap with the QD emission, and FRET interactions are promoted/enhanced; lucigenin has a blue absorption and does not engage in FRET interactions with the QDs because there is little overlap with the QD emission. The fluorophores were embedded into the porous polyacrylic matrix (bead) through photo-initiated suspension polymerization. In this construct, response to change in Cl^- ions was accounted for directly by measuring changes in the lucigenin emission, with little interference from the QD. In comparison, when K^+ ions are present, a change in the Cm I fluorophore emission due to additional contribution from FRET interactions with the QDs takes place. Through the correct choice of QD and ionophore ratio encapsulated inside the particle, the presence of both the K^+/Cl^- ions in low mM concentrations were detected. Dubach and coworkers utilized a modification of this approach to detect mM concentrations of sodium [52]. In this case, a QD donor was similarly overcoated with the Cm I acceptor and a further porous biocompatible coating to create a ~100-nm particle. The Cm I-acceptor overcoating changes color in response to the sodium concentration altering FRET interactions with the central QD donor. The change in QD PL forms the basis for signaling in this one-color sensor. The drawbacks to this strategy, however, are that sensitivity remains essentially a function of ionophore equilibrium response, which can sometimes be millimolar or higher. Furthermore, there is little control over QD-to-acceptor separation distance and the large overall size of the particles may limit potential intracellular applications.

4.4 Quantum Dots As Sensitizers for Photodynamic Therapy

Photodynamic therapy (PDT) is a process that involves the transfer of excitation energy from an excited photosensitizing agent to a nearby oxygen molecule, resulting in the formation of reactive singlet oxygen ($^1O_2$). Being highly reactive species, single oxygen initiates cytotoxic reactions in cells and tissues. This has made PDT a useful therapeutic tool to treat cancerous tissue and cells. The technique is also highly selective because only tissues that are simultaneously exposed to the photosensitizer agent and photoexcitation in the presence of oxygen are affected [53]. Most conventional PDT agents have low extinction coefficient and poor solublity in biological media (in vivo). It is in addressing these issues that QDs can uniquely improve the effectiveness of these agents. First, each QD provides a nanoscaffold for the attachment of several PDT molecules together with anticancer antibodies, which could allow specific homing onto targeted tumor cells; see schematic Figure 4.11(a) [53]. By attaching multiple PDT molecules to a single QD, one can also increase the PDT flux. Second, due to their large absorption cross-sections QDs can function as “energy-harvesting antennas” to enhance the effective photoexcitation of the PDT agent via FRET. Furthermore, because QDs have high two-photon action cross sections, they can allow excitation using NIR irradiation, which is desired for reaching agents in deep tissues.

As this application is really in its initial phases, most of the work has focused on gaining an understanding of the basic aspects of QD sensitization of different PDT agents. Examples reported to date include QD donors coupled to pthalocyanine acceptors [54, 55], peptides labeled with either of the PDT agents rose bengal or chlorin e6 [56], iridium-complex conjugated ligands [57], and *meso*-tetra(4-sulfonatophenyl)- porphine dihydrochloride (TSPP) [58]. In a related study, Neuman and coworkers investigated the use of QD-FRET as means to gener-

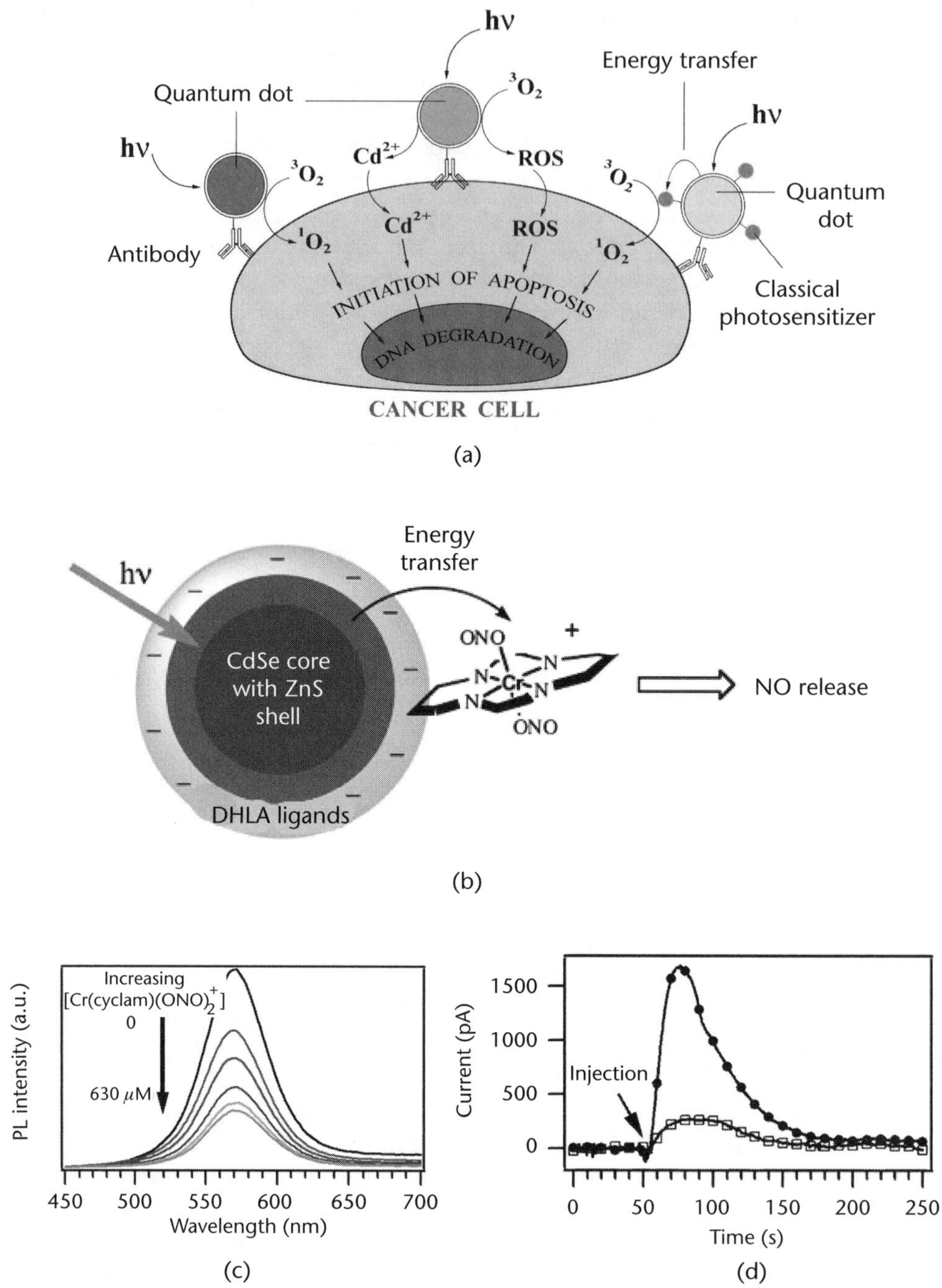

Figure 4.11 (a) Schematic of how QD photosensitizers functionalized with cancer cell–specific antibodies would bind and specifically kill a cancer cell in vivo. The antibodies direct the conjugates to cancer cells and QDs then harvest either UV or IR energy (via 2-photon excitation) to generate reactive oxygen species; the latter initiate cell death. Alternatively, the QDs sensitize PDT agents, which cannot be directly excited within tissues. Figure provided by R. Bakalova and published with permission of the NPG. (b) Schematic of how QDs generate nitrous oxide (NO) species when complexed with Cr(tetraazacyclotetradecane)$(ONO)_2$. (c) Normalized PL spectra (ex 366 nm) of water-soluble QDs (~130 nM) in phosphate buffer with various concentrations of chromium compound added. (d) Detection of NO photochemically produced from Cr(tetraazacyclotetradecane) $(ONO)_2$ injected into stirred buffer solutions with (circles) and without (squares) added QDs. Figure provided by P.C. Ford, U.C. Santa Barbara, and reprinted with permission of the ACS [59].

ate nitric oxide (NO) species; see Figure 4.11(b) [59]. NO species are involved in cardiovascular regulation, and similar to reactive oxygen species (ROS), are sensitized by photoirradiation. CdSe-ZnS QDs donors were electrostatically paired with the oppositely charged chromium compound *trans*-Cr(tetraazacyclotetradecane)$(ONO)_2^+$. Increasing ratios of this compound added to the soluble QDs effectively quenched the QD PL (by FRET) and generated far higher amounts of NO than the compound alone (Figure 4.11(c, d)). The high QD absorption allowed harvesting ~2 to 10 times as much energy (depending upon wavelength) as was generated using a sample containing *2,000-fold more* concentrated chromium compound alone.

Moving beyond an in vitro format, Bakalova and coworkers conjugated CdSe core only QDs with an antibody specific to leukemic cells [60]. The QD conjugates were directed against the Jurkat leukemia cell line, and binding was confirmed with fluorescent microscopy. The cells were then diluted with normal lymphocytes and subjected to UV irradiation in the presence or absence of two PDT agents, trifluoperazine and sulfonated aluminum pthalocyanine. Flow cytometry along with cell viability tests indicated that the QD-antibody conjugates specifically sensitized the attached leukemic cells and resulted in their selective destruction. These preliminary results highlight the potential for QD assemblies to serve as photochemically active drugs. Further, in the appropriate format the QD-photosensitizer-antibody complexes can be considered a relatively "inert prodrug," meaning that it is inactive until photoexcited.

4.5 Special Sensing Configurations

In all the configurations discussed here, the QDs served as donor fluorophores paired with a variety of dye- or sensitizable-acceptors. Metallic and, in particular, Au nanoparticles have also been explored as acceptors with luminescent QDs. Since the quenching of QD emission in the presence of these metallic nanoparticles tends to extend over larger separation distances than what is allowed under exclusive dye-to-dye FRET, phenomena driven by interactions occurring over larger scales become accessible [2, 61]. Examples describing the use of small Au nanoparticle acceptors with QD donors are provided in Chapter 8 of this volume.

Reverse FRET configurations exploring the use of QDs as energy acceptors with organic dyes have been rather limited. This has been attributed primarily to the inability of selectively exciting the dye but not the nanocrystal, due to the rather large QD extinction coefficients combined with their broad absorption spectra [62]. However, in a configuration where fluorescence emission of the potential donor is driven by a natural chemical process (e.g., bioluminescence) and direct photoexcitation of the nanocrystal is removed, QDs can effectively be used as energy acceptor.

Bioluminescence resonance energy transfer (BRET) involves the nonradiative transfer of excitation energy (induced by a natural photon-generating chemical process) to a proximal fluorescent acceptor [63, 64]. A conventional BRET configuration could consist of a donor enzyme that chemically catalyzes the reaction of a substrate, such as oxidation of coelenterazine mediated by *Renilla reniformis* luciferase, paired with an emitting acceptor fluorophore. A representative BRET study using QD acceptors was reported by Rao and coworkers. [64]. They selected an optimized eight-mutation variant of luciferase (Luc8) with improved catalytic efficiency to facilitate BRET. An average of six copies of Luc8 were coupled, via EDC condensation, to carboxyl-modified 655-nm emitting QDs. Upon addition of coelenterazine substrate to the complex, a strong emission peak from the QDs was detected in addition to the 480-nm Luc8 donor emission; see schematics in Figure 4.12. To estimate the efficiency of these interactions, a BRET ratio (similar to a FRET efficiency) defined as QD (A) emission-to-Luc8 (D) emission was used. By using different emissions/colors of QDs and varying the center-to-center separation distance, the authors found that the BRET ratio was sensitive to both changes in D-A separation distance and the overall "spectral overlap" between Lu8 emission and QD absorption, with redder emitting QDs providing more efficient energy transfer. Furthermore, the authors coupled Luc8 to QDs with emissions ranging from 605 nm to 800 nm and observed distinct emissions from each or all when mixed together in a multiplex format. Testing these conjugates in cell lines and in vivo within mice tissues, they showed that after addition of the substrate complex, luminescence spectra characteristic of the QD combination used could be collected and deconvolution of each QD color can be performed. Additionally, enhanced sensitivity and high signal-to-background ratios were measured when performing in vivo imaging in mice for comparatively small amounts of QD-Luc8 conjugates; see Figure 4.12(c).

The same authors further explored the effects of modifying the BRET enzymatic catalyst by utilizing a HaloTag protein (HTP)–Luc8 fusion [65]. HTP is a haloalkane dehalogenase enzyme that normally cleaves carbon halogen bonds in aliphatic halogenated compounds [2, 65]. However, the protein version utilized for this study contains a critical mutation in the catalytic site that allows an ester bond to form with an appropriate HTP-ligand but not the further hydrolysis step. The net result is an irreversible attachment of the HTP-Luc8 fusion to the substrate. QDs were surface modified with a halogenated alkane HTP-ligand using EDC condensation to facilitate binding to HTP-Luc8 and formation of QD-Luc8 conjugates. Similar to the original configuration, they found that addition of coelenterazine generated efficient BRET interactions between Luc8 and QDs, and resulted in a pronounced QD-sensitized signal. Rao and coworkers further developed BRET interactions and tested the ability of such conjugates to sense proteolytic activity. They recombinantly modified Luc8 protein by expressing a C-terminal protease-recognized cleavage sequence followed by a His_6-tag for self-assembly on CdSe-ZnS QDs [66]. After purification and self-assembly onto QDs, addition of the substrate resulted in efficient QD signal due to energy transfer from Luc8. More importantly, they found that further addition of a specific protease, matrix metalloproteinase-2, significantly reduced the BRET ratio/efficiency. This was attributed to cleavage of the appended peptidyl-linkage removing the Luc8 away from the QD and thus reducing BRET interactions, similar to the configuration discussed earlier using FRET and peptide-dye substrates [20]. Additional reports confirmed these findings and expanded the assemblies to include horseradish peroxidase enzyme coupled to the chemical substrate luminol as the light-generating donor while paired with CdTe QD acceptors [67].

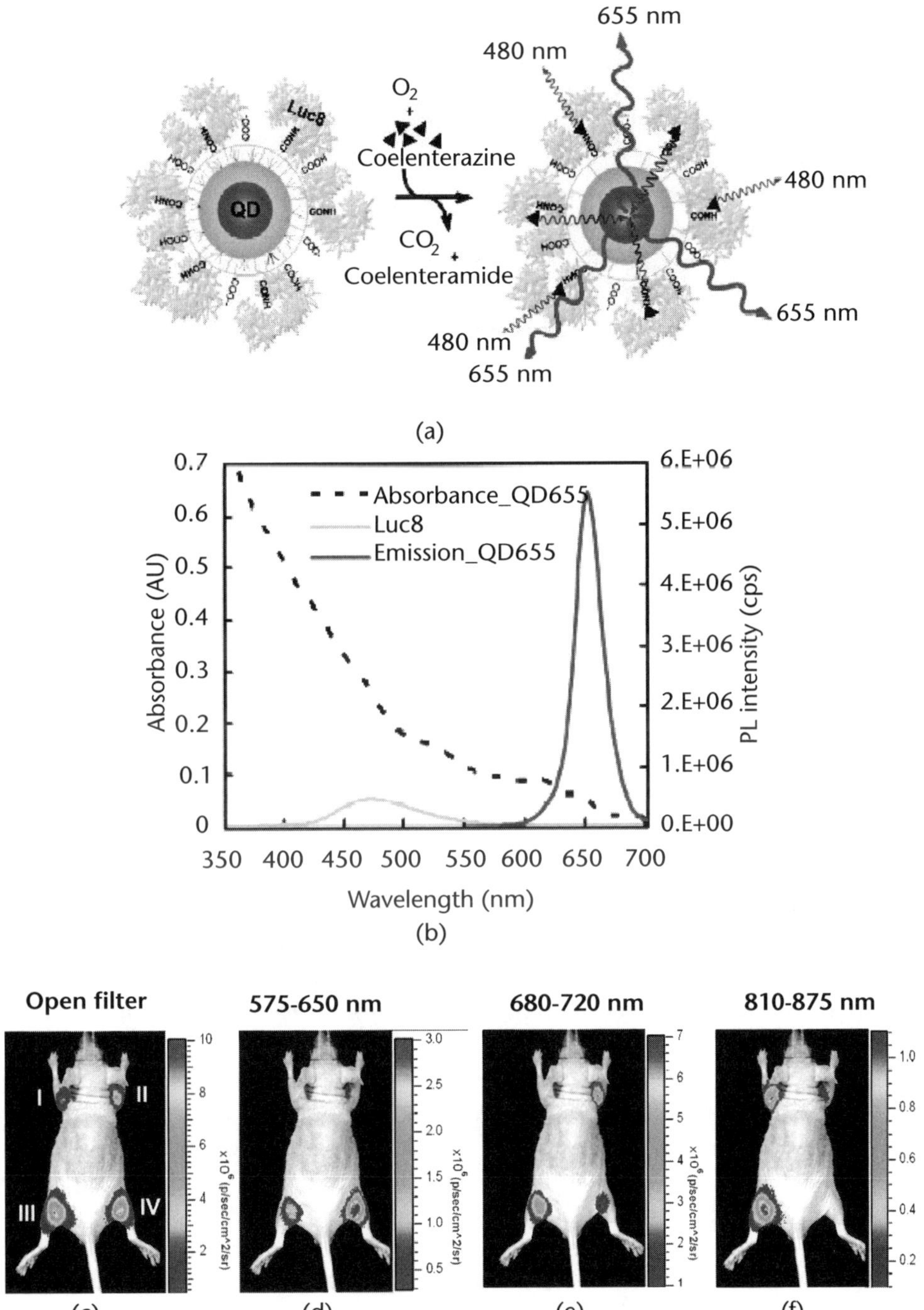

Figure 4.12 (a) Schematic of QD-Luc8 BRET assemblies. The bioluminescent energy from Luc8-catalyzed oxidation of coelenterazine is transferred to the QDs resulting in their emission. (b) Absorption and emission spectra of QD655 (ex = 480 nm) and spectrum of the bioluminescent light emitted in the oxidation of coelenterazine substrate by Luc8. (c) Multiplexed in vivo bioluminescence imaging of the following conjugates intramuscularly injected at the indicated sites in a mouse: (I) QD800-Luc8 15 pmol (II) QD705-Luc8 15 pmol (III) mixture of QD665-Luc8, QD705-Luc8 and QD800-Luc8 (IV) QD665-Luc8 5 pmol. Images (c–f) were collected with the indicated filters . Figures provided by J. Rao, Stanford University, and reprinted with permission of the NPG [64]. (See Color Plate 7.)

From these preliminary studies, it is clear that there are unique benefits to using QD acceptors in BRET configurations. The first arises from the pairing of Luc8-colenterazine, or alternatively HRP-luminol, with a broad range of emitting QDs extending to the near-IR. QDs have very high extinction coefficients (exceeding 2,000,000 M^{-1} cm^{-1}), which make them very effective for "harvesting" nearly all the bioluminescent emission. BRET with QDs could be very useful for in vivo and deep-tissue imaging, as near-IR emission is located in the optimal tissue transparency window, minimizing potential scattering and absorption issues. As the emission is dictated by the QD-enzyme substrate pair, which is conjugated in the steps prior to analysis, there are good multiplexing capabilities available for either in vitro assays or for use in animal models [64]. This format can also benefit from a plethora of mutated Luc enzymes recently reported with control over the emission wavelength of the substrates [68].

4.6 Conclusions and Outlook

The examples discussed in this chapter provide an idea about the progress made in the past five years for developing a variety of sensing assemblies based on the use of QDs and resononce energy transfer. They also detail some of the unique properties offered by luminescent QDs as energy donors and the large potential for developing FRET-based biosensing. Advantages offered by luminescent QDs for implementing FRET-based assays can be summarized in five main facts: (1) tunable QD emission allow one to select a QD color with optimized spectral overlap with a given acceptor; (2) for any QD-dye pair, theyprovide the flexibility to choose an excitation wavelength that minimizes direct excitation contribution to acceptor emission; (3) intraassembly FRET efficiency can be improved by arraying multiple acceptors around a central QD donor; (4) potential access to multiplex FRET sensing, and (5) energy transfer driven by two-photon excitation reduces background contribution to acceptor signal, which can be beneficial to intracellular sensing based on QDs and FRET.

What developments can we expect from FRET-based sensing with QDs in the future? As stated in [11] by Michalet and coworkers, "QDs have a largely untapped potential as customizable donors of a fluorescence resonance energy transfer pair." In the near term, we anticipate that additional FRET-based sensing assemblies targeting a variety of small and large molecules, biological and nonbiological, will continue to be developed. There will be further interest in developing sensors that utilize QDs as acceptors with bioluminescent and chemiluminescent donors. In the longer term, transitioning these in vitro developments to intracellular will certainly be actively pursued. One main hurdle that must be overcome to facilitate such transition is the need for developing reproducible methods that could consistently and controllably deliver QD-assemblies to specific intracellular compartments [69]. These assemblies must be compact to allow for facile transmembrane uptake while permitting large measurable FRET efficiencies. Several delivery techniques have been attempted recently, though with mixed levels of success, including electroporation, chemical, peptide-assisted, and transfection agents [69, 70]. Compactness of hydrophilic QDs and their conjugate assemblies is a very important requirement for achieving high rates of FRET. Strategies for surface functionalization and bioconjugation of QDs and other nanocrystals (such as metallic and magnetic nanoparticles), capable of providing materials that are stable over extended period of time (6–12 months) and over a broad range of biological conditions (broad pH range and in the presence of dissolved salts) will continue to be developed. From a practical perspective, one would like a bioconjugation strategy that allows (1) control over QD-acceptor separation distance, (2) control over the ratio of biomolecules attached per QD or the converse, (3) control over the relative orientation of biomolecules attached to the QDs, and (4) simple conjugation strategies that facilitate formation of any QD-biomolecule pair (QD:DNA, peptide, protein, and so on). The first two criteria are particularly crucial for any FRET applications. The necessary conjugation chemistries involve both the biomolecules in question and the development of new multifunctional surface ligands for the QDs. This remains an area of active research for many different groups, with continuing progress being made in both improving the choices of ligands available [71–73] and the methods for modifying biomolecules to allow attachment to QDs [17, 74]. Additional discussion of these issues is provided in Chapter 1 and Chapter 3 of this volume.

Finally, it's also worth mentioning one unexpected and easily accessible pair that has proven to be a very useful in developing QD FRET sensors. That is pairing commercial ~600–605-nm emitting QDs surface-functionalized with streptavidin with a Cy5 dye-acceptor (absorption maxima ~650 nm, emission maxima 670 nm); see Figure 4.1(b). For this special case, the high QD donor quantum yield ≥ 50 percent, good spectral overlap, the high Cy5 molar absorptivity of 250,000 $M^{-1}cm^{-1}$, and the ability to array multiple Cy5 around a QD have all been combined in a number of different functional assemblies to allow efficient FRET sensing over distances approaching ~100Å [23, 75]. The multiple streptavidin moieties on the QD surface allow easy conjugation to biotinylated DNA, peptides, or proteins, facilitating assembly of many of the sensor configurations.

Acknowledgments

We acknowledge NRL, and the CB Directorate/Physical S&T Division, DTRA for support. We also thank Bing Mei and Kimihiro Susumu for assistance with the preparation of the chapter.

References

[1] Lakowicz, J.R., "Principles of Fluorescence Spectroscopy," New York: Springer; 2006.

[2] Sapsford, K.E., Berti, L., Medintz, I.L., "Materials for fluorescence resonance energy transfer:beyond traditional 'dye to dye' combinations," *Angew. Chem. Int. Ed.*, Vol. 45, 2006, pp. 4562–4588.

[3] Miyawaki, A., "Visualization of the spatial and temporal dynamics of intracellular signaling," *Dev. Cell.*, Vol. 4, No. 3, 2003, 295–305.

[4] Jares-Erijman, E., Jovin, T., "FRET imaging," *Nat. Biotechnol.*, Vol. 21, 2003, pp. 1387–1395.

[5] Watrob, H.M., Pan, C.P., Barkley M.D., "Two-step FRET as a structural tool," *J. Am. Chem. Soc.*, Vol. 125, 2003, pp. 7336–7343.

[6] Stryer, L., Haugland R.P., "Energy Transfer - a Spectroscopic Ruler," *P.N.A.S. (USA)*, Vol. 58, 1967, pp. 719–726.

[7] Majumdar, Z.K., et al., "Measurements of internal distance changes of the 30 S ribosome using FRET with multiple donor-acceptor pairs: Quantitative spectroscopic methods," *J. Mol. Biology*, Vol. 351, 2005, pp. 1123–1145.

[8] Wallrabe, H., Periasamy A., "Imaging protein molecules using FRET and FLIM microscopy," *Current Opinion in Biotechnology*, Vol. 16, 2005, pp. 19–27.

[9] Galperin, E., Verkhusha, V., Sorkin, A., "Three-chromophore FRET microscopy to analyze multiprotein interactions in living cells," *Nat. Methods*, Vol. 1, 2004, pp. 209–217.

[10] Clapp A.R., Medintz I.L., Mattoussi, H., "Förster resonance energy transfer investigations using quantum dot fluorophores," *ChemPhysChem.*, Vol. 7, 2005, pp. 47–57.

[11] Michalet, X., et al., "Quantum dots for live cells, in vivo imaging, and diagnostics," *Science* Vol. 307, 2005, pp. 538–544.

[12] Murray, C.B., Kagan, C.R., Bawendi, M.G., "Synthesis and characterization of monodisperse nanocrystals and close-packed nanocrystal assemblies," *Ann. Rev. Mater. Sci.*, Vol. 30, 2000, pp. 545–610.

[13] Alivisatos, A.P., Gu, W., Larabell, C.A., "Quantum dots as cellular probes," *Ann. Rev. Biomed. Eng.*, Vol. 7, 2005, pp. 55–76.

[14] Chan, W.C.W., Nie, S., "Quantum dot bioconjugates for ultrasensitive nonisotopic detection," *Science*, Vol. 281, 1998, pp. 2016–2018.

[15] Bruchez, M., et al., "Semiconductor nanocrystals as fluorescent biological labels," *Science*, Vol. 281,1998, pp. 2013–2016.

[16] Dabbousi, B.O., et al., "(CdSe)ZnS Core-Shell Quantum Dots: Synthesis and Optical and Structural Characterization of a Size Series of Highly Luminescent Materials," *J. Phys. Chem. B.*, Vol. 101, 1997, pp. 9463–9675.

[17] Medintz, I.L., et al., "A reactive peptidic linker for self-assembling hybrid quantum dot-DNA bioconjugates," *Nano Lett.*, Vol. 7, 2007, pp. 1741–1748.

[18] Clapp, A.R., et al., "Fluorescence resonance energy transfer between quantum dot donors and dye-labeled protein acceptors," *J. Am. Chem. Soc.*, Vol. 126, 2004, pp. 301–310.

[19] Medintz, I.L., et al., "Quantum dot bioconjugates for imaging, labeling and sensing," *Nat. Mater.*, Vol. 4, 2005, pp. 435–446.

[20] Medintz, I.L., et al., "Proteolytic activity monitored by fluorescence resonance energy transfer through quantum-dot-peptide conjugates," *Nat. Mater.*, Vol. 5, 2006, pp. 581–589.

[21] Medintz, I.L., et al., "Self-assembled nanoscale biosensors based on quantum dot FRET donors," *Nat. Mater.*, Vol. 2, 2003, pp. 630–638.

[22] Goldman, E.R., et al., "A hybrid quantum dot-antibody fragment fluorescence resonance energy transfer-based TNT sensor," *J. Am. Chem. Soc.*, Vol. 127, 2005, pp. 6744–6751.

[23] Zhang, C.Y., et al., "Single-quantum-dot-based DNA nanosensor," *Nat. Mater.*, Vol. 4, 2005, pp. 826–831.

[24] Zhang, C.Y., Johnson L.W., "Quantum-dot-based nanosensor for RRE IIB RNA-Rev peptide interaction assay," *J. Am. Chem. Soc.*, Vol. 128, 2006, pp. 5324–5325.

[25] Clapp, A.R., et al., "Quantum dot-based multiplexed fluorescence resonance energy transfer," *J. Am. Chem. Soc.*, Vol. 127, 2005, pp. 18212–1821.

[26] Denk, W., Strickler, J.H., and Webb, W.W., "2-Photon Laser Scanning Fluorescence Microscopy," *Science*, Vol. 248, 1990, pp. 73–76.

[27] Clapp. A.R., et al., "Two-photon excitation of quantum dot-based fluorescence resonance energy transfer and its applications," *Adv. Mater.*, Vol. 119, 2007, pp. 1921–1926.

[28] Larson, D.R., et al., "Water-soluble quantum dots for multiphoton fluorescence imaging in vivo," *Science*, Vol. 300, 2003, pp. 1434–1437.

[29] Sapsford. K.E., et al., "Kinetics of metal-affinity driven self-assembly between proteins or peptides and CdSe-ZnS quantum dots," *J. Phys. Chem. C.*, Vol. 111, 2007, pp. 11528–11538.

[30] Medintz, I.L., et al., "A reagentless biosensing assembly based on quantum dot donor Förster resonance energy transfer," *Adv. Mater.*, Vol. 17, 2005, pp. 2450–2455.

[31] Pons, T., et al. "Solution-phase single quantum dot fluorescence resonant energy transfer sensing," *J. Am. Chem. Soc.*, Vol. 128, 2006, pp. 15324–15331.

[32] Wei, Q., et al., "Development of an open sandwich fluoroimmunoassay based on fuorescence resonance energy transfer," *Anal. Biochem.*, Vol. 358, 2006, pp. 31–37.

[33] Puente, X.S., and Lopez-Otin C. "A genomic analysis of rat proteases and protease inhibitors," *Genome Researc,* Vol. 14, 2004, pp. 609–622.

[34] Puente, X.S., et al., "Human and mouse proteases: A comparative genomic approach," *Nature Reviews Genetics*, Vol. 4, 2003, pp. 544–558.

[35] Shi, L.F., et al., "Luminescent quantum dots fluorescence resonance energy transfer-based probes for enzymatic activity and enzyme inhibitors," *Anal. Chem.*, Vol. 79, 2007, pp. 208–214.

[36] Shi, L.F., et al., "Synthesis and application of quantum dots FRET-based protease sensors," *J. Am. Chem. Soc.,* Vol. 128, 2006, pp. 10378–10379.

[37] Xu, C.J., et al., "A self-assembled quantum dot probe for detecting beta-lactamase activity," *Biochemical and Biophysical Research Communications*, Vol. 344, 2006, pp. 931–935.

[38] Zlokarnik, G., et al., "Quantitation of transcription and clonal selection of single living cells with beta-lactamase as reporter," *Science*, Vol. 279, 1998, pp. 84–88.

[39] Tyagi, S., and Kramer F.R., "Molecular beacons: Probes that fluoresce upon hybridization," *Nat. Biotechnol.,* Vol. 14, 1996, pp. 303–308.

[40] Didenko, V.V., "DNA probes using fluorescence resonance energy transfer (FRET): Designs and applications," *Biotechniques*, Vol 31, 2001, pp. 1106–1121.

[41] Ellington, A.D., and Szostak J.W., "Selection of in vitro single-stranded-DNA molecules that fold into specific ligand-binding structures," *Nature*, Vol. 355, 1992, pp. 850–852.

[42] Gill, R., et al., "Fluorescence resonance energy transfer in CdSe/ZnS-DNA conjugates: Probing hybridization and DNA cleavage," *J. Phys. Chem. B.*, Vol. 109, 2005, pp. 23715–23719.

[43] Bakalova, R., et al., "Quantum dot-conjugated hybridization probes for preliminary screening of siRNA sequences," *J. Am. Chem. Soc.*, Vol. 127, 2005, 21, pp. 11328–11335.

[44] Algar, W.R. and Krull, U.J., "Towards multi-colour strategies for the detection of oligonucleotide hybridization using quantum dots as energy donors in fluorescence resonance energy transfer (FRET)," *Analytica Chimica Acta*, Vol. 581, 2007, pp. 193–201.

[45] Levy, M., et al., "Quantum-dot aptamer beacons for the detection of proteins," *Chembiochem*, Vol. 6, 2005, pp. 1–4.

[46] Alberts, B., et al., *Molecular Biology of the Cell*, 4th Edition, New York, NY: Garland Science, 2002.

[47] Watson, J.D., et al., *Molecular Biology of the Gene*, 5th Editon. Reading, MA: The Benjamin Cummings Publishing Co Inc., 2004.

[48] Snee, P.T., et al., "A ratiometric CdSe/ZnS nanocrystal pH sensor," *J. Am. Chem. Soc.,* Vol. 128., 2006, pp. 13320–13321.

[49] Tomasulo, M., et al., "pH-sensitive ligand for luminescent quantum dots," *Langmuir*, Vol. 22, 2006, pp. 10284–10290.

[50] Tomasulo, M., et al., "pH-Sensitive quantum dots," *J. Phys. Chem. B.*, Vol. 110, 2006, pp. 3853–3855.

[51] Ruedas-Rama, M.J., et al., "A multi-ion particle sensor," *Chem. Comm.*, Vol. 15, 2007, pp. 1544–1546.

[52] Dubach, J.M., et al., "Ion-selective nano-optodes incorporating quantum dots," *J. Am. Chem. Soc.*, Vol. 129, 2007, pp. 8418–8419.

[53] Bakalova, R., et al., "Quantum dots as photosensitizers," *Nat. Biotechnol.*, Vol. 22, 2004, pp. 1360–1361.

[54] Samia, A.C.S. et al., "Semiconductor quantum dots for photodynamic therapy," *J. Am. Chem. Soc.*, Vol. 125, 2003, pp. 15736–15737.

[55] Samia A.C.S., et al., "Quantum dot-based energy transfer: Perspectives and potential for applications in photodynamic therapy," *Photochemistry and Photobiology*, Vol. 82, 2006, pp. 617–625.

[56] Tsay, J.M., et al., "Singlet oxygen production by peptide-coated quantum dot-photosensitizer conjugates," *J. Am. Chem. Soc.,* Vol. 129, 2007, pp. 6865–6871.

[57] Hsieh, J.M., et al., "Iridium-complex modified CdSe/ZnS quantum dots; a conceptual design for bifunctionality toward imaging and photosensitization," *Chem. Comm.*, Vol. 14, 2006, pp. 615–617.

[58] Shi, L.X., et al., "Singlet oxygen generation from water-soluble quantum dot-organic dye nanocomposites," *J. Am. Chem. Soc.*, Vol. 128, 2006, pp. 6278–6279.

[59] Neuman, D., et al., "Photosensitized NO release from water-soluble nanoparticle assemblies," *J. Am. Chem. Soc.*, Vol. 129, 2007, pp. 4146–4147.

[60] Bakalova, R., et al., "Quantum dot anti-CD conjugates: Are they potential photosensitizers or potentiators of classical photosensitizing agents in photodynamic therapy of cancer?," *Nano Lett.*, Vol. 4, 2004, pp. 1567–1573.

[61] Pons, T., et al., "On the quenching of semiconductor quantum dot photoluminescence by proximal gold nanoparticles," *Nano Lett.*, Vol. 7, 2007, pp. 3157–3164.

[62] Clapp, A.R., et al., "Can luminescent quantum dots be efficient energy acceptors with organic dye donors," *J. Am. Chem. Soc.*, Vol. 125, 2005, pp. 1242–1250.

[63] Wilson, T., and Hastings J.W., "Bioluminescence," *Ann. Rev. Cell. Dev. Biol.*, Vol. 14, 1998, pp. 197–230.

[64] So, M.K., et al., "Self-illuminating quantum dot conjugates for in vivo imaging," *Nat. Biotechnol.,* Vol. 24, 2006, pp. 339–343.

[65] Zhang, Y., et al., "HaloTag protein-mediated site-specific conjugation of bioluminescent proteins to quantum dots," *Angew. Chem. Int. Ed.*, Vol. 45, 2006, pp. 4936–4940.

[66] Yao, H. et al., "Quantum dot/bioluminescence resonance energy transfer based highly sensitive detection of proteases," *Angew. Chem. Int. Ed.*, Vol. 46, 2007, pp. 4346–4649.

[67] Huang, X.Y., et al., "A resonance energy transfer between chemiluminescent donors and luminescent quantum-dots as acceptors (CRET)," *Angew. Chem. Int. Ed.,* Vol. 45, 2006, pp. 5140–5143.

[68] Loening, A.M., et al., "Red-shifted *Renilla reniformis* luciferase variants for imaging in living subjects," *Nat. Methods*., Vol. 4, 2007, pp. 641–643.

[69] Delehanty, J.B., et al., "Self-assembled quantum dot-peptide bioconjugates for selective intracellular delivery," *Bioconj. Chem.*, Vol. 17, 2006, pp. 920–927.

[70] Derfus, A.M., et al., "Intracellular delivery of quantum dots for live cell labeling and organelle tracking," *Advanced Materials*, Vol. 16, 2004, pp. 961–966.

[71] Gao, X., et al., "In vivo cancer targeting and imaging with semiconductor quantum dots," *Nat. Biotechnol.*, Vol. 22, 2004, pp. 969–976.

[72] Pinaud, F., et al., "Bioactivation and cell targeting of semiconductor CdSe/ZnS nanocrystals with phytochelatin-related peptides," *J. Am. Chem. Soc.*, Vol. 126, 2004, pp. 6115–6123.

[73] Uyeda, H.T., et al., "Synthesis of compact multidentate ligands to prepare stable hydrophilic quantum dot fluorophores," *J. Am. Chem. Soc.,* Vol. 127, 2005, pp. 3870–3878.

[74] Howarth, M., et al., "Targeting quantum dots to surface proteins in living cells with biotin ligase," *P. N. A. S. (U.S.A.)*, Vol. 102, 2005, pp. 7583–7588.

[75] Zhang, C.-Y. and Johnson, L.W., "Microfluidic control of fluorescence resonance energy transfer:breaking the FRET limit," *Angew. Chem. Int. Ed.*, Vol. 46, 2007, pp. 3482–2485.

CHAPTER 5

Use of Luminescent Quantum Dots to Image and Initiate Biological Functions

Elizabeth A. Jares-Erijman, Avishay Pelah, María Julia Roberti, Valeria Sigot, Lía Pietrasanta, Guillermo Menéndez, María H. Etchehon, and Thomas M. Jovin

5.1 Introduction

Quantum dots (QDs) possess unique properties (brightness, photostability, narrowband emission, and broadband absorption), and excellent bio(chemical) compatibility for imaging structures and functions of living cells. The reader is referred to Chapter 1 for a description of the synthesis, photophysical properties, and biofunctionalization strategies of quantum dots, and to Chapter 3 for an account of peptide-functionalized quantum dots for live diagnostic imaging and therapeutic applications. QDs conjugated with ligands are able to recognize and track multiple targets and visualize dynamic processes. Such QDs can be directed to precise cellular targets [1–9], detecting biomolecules with a sensitivity extending to the single molecule level. Thus, one can study the essential processes underlying the functions and regulation of *living* cells with probes providing "partial molecular derivatives" (i.e., views of individual processes embedded in the totality of the cellular machinery). Without such information, a "dissection" of complex networks is impossible.

Besides the brilliance and photostability of QDs that allow prolonged imaging and tracking of individual nanoparticles (NPs), other characteristics related to the local density and nature of molecular components can be exploited in cells and tissues for purposes other than mere detection. In particular, the systematic "engineering" of the molecular composition on the surface of QDs has been a central feature in numerous applications ranging beyond biosensing to cell delivery and release and to the activation of individual reactions and entire pathways.

A widespread tendency is to consider the existence of multiple groups on the surface of NPs as disadvantageous in comparison with single attachment or reactive points. The rationale behind this assertion is that a high number of molecules would provide multiples sites of conjugation leading to a distribution of NP subpopulations differing in particle-label stoichiometries, to undesirable and unphysiological cross-linking and to other effects. Procedures for achieving precise control of the number of sites (down to single moieties) have been developed [10]. We will maintain in this presentation, however, that under certain circumstances the presence of a *large* number of sites may offer distinct advantages. In fact, numerous studies demonstrate that multiple identical or different molecules on the surface of NPs can be exploited for a wide variety of purposes, ranging from the control of optical or physical properties to the concurrent regulation of different functions.

Commercially available NPs coated with a polymeric layer to isolate the core-shell structure from the aqueous environment have diameters of 15–20 nm and may extend to double these values if covered with PEG. Is this considerable size important such that QDs operate more as *platforms* rather than as single molecular entities? The distinction is subtle. For example, QDs have been shown to be useful as FRET donors and acceptors in numerous applications [11, 12], although there have been relatively few reports of experiments based on imaging [1, 3, 4, 6, 13–17]. In our own studies of cellular signaling mediated by growth factors [5, 18–20] and their receptors, QDs conjugated with ligands have revealed the existence of novel transport and trafficking mechanisms. Figure 5.1 depicts a strategy QDs attached to ligands as in this case the epidermal growth factor (EGF) vehicles for specific targeting of cell surface receptors based on [20]. Luminescent QDs allowed the visualization of the displacement of complexes of EGF-EGFR on filopodia cellular extensions with a core of actin filaments toward the body of living A431 cells, and their subse-

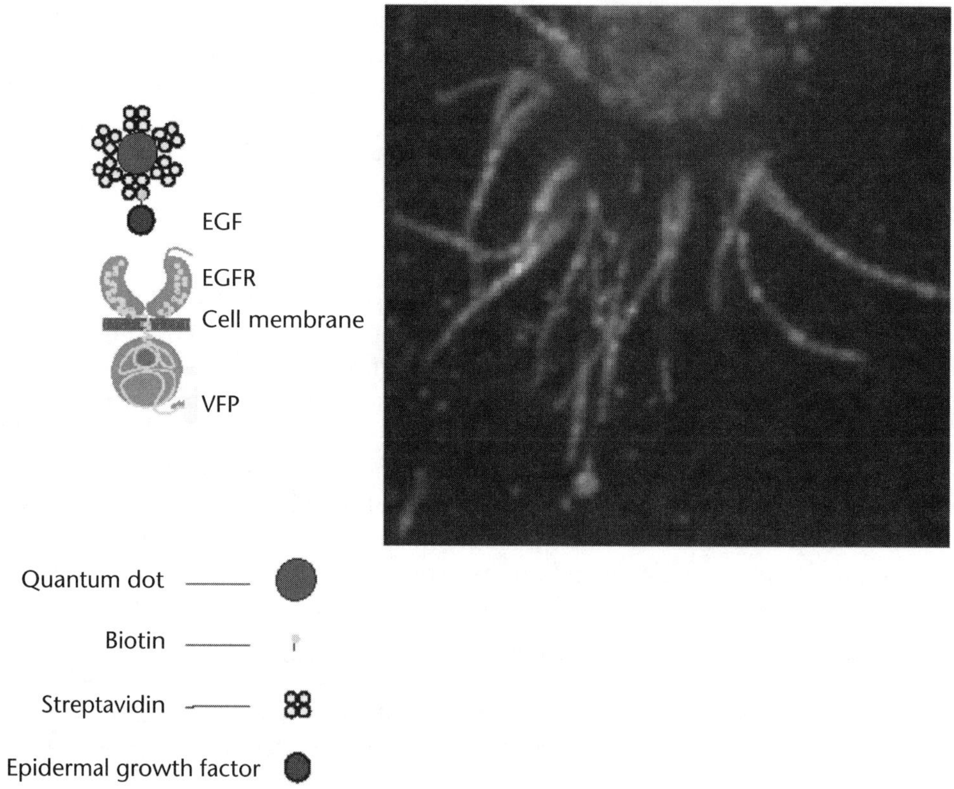

Figure 5.1 Strategy to study the binding of QD-EGF to the EGF receptor (EGFR), and the resultant activation and endocytosis of the receptor into living cells. The image displays A431 cells expressing ERB1-EGFP 20 min after addition of biotinylated EGF bound to Streptavidin QD-605. For further details, see [20]. (See Color Plate 8.)

quent internalization by endocytosis [5]. For this purpose biotin-EGF was bound to streptavidin QDs. An important question was whether the QDs bound to the filopodia were first taken up into the filopodia and thus transported *within* the cell or instead were transported while remaining outside the plasma membrane. This question was addressed by externally adding a nonpermeable biotinylated FRET acceptor of the QDs that could bind to the nanoparticles only if they were acessible to the medium (i.e., on the outside of the cell). Rapid and extensive FRET signals were observed, attesting that the latter situation prevails [5]. Thus, the QD-EGF reagents served not only as tags of the EGF receptor but also provided insight into the molecular disposition of this prototypic family of receptor tyrosine kinases (RTKs) during the early stages of activation and processing.

QD donors have been applied extensively in FRET-based assays of enzymatic activities, with the systematic introduction of multifunctionality being a major issue ([21] and references therein). For a detailed description of FRET-based biosensors, see Chapter 4 of this book, "Resonance Energy Transfer-Based Sensing Using Quantum Dot Bioconjugates." The distance dependence of FRET operating via surface-bound or nearby small-molecule acceptors reflects the complex interplay between factors such as stoichiometry, spatial distribution and orientation, composition (passivation shell, capping moieties), and shape. (QDs emitting at > 600 nm tend to be nonspherical and demonstrate finite emission polarization, [22]).

Optical properties such as fluorescence intensity or lifetime can also be tailored with FRET acceptors. The design of FRET-based biosensors required for recording given states also requires control of the number of acceptors associated with each QD donor [23].

5.2 Multivalency Allows Multifunctionality

An illustrative example of how multiple sites can be advantageous for multifunctionality is given by the application of QDs as "torch bearers" into cells [24]. In this study, we used QDs as tools for enabling and at the same time monitoring the internalization of liposomes (with a given cargo) into cells. The strategy (Figure 5.2) takes advantage of the fact that the EGFR is overexpressed in a broad spectrum of malignant tumors and thus represents a suitable target for delivery of therapeutic liposomes. Streptavidin QDs prelabeled with biotin-EGF were bound to biotinylated liposomes stabilized with polyethyleneglycol (PEG). In the two alternative schemes featured in the cited study, QDs of a second color were used to monitor internalization and delivery. In the first approach, the second QD was attached to the surface of the liposomes via links provided by biotinylated lipids incorporated in the bilayer. The internal liposomal space was available for loading with cargo (drugs, DNA, and so on). In the other approach one or more QDs of the second color was (were) encapsulated within the liposome. In both procedures, the QDs served to monitor endosomal escape after cellular uptake [24].

A related strategy has been designed to provide the delivery of a target siRNA sequence attached to a scaffold-based PEGylated-QDs bearing F3 tumor-homing peptides promoting internalization by tumor cells. The attached siRNA did not interfere with the activity of the F3 peptide. The study was performed on the expres-

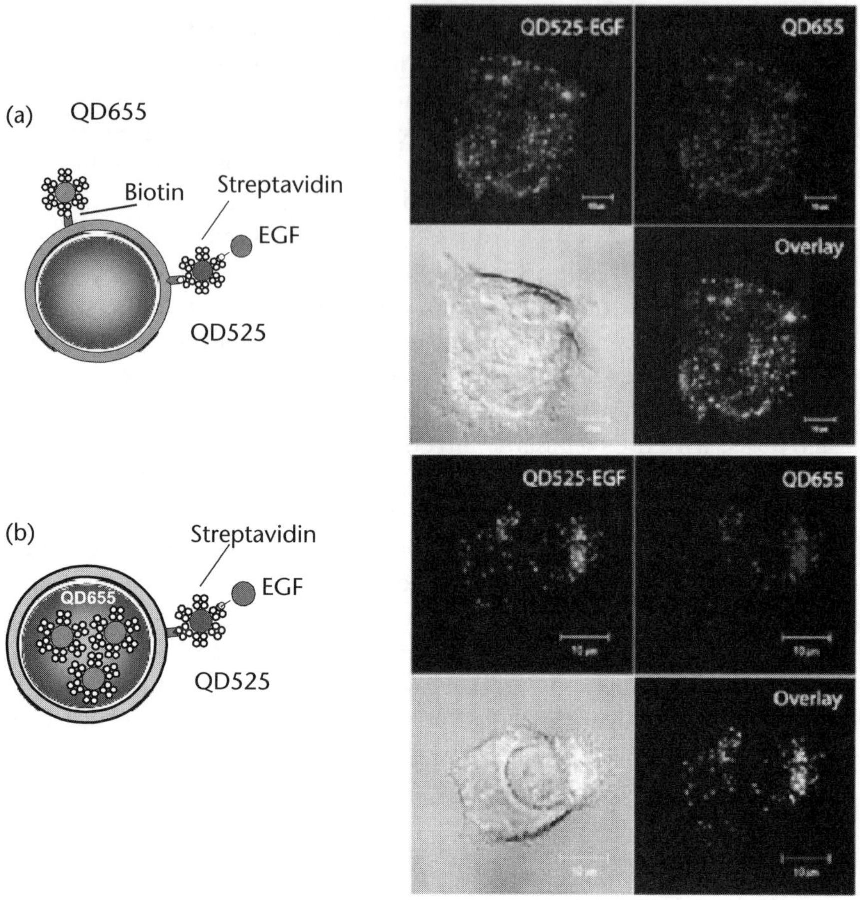

Figure 5.2 Preparation of liposomes attached to and/or containing QDs: (a) Surface labeling of lipid particles with QD525-EGF and untargeted QD655. (b) Lipid particles with encapsulated QD655 and surface labeled with QD525-EGF. QD-655 are either encapsulated or decorate the liposome surface. In a second conjugation step, preformed QD525-EGF complexes in 1:2 molar ratio target the liposomes for specific cell delivery. The images depict the cellular uptake of dual QD-labeled liposomes by live A431 cells, detected as colocalized dots in endosomal vesicles after 2h incubation at 37 degrees C according to strategies (a) and (b). (See Color Plate 9.)

sion of a model EGFP molecule, adjusting the ratio of F3 peptide and siRNA so as to optimize internalization and suppression of EGFP expression [25].

In addition to the engineering of complex functionality, a multiplicity of sites on nanoscale surfaces enables further possibilities. Since kinetic and thermodynamic parameters are dependent on the nanoscaled architecture, it is possible to conceive of strategies for taking advantage of such special characteristics in order to exert a desired biological effect. For example, multivalent NPs have been applied extensively for in vitro assays based on the modification of certain properties arising as a consequence of self-assembly. DNA hybridization (Figure 5.3, upper panel), biotin-avidin (Figure 5.3, lower panel) and other systems have been used as the "glue" for interparticle interactions. The changes in optical [26, 27] or magnetic properties were used for monitoring either nucleic acid hybridization or protease activity. A very elegant example [28] of the control of self-assembly of superparamagnetic NPs

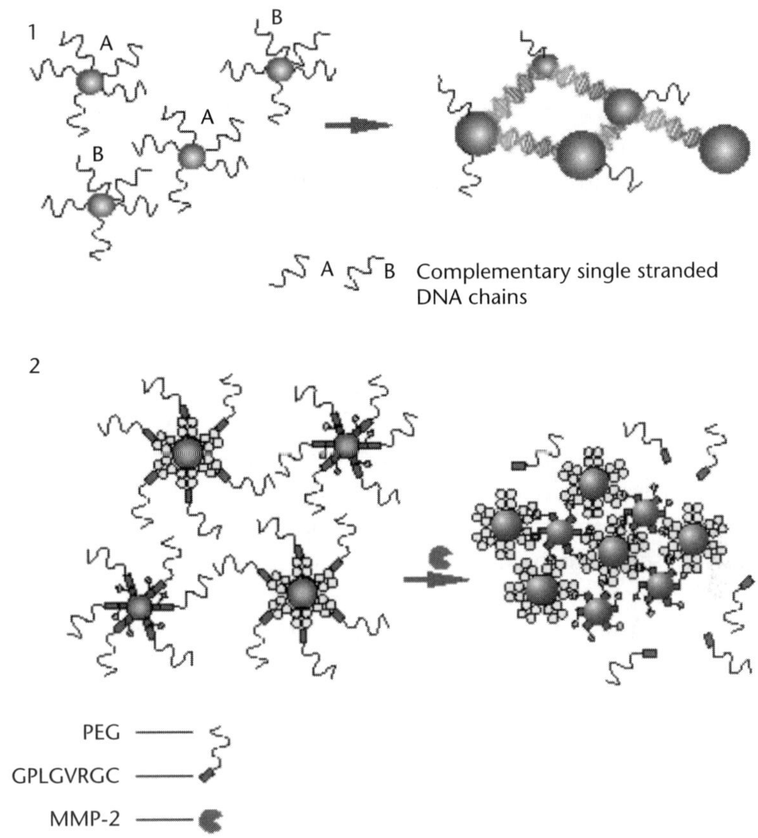

Figure 5.3 Biosensing based on the association of metal nanoparticles: (1) Self-assembly of metal nanoparticles bearing complementary single-stranded DNA chains. The aggregation is detected by the shift in the exciton band of the nanoparticles. (2) Schematic representation of a proteolytic actuation of self-assembly. Neutravidin- and biotin-functionalized superparamagnetic iron oxide nanoparticles are functionalized by the attachment of 10-Kd PEG chains anchored by MMP-2 cleavable peptide substrates (GPLGVRGC). Upon proteolytic removal of PEG through cleavage of the peptides, the particles self-assemble into nanoassemblies with enhanced magnetic susceptibility, T2 magnetic resonance relaxation, and lowered diffusivity.

involved the conjugation of a protease target peptide GPLGVRGC to PEG. A 10-kD ethylene-glycol polymer prevented the interaction of biotins bound to the surface of one NP type with the neutravidin on the surface of a second NP type (see Figure 5.3, lower panel). The proteolytic activity of metalloproteinase-2 (MMP-2), which correlates with cancer invasion, angiogenesis, and metastasis, removed the PEG and initiated the self-assembly of NPs. The protease activity was easily detected by MRI via changes in the transverse T2 relaxation times of the NP aggregates. In addition, the aggregation of nanoparticles led to the manifestation of an amplified magnetic dipole, allowing their manipulation with magnets that failed to attract free NPs.

Another interesting approach was featured with an NP system in which self-assembly was dynamically coupled to the balance between two antagonistic actions of a tyrosine kinase and a phosphatase [29]. The system was designed to produce coalescence of NPs in the presence of the kinase and redispersion in the presence of the phosphatase. The strategy involved the design of two NP populations. The first was modified with peptide substrates able to be phosphorylated by the Ab1 tyrosine kinase and dephosphorylated by a phosphatase. The second population was modified with Src Homology 2 (SH2) domains that recognize and bind the phosphorylated Ab1 kinase substrate in a sequence-specific manner. In combination, these NPs reported kinase and phosphatase activities by self-assembling as peptides became phosphorylated and disassembling as the phosphate groups were removed.

Engineering the surface of NPs can also be applied for the initiation and control of the self-assembly of biomolecules. In the case of the amyloid-forming proteins involved in most neurodegenerative diseases, such tools can provide important insights into the mechanism of fibrillation in living cells and organisms and also have great potential for very sensitive readouts in drug discovery efforts.

The self-assembly of natively unfolded or misfolded proteins into ordered fibrillar aggregates known as amyloid is a feature common to numerous human diseases. These conditions are often neurodegenerative, such as in Alzheimer's and Parkinson's diseases and spongiform encephalopathies, as well as nonneuropathic, as in type II diabetes and different forms of cancer. A ubiquitous cytopathological finding is the presence of intracellular or extracellular highly organized fibrillar aggregates. Although the polypeptide chains involved in these diseases lack sequence homology or strong similarities in amino acid composition and size, the resultant amyloid fibrils are remarkably uniform with respect to both external morphology and internal structure. Despite an increasing number of proteins and peptide fragments being recognized as amyloidogenic, how these amyloid aggregates assemble remains unclear. In particular, the identity of the nucleating species, an ephemeral entity that defines the rate of fibril formation, remains a key outstanding question. In addition, evidence points to transient oligomeric intermediates along the fibrillation pathway as the predominant molecules species responsible for cytotoxicity (i.e., neuronal death).

Thus both in vitro and in living cells, the question of what structures act as a nucleation centers triggering the onset of pathologic aggregation is central to the understanding of underlying disease mechanism(s).

The aggregation of amyloid proteins is a process highly dependent on protein concentration. In fact, experiments in vitro typically require protein concentrations in excess of 100 μM, in order to observe the formation of aggregates in 3–10 days at 37 degrees C. Thus, a central, practical consideration is whether nanoparticles can be employed to influence the nucleation process, generally regarded as the rate-determining step, in a deterministic and consistent manner. A nonspecific approach that takes advantage of the large surface area offered by most nanostructures was introduced recently [30]. Copolymer particles, cerium oxide particles, QDs, and nanotubes were tested as nucleation agents for the aggregation of the protein human β2-microglobulin. The authors reported an acceleration of nucleation that depended on the extent and nature of the particle surface. The disadvantage of this procedure is that it lacks specificity (i.e., it cannot discriminate between different molecules with the tendency to form aggregates or molecules exhibiting affinities for such structures). In addition, aggregation under such conditions requires high concentrations of the nanostructures (100 nM in the case of QDs). Such concentrations can seriously perturb the biological systems under study.

Nanoparticles can, however, can be employed in a more specific manner in such studies. Several of the other chapters in this volume discuss methods for controlling the density of molecules on the surface of QDs and other nanoparticles, ranging from the use of small molecules to nucleic acids, peptides, and proteins. In our case, attaching a controlled number of molecules of α-synuclein (AS)—a protein involved in the pathogenesis of Parkinson's disease—on the surface of QDs led to a high local concentration of the protein. This condition provided the condition required for the facile initiation of aggregation in a completely specific manner (i.e., restricted to the protein in question). With this strategy, very low concentrations of QDs (1–5 nM, Roberti et al., submitted manuscript) suffice for significantly accelerating the fibrillation of 100-μM AS in vitro as well as in living cells. That is, luminescent QDs bearing a controlled number of AS molecules combined a specific induction and efficient detection of amyloid aggregation in living cells. The nucleation capacity of QDs increased with the number of AS molecules attached to their surface. Control QDs (i.e., preparations without added biotinylated AS) were ineffective either as initiators or biosensors of aggregation. The experiments are described in further detail in the ensuing paragraphs.

Great efforts have been devoted to elucidating the mechanisms underlying the physiological function(s) of AS and the conditions leading to its pathological self-association [31]. In living cells and organisms, oxidative stress conditions can be created by exposure to a variety of chemical agents such as $FeCl_2$ or H_2O_2. These compounds initiate a complex cascade of events leading to different disfunctions, including that of amyloid protein aggregation. In the case of the AS-modified QDs acting as specific nucleation sites, AS aggregation was initiated by a physical-chemical process inherent to the nanoparticle rather than a consequence of complex mechanisms involving a plethora of molecular entities.

External stimulation, such as by oxidative stress, was required in the case of other expression probes for AS. For example, we have recently created an AS mutant (AS-C4) fused to a 12-amino-acid tag with the tetracysteine motif that specifically binds fluorogenic biarsenical compounds (e.g., FlAsH, ReAsH) [32]. In such a mutant, the functional properties of wild type AS protein were retained. Fibril formation induced by oxidative stress (e.g., exposure to $FeCl_2$) could be readily detected and characterized both in vitro and in live cells. The availability of a specifically labeled protein that can be expressed in live cells or in tissues represents an important advance for the study of the mechanism of aggregation. However, such processes ocurring under "classical" conditions of oxidative stress condition are poorly understood. Our newly developed QDs, useful as nucleation sites and as markers, served to avoid the use of such chemicals and yet led to protein aggregation. The combination of AS-C4 with the QD reagents described earlier was particularly useful, as demonstrated in studies of living cells (HeLa, Figure 5.4). Variable (0–20 nM) concentrations of AS-QDs were microinjected together with 100 mM of AS-C4. In the presence of 2 nM QDs (Figure 5.5, upper panel), cells displayed a markedly increased incidence of aggregates, observed 24 hours after microinjection, compared to the controls (lower panel) lacking QDs. In this strategy, the QDs functioned in a dual manner (i.e., both as biomarkers and "nanoactuators," or specific

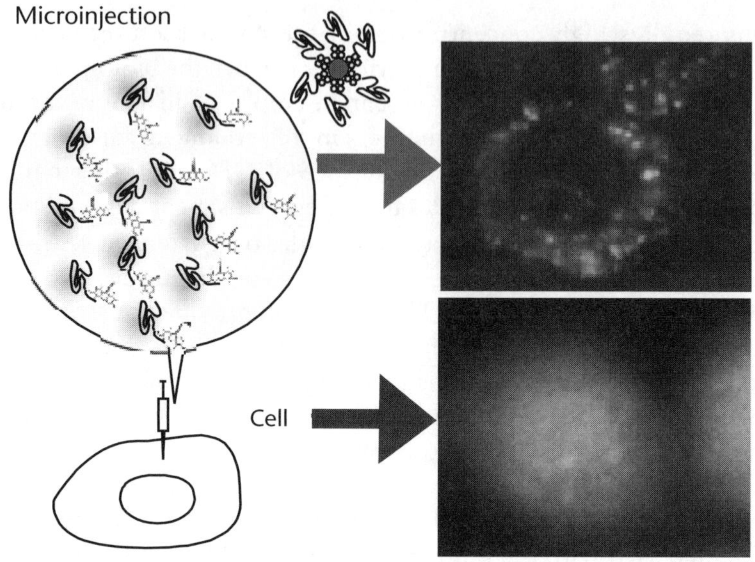

Figure 5.4 QDs acting as specific nucleation sites for ∝-synuclein (AS) in living cells. Cells were microinjected with AS in the presence or absence of AS-QDs-605 (40:1 protein:QD ratio) and observed after 24h of incubation. A mixture 2 nM AS-QDs-605 and 100 mM of AS-TC labeled with FlAsH was microinjected into HeLa cells (upper panel, red arrow). QDs were detected, colocalizing to a pronounced degree with AS aggregates. Lower panel, blue arrow, microinjection of 100 mM of AS-TC labeled with FlAsH in the absence of QDs; little or no aggregation was observed. (See Color Plate 10.)

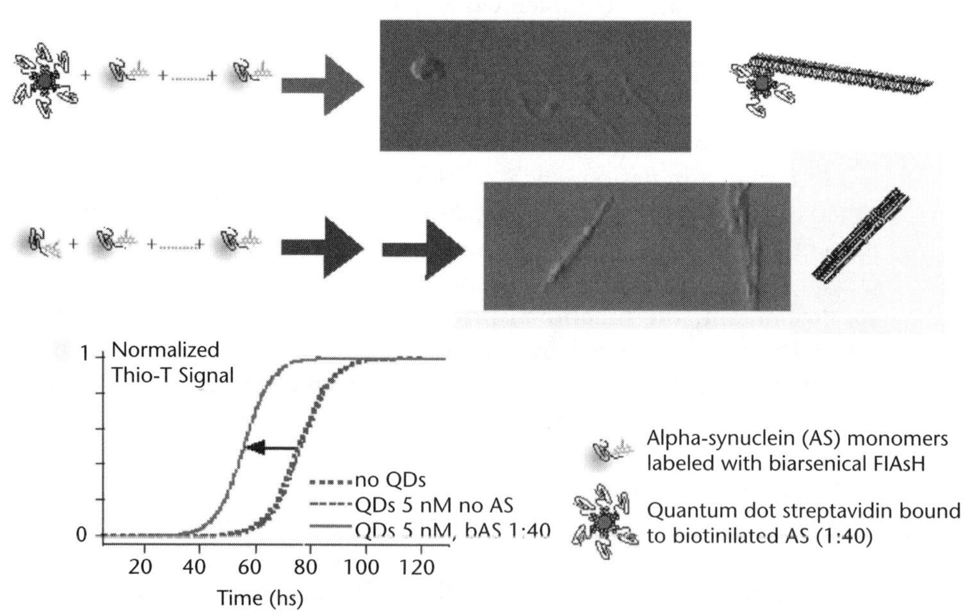

Figure 5.5 QDs acting as specific nucleation sites for ∝-synuclein (AS) in vitro. The aggregation of AS was monitored by Thio-T fluorescence and by AFM; 5 nM (40:1 protein:QD ratio) AS-QDs605 incubated together with 100 mM of AS displayed a shorter lag and faster aggregation than in absence of QDs. The upper arrow indicates the aggregation course leading to fibrils attached to NPs, as confirmed by AFM (upper panel). The second row including two consecutive arrows to indicate a slower process show fibril morphologies after aggregation in the absence of the QD nucleation centers.

nucleation agents). As biomarkers at very low concentrations, they allowed the facile detection of AS molecules in fibrils, despite the presence of a vast excess of monomeric protein. The dual labeling with the biarsenical compounds provided a further "photophysical" enhancement of sensitivity (Roberti et al., manuscript in preparation). These techniques will also benefit from improved biarsenicals that we have synthesized as an associated activity of these investigations [33]. In addition, we anticipate that dual-function NPs will undoubtedly be exploited in numerous other systems.

Figure 5.5 depicts the function of AS-QDs in vitro. The aggregation kinetics were monitored in the presence and in the absence of the NPs. The association of QDs with nascent fibers was confirmed by AFM (upper panel), and the acceleration of aggregation (shorter lag phase) was demonstrated by the standard Thioflavin T assay.

5.3 Stimuli-Responsive Polymers and Qds As Tools for Imaging

Stimuli-responsive polymers present attractive nanoactuation possibilities due to the controlled reversible alteration of their physical characteristics upon induction of the stimulus. One such material is the well-known temperature responsive polymer, poly (N-isopropylacrylamide), PNIPAM. PNIPAM is a water-soluble polymer with a lower critical solution temperature (LCST) of 32 degrees C [34]. Heating an aqueous solution of this polymer above the LCST leads to dehydration of the polymer chains, resulting in a thermoreversible coil-to-globule phase transition and hydrophobically driven chain aggregation. In a cross-linked hydrogel form, PNIPAM is water swollen below the LCST, whereas above the LCST the gel ejects water and collapses, which leads to its dramatic reduction in size. This reversible property renders PNIPAM useful in numerous biology-related applications, such as switching enzyme activity [35, 36] and dynamically controlling microtubule motility [37]. The versatility of such stimuli-responsive polymers, in both their linear and cross-linked hydrogel forms, allows the construction of diverse actuators for specific needs.

Proteins, or NPs such as QDs coated with specific proteins, may be used to link the polymeric actuator with a target of choice, relaying the swell/collapse forces to the target. The example of biotinylated PNIPAM beads bound to fluorescent streptavidin and streptavidin-coated QDs is shown in Figure 5.6 [38]. The volume of "naked" beads as well as that of a "giant" fluorescently labeled beads changed reversibly with temperature (Figure 5.7(a, b)). Evidence that such hydrogels are able to generate forces was demonstrated by attaching biotinylated PNIPAM beads to streptavidin-coated magnetic microspheres (Figure 5.7(c)) [38, 39]. Upon cycling the temperature, the volume of the bead changed and the force generated by this alteration was able to displace the magnetic microspheres. Physical forces play critical roles in cell, tissue, and organ development. Such forces are transduced into biochemical responses, and their investigation is of utmost importance. Internal rather than external polymeric force generators may also be conceived, leading toward new approaches for the manipulation of the cellular machinery. For example, inserting smart polymer-antibody conjugates into a cell can serve to reversibly

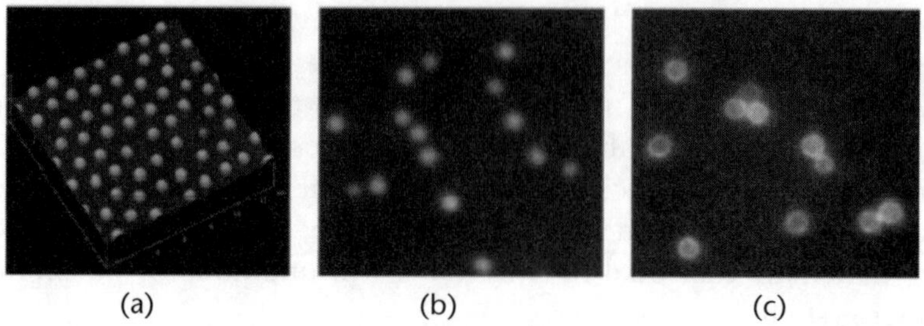

Figure 5.6 Poly (N-isopropylacrylamide, PNIPAM) temperature-responsive microbeads: (a) Beads imaged by an AFM. (b) Biotinylated beads conjugated to streptavidin Alexa 546. (c) Biotinylated beads conjugated to 605-nm QDs. Beads were ~1 mM in diameter.

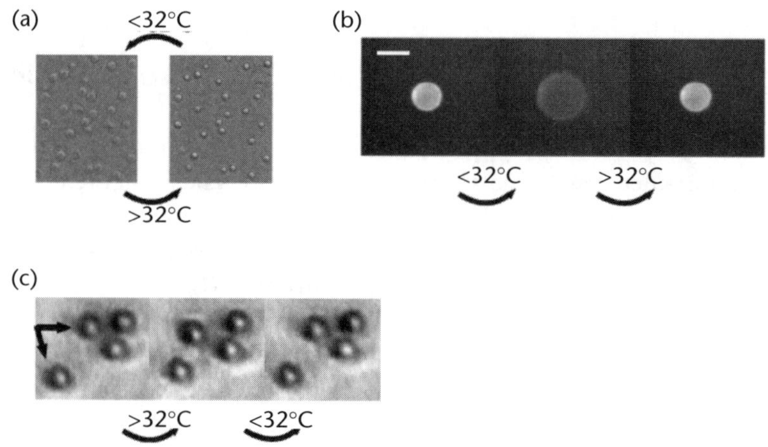

Figure 5.7 Volume change of PNIPAM beads and subsequent force generation upon temperature cycle: (a) "Naked" micrometer-sized beads. (b) "Giant" fluorescently labeled PNIPAM beads. Scale bar: 6 mm. (c) Displacement of strepavidin-coated magnetic spheres by micrometer-sized biotinylated PNIPAM beads.

aggregate/disaggregate a target protein or shield it from proteolytic degradation, thus manipulating its cellular functionality. Stimuli-responsive polymers, other than PNIPAM, sensitive to pH, light, or other factors should further extend the versatility of polymeric actuators. Additional functionalities, such as local heating or sensing capabilities may be incorporated into such actuators by the addition of various NPs.

5.4 Conclusions

In this report we have emphasized the increasing potential offered by the multifunctionality derived from introducing multiple sites on QDs. Such reagents offer unique opportunities for combining different functions, such as sensing, targeting, cell penetration, and delivery. In addition, by taking advantage of the particular chemistry at the surface of NPs, "smart" actuators can be devised and employed. Further combination with programmable inorganic and organic materials that demonstrate properties responsive to manipulation of temperature, light, electric and magnetic fields, pH, and ionic strength will enable a still greater increase in design complexity and utility. A golden age of smart nanodevices and nanomachines is in sight.

Acknowledgments

This work was supported in part by the UBA, CONICET, ANPCyT, the Toxic Protein Conformation Project of the Max Planck Society, and the Nanomicroscopy Cluster of Excellence of the National Center of the Molecular Physiology of the Brain. EAJ is the head of a PartnerGruppe of the Max Planck Institute for Biophysical Chemistry.

References

[1] Cambi, A., et al., "Ligand-conjugated quantum dots monitor antigen uptake and processing by dendritic cells," *Nano Letters*, Vol. 7, No. 4, 2007, pp. 970–977.

[2] Fountaine, T. J., et al., "Multispectral imaging of clinically relevant cellular targets in tonsil and lymphoid tissue using semiconductor quantum dots," *Modern Pathology*, Vol. 19, No. 9, 2006, pp. 1181–1191.

[3] Li, Z. B., Cai, W., Chen, X. Y., "Semiconductor quantum dots for in vivo imaging [Review]," *Journal of Nanoscience & Nanotechnology*, Vol. 7, No. 8, 2007, pp. 2567–2581.

[4] Lidke, D. S.; D. J. Arndt-Jovin, "Imaging takes a quantum leap," *Review of Medical Physiology*, Vol. 19, 2004, pp. 322–325.

[5] Lidke, D. S., et al., "Reaching out for signals: filopodia sense EGF and respond by directed retrograde transport of activated receptors," *Journal of Cell Biology*, Vol. 170, 2005, pp. 619–626.

[6] Rhyner, M. N., et al., "Quantum dots and multifunctional nanoparticles: new contrast agents for tumor imaging [Review]," *Nanomedicine*, Vol. 1, No. 2, 2006, pp. 209–217.

[7] Pinaud, F., et al., "Advances in fluorescence imaging with quantum dot bio-probes," *Biomaterials*, Vol. 27, No. 9, 2006, pp. 1679–87.

[8] Gao, X., et al., "In vivo cancer targeting and imaging with semiconductor quantum dots," *Nature Biotechnology*, Vol. 22, No. 8, 2004, pp. 969–76.

[9] Lidke, D. S., et al., "Quantum dot ligands provide new insights into erbB/HER receptor-mediated signal transduction," *Nature Biotechnology*, Vol. 22, No. 2, 2004, pp. 198–203.

[10] Sperling, R., et al., "Electrophoretic Separation of Nanoparticles with a Discrete Number of Functional Groups," *Advanced Functional Materials* , Vol. 16, 2006, pp. 943–948.

[11] Sapsford, K. E., Berti, L., Medintz, I. L., "Materials for fluorescence resonance energy transfer analysis: Beyond traditional donor-acceptor combinations [Review]," *Angewandte Chemie-International Edition*, Vol. 45, No. 28, 2006, pp. 4562–4588.

[12] Sapsford, K. E., et al., "Sensors for detecting biological agents [Review]," *Materials Today*, Vol. 11, No. 3, 2008, pp. 38–49.

[13] Medintz, I. L., et al., "Quantum dot bioconjugates for imaging, labelling and sensing [Review]," *Nature Materials*, Vol. 4, No. 6, 2005, pp. 435–446.

[14] Lidke, K. A., et al., "The role of photon statistics in fluorescence anisotropy imaging," *IEEE Transactions of Image Processing*, Vol. 14, No. 9, 2005, pp. 1237–1245.

[15] Jaiswal, J. K., et al., "Long-term multiple color imaging of live cells using quantum dot bioconjugates," *Nature Biotechnology*, Vol. 21, 2003, pp. 47–51.

[16] Jaiswal, J. K., et al., "Use of quantum dots for live cell imaging," *Nature Methods*, Vol. 1, No. 1, 2004, pp. 73–78.

[17] Inoue, Y., et al., "In vivo fluorescence imaging of the reticuloendothelial system using quantum dots in combination with bioluminescent tumour monitoring," *European Journal of Nuclear Medicine & Molecular Imaging*, Vol. 34, No. 12, 2007, pp. 2048–2056.

[18] Echarte, M., et al., "Quantitative single particle tracking of NGF-receptor complexes: transport is bidirectional but biased by longer retrograde run lengths," *FEBS Letters*, Vol. 581, No. 16, 2007, pp. 2905–2913.

[19] Lidke, D. S., et al., "Imaging molecular interactions in cells by dynamic and static fluorescence anisotropy (rFLIM and emFRET)," *Biochemical Society Transactions,* Vol. 31, 2003, pp. 1020-1027.

[20] Lidke, D. S., et al., "Quantum dot ligands provide new insights into erbB/HER receptor-mediated signal transduction," *Nature Biotechnology*, Vol. 22, 2004, pp. 198–203.

[21] Susumu, K., et al., "Enhancing the stability and biological functionalities of quantum dots via compact multifunctional ligands," *Journal of the American Chemical Society*, Vol. 129, 2007, pp. 13987–13996.

[22] Grecco, H., et al., "Ensemble and single particle photophysical properties (two-photon excitation, anisotropy, FRET, lifetime, spectral conversion) of commercial quantum dots in solution and in live cells," *Microscopy Research and Technique*, Vol. 65, No. 4-5, 2005, pp. 169–179.

[23] Medintz, I. L., et al., "A fluorescence resonance energy transfer-derived structure of a quantum dot-protein bioconjugate nanoassembly," *Proceedings of the National Academy of Sciences of the United States of America*, Vol. 101, No. 26, 2004, pp. 9612–9617.

[24] Sigot, V.; T. Jovin, "Quantum Dot Torch Bearers into Cells. Dual Labeled Liposomes for EGFR Mediated Cellular Delivery," *Imaging and Microscopy*, Vol. 1, 2008, pp. 40–43.

[25] Derfus, A. M., et al., "Targeted quantum dot conjugates for siRNA delivery," *Bioconjugate Chemistry*, Vol. 18, No. 5, 2007, pp. 1391–1396.

[26] Thaxton, C. S., Georganopoulou, D. G., Mirkin, C. A., "Gold nanoparticle probes for the detection of nucleic acid targets [Review]," *Clinica Chimica Acta*, Vol. 363, No. 1-2, 2006, pp. 120–126.

[27] Chang, M. M. C., et al., "Nanotechnologies for biomolecular detection and medical diagnostics [Review]," *Current Opinion in Chemical Biology*, Vol. 10, No. 1, 2006, pp. 11–19.

[28] Harris, T. J., et al., "Proteolytic actuation of nanoparticle self-assembly," *Angewandte Chemie-International Edition*, Vol 45, 2006, pp. 3161–3165.

[29] von Maltzahn, G., et al., "Nanoparticle Self-Assembly Directed by Antagonistic Kinase and Phosphatase Activities," *Advanced Materials*, Vol. 19, 2007, pp. 3579–3583.

[30] Linse, S., et al., "Nucleation of protein fibrillation by nanoparticles," *Proceedings of the National Academy of Science USA*, Vol. 104, No. 21, 2007, pp. 8691–8696.

[31] Chandra, S., et al., "Alpha-synuclein cooperates with CSPalpha in preventing neurodegeneration," *Cell*, Vol. 123, No. 3, 2005, pp. 383–396.

[32] Roberti, M., et al., "Fluorescence imaging of amyloid formation in living cells by a functional, tetracysteine-tagged alpha-synuclein," *Nature Methods*, Vol. 4, No. 4, 2007, pp. 345–351.

[33] Spagnuolo, C., Vermeij, R., Jares-Erijman, E.,, "Improved Photostable FRET-Competent Biarsenical-Tetracysteine Probes Based on Fluorinated Fluoresceins," *Journal of the American Chemical Society*, Vol. 128, No. 37, 2006, pp. 12040–12041.

[34] Schild, H. G., "Poly (N-isopropylacrylamide) - experiment, theory and application," *Progress in Polymer Science,* Vol. 17, No., 1992, pp. 163–249.

[35] Shimoboji, T., et al., "Temperature-Induced Switching of Enzyme Activity with Smart Polymer-Enzyme Conjugates," *Bioconjugate Chemistry*, Vol. 14, 2003, pp. 517–525.

[36] Stayton, P. S., et al., "Control of protein-ligand recognition using a stimuli-responsive polymer," *Nature*, Vol. 378, 1995, pp. 472–474.

[37] Ionov, L., Stamm, M., Diez, S., "Reversible switching of microtubule motility using thermoresponsive polymer surfaces," *Nano Letters*, Vol. 6, No. 9, 2006, pp. 1982–1987.

[38] Pelah, A., T. M. Jovin, "Polymeric Actuators for Biological Applications," *ChemPhysChem*, Vol. 8, No. 12, 2007, pp. 1757–1760.

[39] Pelah, A., Seemann, R., Jovin, T. M., "Reversible cell deformation by a polymeric actuator," *Journal of the American Chemical Society*, Vol. 129, No. 3, 2007, pp. 468–469.

CHAPTER 6

Single Particle Investigation of Biological Processes Using QD-Bioconjugates

Thomas Pons and Hedi Mattoussi

6.1 Introduction

Single molecule detection has become a widely used tool for investigating a broad range of physical, chemical, and biological processes [1, 2]. Because ensemble measurements are macroscopic in nature, they provide only information about the average properties of a sample (e.g., average size, conformation, or orientation of proteins). In comparison, single molecule measurements are able to resolve molecular-scale heterogeneities and the fate of individual molecules. Fluorescence detection is a powerful, versatile, and relatively easy-to-use technique. When applied to single molecules, it gives access to valuable molecular-scale information. Single molecule (or particle) fluorescence is one of the most commonly used single molecule techniques in biological and biophysical research. The ability to detect fluorescence from single fluorophores, enabled by recent progress in optical detection techniques, has allowed the development of a variety of single molecule assays to study ligand-receptor binding, enzymatic activity, changes in macromolecular conformation and single biomolecule diffusion and transport.

Luminescent semiconductor nanocrystals, or quantum dots (QDs), are potentially superior alternatives to traditional organic fluorophores for an array of biological applications, including sensing and cell and tissue imaging [3, 4]. They exhibit high fluorescence quantum yields, a pronounced resistance to photo and chemical degradation, and high photobleaching thresholds [3–5]. These features are particularly appealing for single molecule fluorescence measurements, as QDs may be individually detected with high signal-to-noise ratios and for extended periods of time (several orders of magnitude longer than traditional organic dyes). QDs also exhibit narrow and tunable emission bands along with broad excitation spectra, which permit unambiguous discrimination of different single QD colors and make them particularly suitable for multiplexed fluorescence imaging. These properties combined have naturally led to their use as individual fluorophores in a wide range of biophysical studies.

In this chapter, we will describe some of the progress recently made using single molecule studies employing QD fluorophores and the ability of this technique to gain insights into specific biological processes. We will also discuss the advantages offered and limitations encountered by single QD fluorescence as an effective investigative tool in biology.

6.2 Physical Properties of Single QDs

In addition to the unique size and composition-dependent optical and spectroscopic properties described in Chapter 1 of this volume, colloidal luminescent QDs have another important characteristic that distinguishes them from organic fluorophores: intermittent photoemission (blinking) of individual nanocrystals. The photoluminescence of isolated QDs displays an alternation of "on" (emitting) and "off" (dark) periods, which durations follow a "heavy-tail" power law distribution with time [6, 7]. In particular, there is a nonvanishing probability for the QD to enter a long dark period. This feature becomes especially important for single molecule detection, since a QD will become periodically unavailable for detection. PL blinking is certainly one of the most discussed aspects of QDs and remains an active area of research, as its underlying mechanisms are not yet fully understood (e.g., see [8]). The total size of a QD varies from ~10 to ~50 nm, depending on the type of solubilization and functionalization technique used [3, 4]. This is significantly larger than the average size of an organic fluorophore and will strongly influence the QD-conjugate diffusion and its ability to access certain cellular compartments. Finally, the surface of a single QD often offers multiple functionalization sites, contrary to mono-functional dyes. The ability to conjugate several biomolecules on the surface of a single QD may be particularly advantageous in certain instances (e.g., when enhanced target affinity and energy transfer efficiency are desired). However, this multivalency may also be a limitation in other instances, especially when a strict one-to-one QD-biomolecule conjugation is required; extra purification steps are then necessary to discard QDs conjugated to multiple biomolecules. Overall, the different physical properties of QDs make them particularly attractive fluorescence probes in a wide variety of single molecule assays.

6.3 In Vitro Detection of Biomolecular Interactions Using Single QD Fluorescence

The ability to detect single QD photoemission with a good signal-to-noise ratio and for extended periods of time can benefit an array of in vitro biomolecular assays requiring either high detection sensitivity or data collection over long time intervals. It permits one to examine the properties of individual biomolecules separately from those averaged over macroscopic populations. Because virtually every photon emitted by a QD can be detected within a narrow emission band, the proportion of photons that are rejected by the detection spectral band is substantially reduced, which simplifies the spectral deconvolution of signals from different QD colors. This could be extremely beneficial to single molecule assays, where the number of detected photons is inherently low.

6.3.1 Detection of Biomolecules Using Multicolor Colocalization of QD Probes

The narrow and tunable emission of QDs has been exploited in developing multiplexed "sandwich" assays that rely on the simultaneous interactions of distinct color QD-bioconjugates, each binding to a different site on the same target molecule. For example, if two QDs with distinct emission spectra conjugated to two different DNA probes are mixed in a solution with a target DNA containing complementary sequences for both probes, the target hybridizes simultaneously to the two QD-DNA probes. This hybridization could then be detected optically on a microscope slide using wide field fluorescence microscopy, where simultaneous imaging of the signals from the two QD probes is measured. In [9], Wang and coworkers applied the detection strategy based on the multicolor colocalization of QDs to the genetic analysis of anthrax *pathogenicity*. Positive identification of this bacterium requires the simultaneous presence of three distinct genes, namely, rpoB, pagA, and capC. For this assay, the authors conjugated three pairs of target-specific DNA probes (combinatorially) to three distinct color QDs emitting at 525 nm, 605 nm, and 705 nm. As targets, they used three synthetic oligonucleotides, each derived from conserved sequences from each of the three anthrax-related genes; these were used as simulated targets (in a background of *E. coli* genomic DNA) for analysis. They first used the simultaneous fluorescence signals in the combined pseudocolors of the spots, namely, indigo, magenta, and orange, as an indication of the presence of rpoB, pagA, and capC, respectively (Figure 6.1(a)). They then carried out four sets of experiments, where the specificity of the assay was essentially defined by its

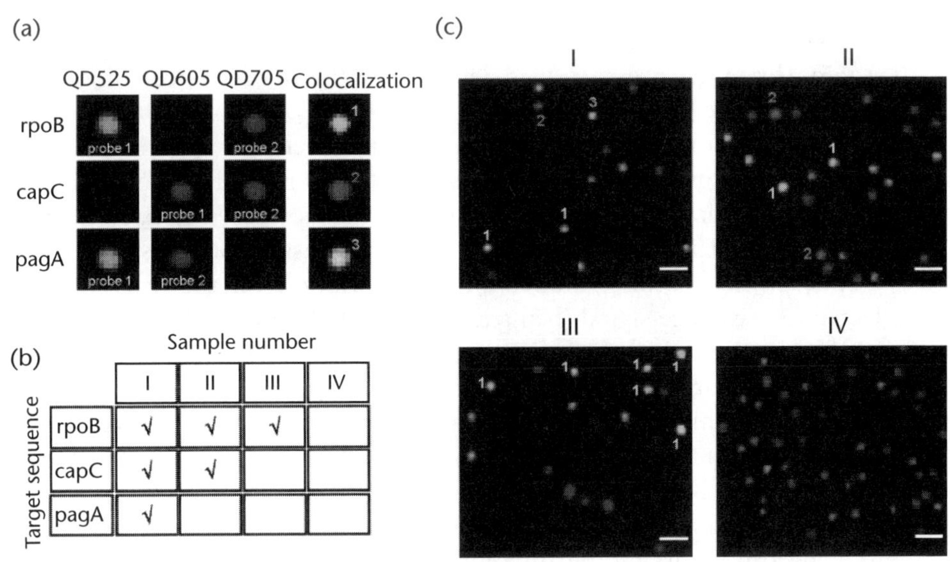

Figure 6.1 Simulated multiplexed analysis of anthrax-related genetic targets: (a) color pallet for the three pairs of target-specific QD nanoprobes and their resulting colocalized fluorescent images upon sandwich hybridization; (b) four samples containing different combinations of the three targets, rpoB, capC, and pagA. Checks represent the existence of certain target sequences. Sample IV does not contain any target and is used as a negative control. (c) Fluorescent images I, II, III, and IV correlate with samples I, II, III, and IV, respectively. (Bar dimension is 1 μm.). Reprinted by permission from the American Chemical Society [9]. (See Color Plate 11.)

capacity to correctly identify and quantify the individual target sequences in a complex mixture of various target combinations (Figure 6.1(b)). In the first experiment, fluorescent spots in all the three combined pseudocolors were detected, verifying the presence of the three targets in the solution (Figure 6.1(c), I). In the next two experiments, the presence of two (Figure 6.1(c), II) or only one (Figure 6.1(c), III) target was also unambiguously determined without false positive or negative results. In the fourth negative control sample, only fluorescent spots stemming from unhybridized blue, green, and red QD probes were observed (Figure 6.1(c), IV); in this particular sample, no specific target was present.

Alternatively, the sample could be injected into a small glass capillary and the QD signals could be detected sequentially as the solution is flowed through the observation volume [10]. In both cases, the size of the total target-DNA probe-QD complex is smaller than the optical resolution of the detection system, and the presence of the target could be detected by the colocalization of two distinct single QD fluorescence signals. This method is fast, as it occurs in solution phase rather than on a solid substrate and does not require separation of the unbound probes, since they are not colocalized. It allows identification of samples without prior polymerase chain reactions (PCRs) amplifications, which are not quantitative and can introduce nonnegligible errors. It also allows detection of low abundance targets and has a higher sensitivity than microbead assays in which weak target signals may be difficult to discriminate against the strong microbead coding signal. Its sensitivity has been demonstrated even in the presence of a strong nonspecific background (i.e., samples mixed with cell extracts) [10]. It could also be applied to more than two QD probe colors. For example, using 10 different QD colors could conceptually provide 45 different QD pair combinations. A similar assay has been demonstrated using QD-antibody conjugates binding different sites of the same target protein [10]. Again, the target presence was detected by the fluorescence colocalization of two different single QD probes.

Other reported assays using this format included QD-conjugate binding two extremities of individual DNA molecules that were stretched on a glass surface, and the identification of single large entities such as viruses or bacteria from different strains in a macroscopic mixture [9–13]. These assays often use QDs with spectrally distinct emissions conjugated to different antibodies. In the virus constructs, the collected fluorescence signal (being a mix of signals emitted by different QD-antibody conjugates bound onto a single scaffold) provided a spectral "bar code" that revealed the nature and number of proteins displayed on the virus surface. This has, for example, allowed a rapid identification of the virus strain [10]. We should emphasize that this assay format to identify viruses could be performed with organic fluorophores, but effective analysis requires complex spectra deconvolution and attendant data analysis. However, QDs offer advantages such as higher sensitivity and spectral unmixing (deconvolution), which enable the multiplexed detection of single small biomolecules carrying only a few fluorescent markers. A limitation to this type of assay, however, resides in the intermittent emission of QDs (blinking) and the related "dark," or nonemitting, QD fraction. This causes some colocalized QD probes to appear as isolated QDs and thus may introduce an unknown number of "false negative" counts.

6.3.2 Colocalization Studies Using Streptavidin-Coupled QD-Dye Pairs

In a seemingly similar study but drastically different in concept and goals, Webb and coworkers investigated the relationship between ensemble fluorescence quantum yields measured for macroscopic samples and the blinking properties of individual QDs [14]. The authors coupled streptavidin-functionalized 525-nm emitting QDs with biotin-functionalized Alexa Fluor 594 dye and used the fluorescence collected from dot and dye to distinguish between dark and bright freely diffusing single nanocrystals. This presents a different configuration from that of surface-immobilized QDs (e.g., dispersed in polymeric films). The bright fractions of QDs were measured by fluorescence coincidence analysis and two-photon fluorescence correlation spectroscopy. In particular, they reported that the bright fraction of QDs was proportional to the measured macroscopic quantum yields of the samples. However, brightness of individual QDs was constant across samples with different quantum yields. They then applied the same measurements to solutions with much higher viscosity, where nanocrystal residence time in the illuminated volume was substantially increased. Their findings clearly indicated that increasing the residence time by as much as tenfold did not change the fraction of "apparently dark" QDs, which they attributed to the presence of two populations of QDs in a sample: one dark nonemitting and one emitting; only the emitting fraction contributed to the measured macroscopic fluorescence yields. These findings are intriguing, but additional work is needed to better understand the correlation between single and ensemble fluorescence properties of QDs.

6.3.3 Fluorescence Energy Transfer from Single QD to Organic Fluorophores

Fluorescence resonance energy transfer (FRET) provides a unique tool to probe intermolecular association dynamics and intramolecular conformation changes in the 1–10-nm range [15, 16]. It relies on the nonradiative transfer of excitation energy from a fluorescent donor to a ground state proximal acceptor. The transfer efficiency strongly depends on the donor-acceptor separation distance and the spectral overlap between the donor emission and the acceptor absorption. FRET provides a powerful means for studying biomolecular interactions involved in drug screening or disease diagnosis and has been a widely used biophysical tool for studying protein and oligonucleotide conformation in vitro and in live cells using dye donor-dye acceptor FRET pairs. QDs offer a few unique advantages (compared to organic dyes) for use as FRET donors [17–19]. Their narrow emission bands can be tuned to precisely match the acceptor absorption spectrum and allow easy deconvolution of the donor and acceptor emissions. In addition, their broad absorption spectra allow excitation of the donor far from the acceptor absorption band, substantially reducing direct excitation contribution to the acceptor signal. Finally, because several acceptors may be conjugated to a single QD donor, the overall FRET rate can be substantially increased, a clear advantage especially with longer separation distances. The use of QD FRET donors has been demonstrated in ensemble assays for detecting DNA hybridization [20], enzyme activity [21], and for elucidating the structure of QD-protein assemblies [22]. Additional details on ensemble steady-state and time-resolved FRET using QD donors applied to biological systems can be found in Chapter 4 of this volume. There has been a strong interest in translating these assays to the single molecule level, which could provide higher sensitivity measurements while reducing materials consumption.

The most obvious single particle (sp-) FRET configuration would use immobilized QD-bioconjugates, which can allow one to collect and resolve time-dependent conformational changes at the single molecule level. In a recent report, single immobilized QD-oligonucleotide conjugates were used to probe DNA Holliday junction dynamics [23]. One of the characteristics of this four-DNA-strand assembly is that it is structurally polymorphic, and its conformation fluctuates between two different forms depending, for example, on salt concentration. At low salt concentration and in the absence of multivalent ions, the junction has an open form, which minimizes the repulsion between charged phosphates at the junction. When the salt concentration increases (or in the presence of multivalent cations), effects of electrostatic repulsions are reduced, and the junction folds into one of two stacked conformers. By labeling one of the DNA strands with a dye acceptor and the other with a QD, the authors showed that these conformational changes induce fluctuations in the FRET efficiency measured between the QD and dye. However, this type of surface-immobilized assay remains particularly difficult to implement due to the weak FRET efficiency for one QD-one dye pair, primarily due to the use of large multilayer functionalization and conjugation schemes (the case with some of the commercially available nanocrystals). Moreover, the intermittent and fluctuating nature of single QD emission remains an important obstacle to quantitatively monitoring the evolution of FRET efficiency with time.

These limitations can be circumvented by probing freely diffusing QD-bioconjugates in solution samples, which limits the specimen excitation to the residence time within the illuminated volume. It also reduces issues associated with intermittent emission and data collection and analysis. Experimentally, solution-phase single particle FRET configuration utilizes a confocal microscope and a laser excitation that provides a highly focused beam for specimen excitation (Figure 6.2). The collected signal consists of simultaneous bursts of PL intensities from the donor (QD), collected on the donor channel, I_D, and the acceptor (dye), collected on the acceptor channel, I_A, corresponding to Brownian diffusion of single QD conjugates in and out of the 3D-restricted confocal volume (see experimental step up, Figure 6.2). The spFRET signature consists of plotting the population fraction of events versus emission ratios, η, defined as $\eta = I_A/(I_A + I_D)$. For a control solution of QD donors only (absence of FRET), the population fraction versus η is reduced to a peak centered at $\eta = 0$. For QD-dye pairs, nonzero contribution from the acceptors due to energy transfer broadens the distribution peak and shifts it to higher η values (Figure 6.2). In what follows, we will describe a few representative examples where spFRET with QD-bioconjugates provided valuable and unique information.

6.3.3.1 spFRET Applied to DNA Hybridization

Zhang and coworkers showed that solution-phase spFRET applied to hybridization assays could allow detection of a target DNA sequence with high sensitivity [25] (Figure 6.3). A "reporter probe" carrying an organic dye acceptor and a biotinylated "capture probe" were mixed with the DNA sample to be analyzed. These two probes were designed to have complementary sequences to two different sections of

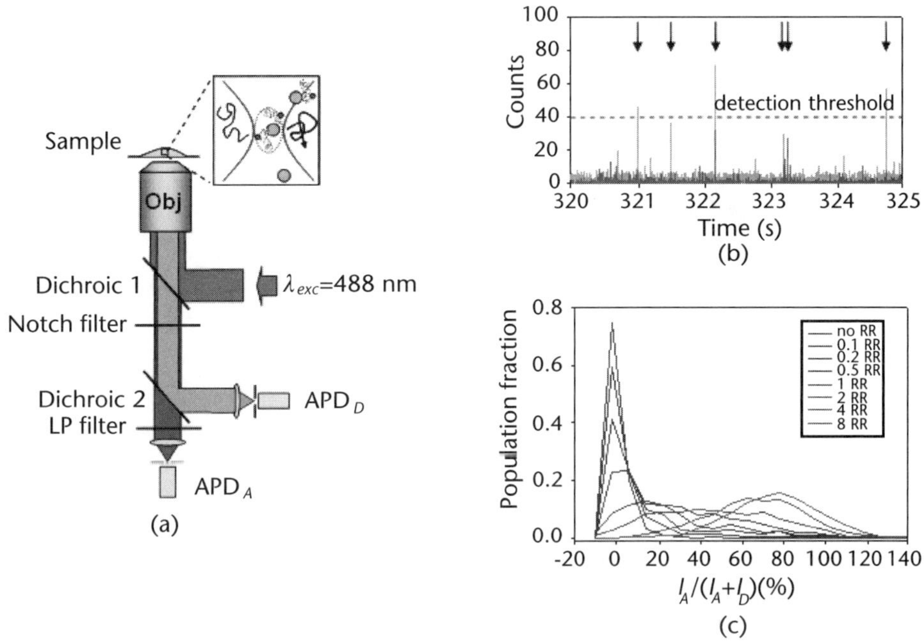

Figure 6.2 (a) Confocal microcopy setup used for implementing solution-phase spFRET. (b) A typical example of superimposed donor and acceptor time traces. Only the bursts with the sum of both signals exceeding the threshold level (indicated by arrows) can be used for analysis. (c) Emission ratio distributions obtained from spFRET measurements as a function of the acceptor-to-QD ratio. Reprinted by permission from the American Chemical Society, [24], © 2006.

the target sequence; they thus can simultaneously hybridize with the target DNA (as shown in Figure 6.3). As a consequence, in the presence of the target, a sandwich hybrid was formed between the capture probe, the reporter probe, and the target sequence. When mixed with streptavidin-coated QDs (commercially available), the sandwich structures bound to the QD surface, which brought several Cy5 in close proximity to the donor center in each conjugate. The sample containing the QD-sandwich complexes was then introduced in a glass capillary and flowed through a small observation volume where fluorescence signals from individual bioconjugates could be detected sequentially (Figure 6.3). Similar to multicolor colocalization assays, the presence of the target was detected by the simultaneous detection of QD emission (I_D) and Cy5 fluorescence (I_A), indicative of the QD-DNA complex formation. This assay has particularly high detection sensitivity (in terms of minimal detectable target concentration) compared to a molecular beacon assay employing organic dyes, due to two features specific to the QD-DNA assemblies. First, direct excitation contribution to the acceptor signal was extremely weak, because the system was excited in a region of minimal acceptor absorbance. As a result, the measured acceptor signal resulted only from FRET contribution, which reduced the detection background to a minimal level. Second, because the QDs were functionalized with several streptravidin groups, each QD-conjugate had several sandwich hybrids arrayed around the nanocrystal surface. This increased the local acceptor concentration around a single donor and allowed for high FRET effi-

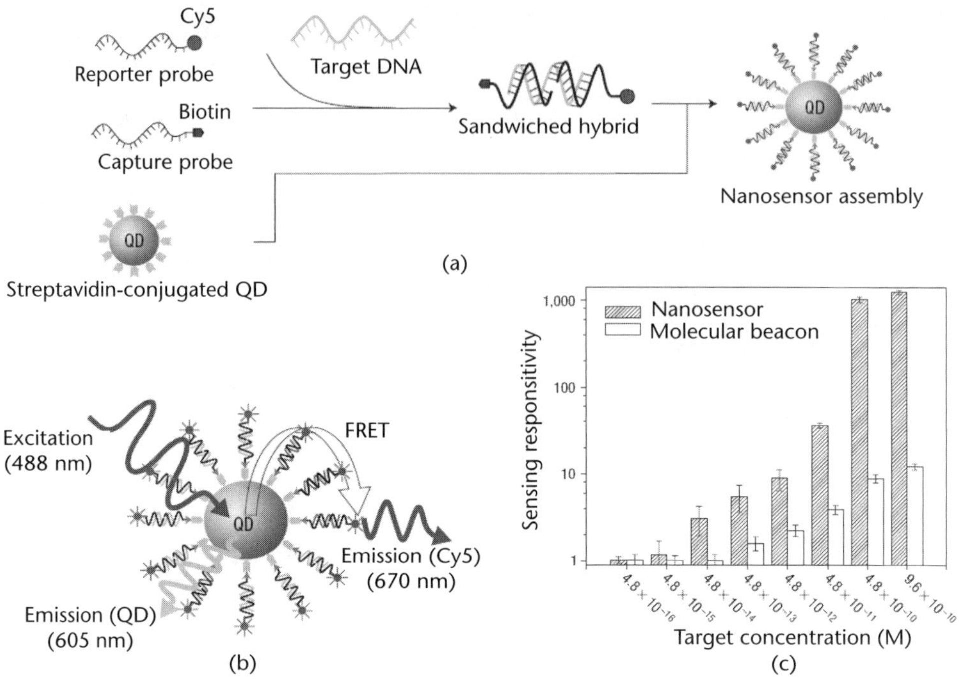

Figure 6.3 Schematic of single QD–based DNA nanosensors. (a) Conceptual scheme showing the formation of a sensing assembly in the presence of targets. (b) Fluorescence emission from Cy5 on illumination of QD caused by FRET between Cy5 acceptors and the QD donor in the assembly. (c) Sensing responsitivity at different target concentrations for nanosensors and molecular beacons. Reprinted by permission from Macmillan Publishers Ltd [25], © 2005.

ciency and bright acceptor fluorescence bursts, further enhancing the detection sensitivity. These QD sensors were successfully applied in conjunction with an oligonucleotide ligation assay to reach single nucleotide mutation detection [25]. In a similar assay, an increase in the flow velocity in the capillary was shown to slightly increase the average FRET efficiency [26]. This effect was attributed to the DNA deformation in the capillary stream that brought the dye acceptor in closer proximity to the QD donor.

In a subsequent study, Zhang and Johnson applied spFRET as a means to quantify the interactions between a specific peptide on the Rev protein (Rev-peptide) and the Rev responsive element within the RNA gene (RRE-RNA) and to identify and characterize potential inhibitors [27]. Interactions between the regulatory protein Rev and a portion of *env* gene within the RNA gene (RRE-RNA) are critical to HIV-1 replication. Rev peptide is a sequence from the basic region of Rev with reported high affinity to RRE. The authors demonstrated that the stoichiometry of Rev-peptide binding to RRE-RNA sequence can be accurately determined using such FRET-based single QD-RRE-RNA sensing assemblies (Figure 6.4). They further used this single particle configuration to potentially quantify the inhibitory effects of proflavin on the affinity between Rev-peptide and RRE. In particular, spFRET permitted them to quantify these inhibitory effects even in the presence of substantial levels of interference fluorescence from high-concentration proflavin;

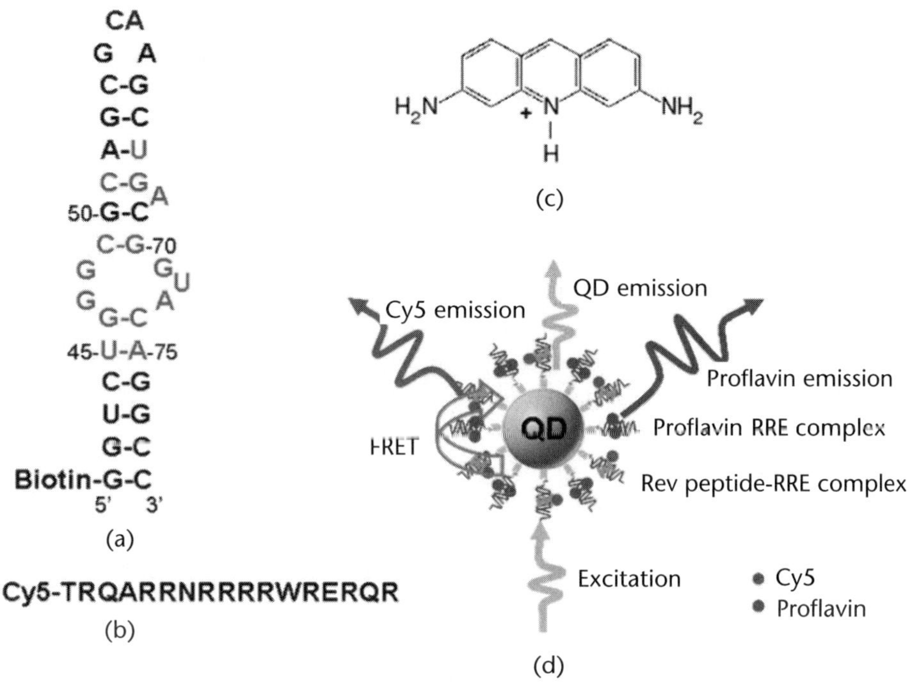

Figure 6.4 (a) Secondary structure of biotin-functionalized RRE IIB RNA. (b) Cy5-labeled Rev peptide used. (c) Proflavin chemical structure. (d) Schematic representation of the single-QD FRET-based sensing assembly utilized for evaluating Rev-peptide-RRE interaction along with the inhibitory efficacy of proflavin; commercial 605QD was used. Reprinted by permission from the American Chemical Society [27], © 2007.

the latter is a blue fluorescent compound that often prevents the discrimination of FRET signals in ensemble measurements. The main factors enabling efficient FRET from a QD donor to acceptors located at the other extremities of long double-stranded DNA and effective signal discrimination remained the high acceptor-to-donor ratio and the flexibility to choose the excitation wavelength far from the dye (and proflavin) absorption bands.

6.3.3.2 spFRET Applied to Determining QD-Bioconjugate Heterogeneity

In the second example, we used single-QD FRET to characterize the heterogeneity of self-assembled QD-bioconjugates and to gain information about the distribution in conjugate valence [24]. These conjugates were formed by attaching (via metal-affinity driven self-assembly) average numbers of maltose binding protein (MBPs) labeled with rhodamine red (RR) onto CdSe-ZnS QDs capped with dihydrolipoic acid (DHLA) ligands; the QDs served as exciton donors and scaffolds for arraying various numbers of dye-labeled proteins. The influence of the acceptor-to-donor ratio was examined by varying the ratio of acceptor dye labeled-to-unlabeled proteins while keeping the same total number of proteins conjugated around a single QD. This study showed that within a macroscopic homogeneous sample, heterogeneity in conjugate valence characterizes individual self-assembled QD-protein conjugates. More importantly it was shown that the number of acceptors per QD followed a Poisson distribution, where the probability of finding a conjugate having exactly n acceptors for sample with a nominal number of protein dye per QD, N, obeys the relation [24]:

$$p(N,n) = N^n \exp(-N)/n! \tag{6.1}$$

In particular, using the distribution plots shown in Figure 6.2(c), spFRET allowed us to determine the fraction of QD-conjugates having zero valence (i.e., QDs that are not conjugated to any MBP dye), $p(N,0)$, for a series of macroscopic samples with increasing nominal valence, N. This was extracted from a very narrow window in the distribution of population fraction centered at $\eta = 0$ (Figure 6.5). Data clearly showed that the zero valence population fraction ($p(N,0)$) decreased exponentially with increasing N, which agrees well with the prediction of (6.1). It is worth mentioning that this study also showed that single QD FRET measurements provided estimates of donor-acceptor separation distance that was compatible with ensemble measurements and the structure of the QD-protein conjugate. Additional details on applying these findings to QD-protein sensors can be found in [24].

6.4 In Vitro and In Vivo Tracking of Protein Using Single QDs

6.4.1 In Vitro Detection of Kinesin and Myosin Motor Movement

Single molecule tracking has played a crucial role in elucidating the characteristics of motor proteins, such as kinesin, myosin, and dynein, that are responsible for active intracellular transport of vesicles, organelles, and protein complexes (as cargos) along microtubules or actin filaments. A number of studies have used either polymer beads of a few hundreds nanometers in size or fluorescent organic dyes to follow the movement of individual motors; determine their velocity, the size, and rate of their steps; and provide unique insights into their structural properties (see, for example, [28, 29]). However, use of QDs to tag molecular motors, instead, could open up new possibilities to study their dynamic properties by extending the observation times, due to the high photobleaching thresholds compared to organic dyes; conventional fluorophores allow observation for only a few seconds to a few tens of seconds depending on the experimental conditions.

QDs have been used to label single fragments of actin or microtubule, the substrate on which the motors move. In these "sliding" assays, motors are adsorbed on a surface and then exposed to substrate fragments. The immobilized motors are able to bind these fragments and induce their transport across the surface. A first "proof-of-principle" study by Mansson and coworkers demonstrated the use of QDs to label actin filaments sliding on a surface of adsorbed myosin motors, where movement of actin filaments was tracked for several seconds [30]. It was then envisioned that the streptavidin-QDs used to label the actin filaments could also be used as anchor points (or a scaffold) to bind and transport large biotinylated cargos. In a more refined study Leduc and coworkers used single QDs to investigate the cooperative interactions between kinesin motors interacting with the same microtubule [31]. Kinesin motors were combined with fluorescent proteins before being immobilized

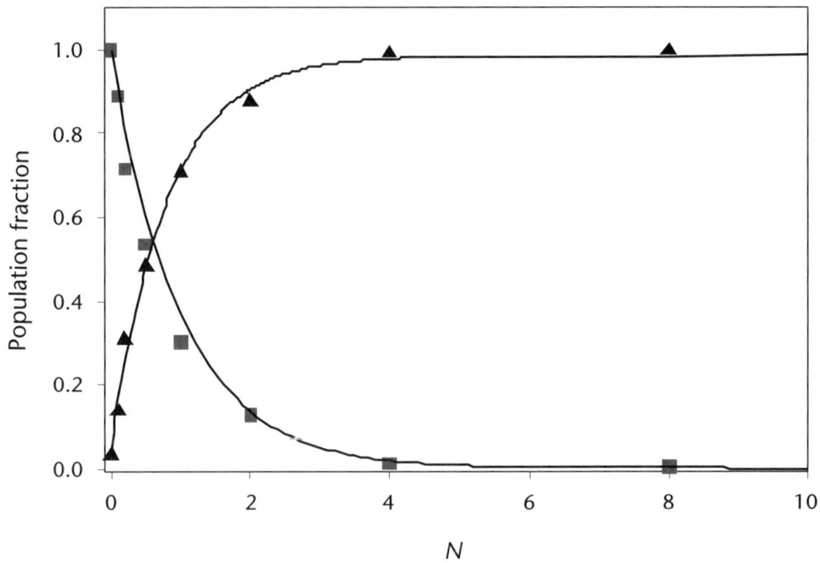

Figure 6.5 Fraction of QDs without any acceptors or "zero valence" ($\eta < 10$ percent; squares) and that engaged in FRET ($\eta > 15$ percent; triangles) as a function of N, the average number of RR acceptors per QD, obtained from spFRET measurements shown in Figure 6.2(c). The fits corresponds to the Poisson distribution $p(N,0) \sim \exp(-N)$ and $1-p(N,0)$. Reprinted by permission from the American Chemical Society [24], © 2006.

on a glass surface, so that their locations could be determined by fluorescence imaging. QD-labeled microtubules were then deposited on the kinesin-functionalized surface, and their motion was tracked by detecting the QD emission with a ~3-nm precision. By analyzing the motion, velocity, and step size of microtubules bound to one, two, or more motors, the authors showed the existence of fractional motion steps and the absence of synchronization between several kinesin motors interacting with the same microtubule.

QDs have also been used to label single motor proteins and track their motion with high precision. For example, individual kinesin motors were labeled with QDs, and their motion characteristics, such as velocity, step length, and dwell time, were determined under different conditions using single QD tracking [32]. In particular, the authors demonstrated that in the presence of obstacles or in crowded conditions, kinesin motors can wait on the microtubule in a strongly bound state. They postulated that this behavior could explain pauses in the motion of kinesin-transported cargos observed in living cells. In another study, the two heads of individual myosin V motors were labeled with two different QD colors [33]. Using two-color single QD tracking, the authors were able to locate the positions of the two heads with ~6-nm precision for several minutes, follow the motion of individual myosin molecules, and probe changes in their intramolecular conformation. They observed that the two heads move alternatively along the actin filament and that the heads were separated by 36 nm during pauses in motion, confirming the predictions of the hand-over-hand model of myosin mode of walking along an actin filament (Figure 6.6).

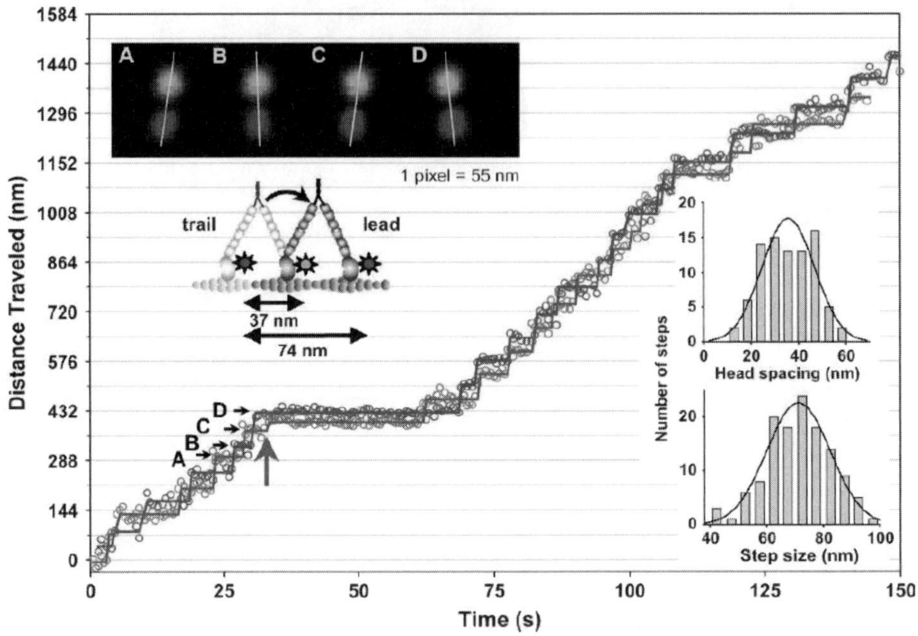

Figure 6.6 Myosin V processive runs with heads labeled with different color QDs. Green and red open circles are the two different QD positions determined by Gaussian fits. Solid lines are the average QD positions between steps, with the onset of steps determined by eye. Upper left are averaged QD images for steps labeled A–D. The yellow lines connect QD centers emphasizing alternating relative head positions. The green arrow identifies the substep. Lower right are histograms of interhead spacing and step size. Reprinted by permission from the Biophysical Society [33], © 2005. (See Color Plate 12.)

6.4.2 Tracking of Protein Receptors in Live Cells

Transposing single QD conjugate tracking from in vitro conditions to living cells has the potential to unravel complex biomolecular interactions underlying specific cellular activities. However, tracking of individual proteins in live cells using single QD fluorescence encounters difficulties that are often shared with other single particle tags (e.g., latex beads, gold nanoparticles, and so on) or single fluorophore tracking techniques. The first difficulty is caused by nonspecific interactions of QDs and their conjugates with their environment, either due to steric hindrance ("crowding" effects, limited access to particular cellular compartments, and so on) or to undesired adsorption of endogenous molecules onto the QD surface. The second major hurdle to the effective use of QDs for single molecule tracking in live cells derives from the difficulties of crossing of the plasma membrane and the delivery of isolated QD-conjugates into the cytoplasm. For these reasons, single QD tracking of receptor proteins in cell media have been successfully reported primarily for easily accessible targets. These include transmembrane proteins to investigate membrane-bound receptor diffusion or endosomal trafficking.

Spatial organization of the cellular membrane components (lipids, proteins, carbohydrates, and so on) plays a critical role in their interactions with other membrane components, and in the cell signaling and communication with the extracellular environment and surrounding tissue. Understanding when and how the cell reorganizes these membrane components is therefore a key challenge in the study of cellular activity. In particular, trafficking of neurotransmitter receptor proteins within membrane compartments and between membrane and intracellular space plays an important role in the regulation of neuronal activity. The QD resistance to photobleaching has given researchers the opportunity to track single transmembrane neurotransmitter receptors for long periods of time and led to a better understanding of receptor trafficking in neurons. Dahan and coworkers reported the first use of QD for single receptor tracking in cultured neurons in 2003 [34]. The authors labeled individual glycine receptors with single QD-streptavidin conjugates via primary and secondary antibodies. Single QDs were identified and tracked by their blinking properties. They observed a considerably higher fluorescence signal compared to standard fluorophores, resulting in a spatial resolution reaching 5–10 nm, compared with 40 nm with an organic dye. Even more impressing was the duration for which they were able to follow the trajectory of single QD-labeled receptors—more than 20 minutes, compared to ~5s for a standard organic fluorophore. This allowed the visualization of receptor trajectories on a time scale that was not accessible before and revealed new diffusion dynamics. In particular, the authors showed the existence of several membrane domains corresponding to synaptic, perisynaptic, and extrasynaptic regions with different receptor diffusion behaviors. Since then, numerous studies have since used QDs to track trajectories of individual membrane receptors, in neurons [35–39], or other cell types [40, 41]. Single QD tracking will likely become one of the methods of choice for studying transmembrane protein dynamics, accessible to both specialists and nonspecialists.

QDs have also given access to new information regarding endosomal trafficking of transmembrane receptors. A study by Lidke and coworkers in 2004 demonstrated that QDs conjugated to the epidermal growth factor (EGF) using streptavidin-biotin binding could be used to monitor the binding of EGF to specific membrane receptors and track their intracellular fate [42] (Figure 6.7). EGF-QDs were shown to correctly bind and activate the targeted erbB1 receptor, followed by

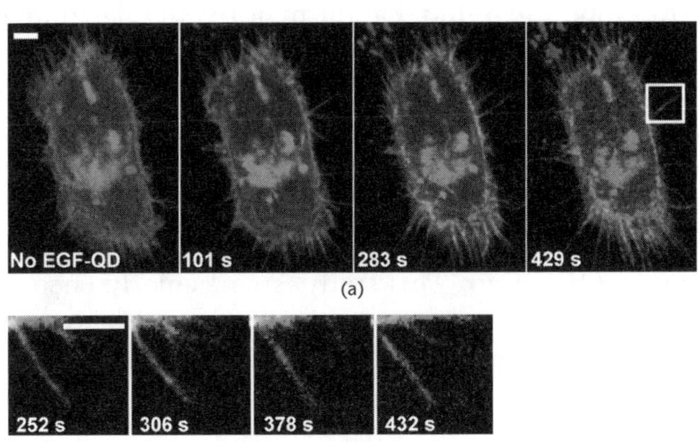

Figure 6.7 Retrograde transport of EGF-QDs (red) on filipodia. (a) A431 cell expressing receptor erbB3-mCitrine (green); maximum intensity projection of four 0.5-μm confocal sections as a function of time. (b) Magnified image of filipodium indicated in the last panel of (a), showing the uniform migration of the EGF-QDs toward the cell body with a velocity of ~10 nm/s. All scale bars, 5 μm. Reprinted by permission from Macmillan Publishers Ltd [42], © 2004. (See Color Plate 13.)

endocytotic uptake of the EGF-QD-receptor complex. The authors were then able to track the trajectories of individual EGF-QD-receptors and show the existence of a new retrograde transport mechanism in filopodia from the cell surface to the cell body. In a subsequent study, the authors used single EGF-QD tracking to examine the nature of this retrograde transport in detail [43]. In particular, analysis of single QD trajectories and their mean square displacements showed a behavior consistent with active transport and not a Brownian motion. The authors showed that this transport was supported by the actin network, as indicated by analysis of transport velocities and the effects of pharmacological agents. They next exposed the cells to two different colors of EGF-QD conjugates and observed that the onset of active transport correlated with merging of two EGF-QD conjugates. This showed that dimerization of EGF-activated receptors was necessary to trigger the active transport. Finally, they examined whether retrograde transport occurred before or after endocytosis of the EGF-QD-receptors conjugates using FRET between QD donors and organic dyes. Membrane-impermeable biotinylated dyes were able to bind the remaining biotin-binding sites on QD-EGF conjugates, resulting in efficient FRET, even after the onset of retrograde transport. This demonstrated that these conjugates were still available to the extracellular medium and that receptor endocytosis occurred only after retrograde transport along the filopodia, when reaching the cell body. In another study, Vu and coworkers used antibody-conjugated QDs to target specific membrane receptors to the nerve growth factor [44]. The authors showed that QDs allowed monitoring not only of the receptor cellular uptake, but also of its intracellular fate. QD-labeled receptor processing by the cells was consistent with that of unlabeled receptors, including active shuttling of QD-receptors conjugates to new neural processes.

Circumventing issues of effective transmembrane delivery of QD-bioconjugates, Courty and coworkers used osmotic lysis of pinosomes to deliver individual QD-kinesin motor conjugates into the cell cytoplasm. This mode of delivery involves exposure of the cells to first a hyper-osmotic solution to induce QD pinocytosis, then to a hypo-osmotic solution to break the pinosomes and release their content into the cytoplasm. The authors were then able to follow the QD trajectories over time and found that the majority of QD-conjugates exhibit trajectories typical of freely diffusing Brownian motion, but a smaller fraction (~ 10 percent) of conjugates exhibited a rather linear directed motion. This directed motion was never observed when using unconjugated QDs or when inhibiting kinesin motor transport by a chemically induced depolymerization of the actin filaments. When analyzing the directed motion of this fraction of QD-conjugates, the authors observed a velocity consistent with in vitro observations, which show that kinesin movement was not affected by its QD cargo. This study is particularly encouraging for future use of QDs to track individual biomolecules in the cytoplasm, even though systematic studies will be needed to validate this type of cellular delivery and to ensure the absence of nonspecific interactions of the QDs with the complex intracellular environment.

These studies, and others, clearly indicate that QDs may offer precious insights into intracellular trafficking of membrane receptors and reveal previously inaccessible transport mechanisms. In general, the main limitations of these techniques originate from the still relatively large size of the QD conjugates, which may influence the

QD-labeled protein diffusion in confined spaces like synaptic clefts or from nonspecific interactions with endogenous molecules. The size limitation adds constraints even to probing extracellular transmembrane protein tracking (e.g., due to the presence of large transmembrane carbohydrates). Blinking of QD fluorescence causes intermittent interruption of the reconstructed trajectories, but it appears that this is not a major obstacle to the use of QDs as long as the density of labeled receptors is low enough that the same QD can be identified again during the next emitting period. However, it may be necessary to correct quantitative transport measurements from QD blinking effect in certain applications [45].

6.5 Conclusion

QDs are finding increasing utility in a variety of applications, including biological sensing and imaging, due to several unique intrinsic photophysical properties. By allowing easy measurements with high signal-to-noise ratios and extended observation times, QDs have also opened up new possibilities for studying biomolecular interactions at the single molecule level. For example, they allowed tracking of single biomolecule trajectories over several tens of minutes with high signal-to-noise ratios and consequently high spatial resolution. The set of single molecule studies summarized in this chapter constitute only a fraction of what use of luminescent QDs promises in biology. These materials have the potential not only to improve existing single biomolecule assays, but more importantly to provide previously inaccessible information about biomolecular interactions, as has been demonstrated in a few preliminary in vitro and live cell studies. Optical techniques for the tracking of single molecules, in particular, will continue to benefit from using QDs [45-47], as further progress will potentially bring even better spatial and temporal resolution of reconstructed trajectories in living cells.

However, further progress will be required in several domains to take advantage of the full potential of QDs use in single molecule studies. In particular, more systematic studies are needed to characterize the effects of surface coating and conjugation strategies on the long-term stability of hydrophilic QDs and QD-bioconjugates in buffers and in intracellular environments. These issues are further discussed in Chapter 1 of this volume. Intracellular compartments are complex and usually rich in ionic materials, and nonspecific interactions often affect the QD movements in these media. Since QDs offer real advantages for single molecule studies compared to other fluorescent markers, we can expect that as the surface properties, stability, and conjugation strategies continue to progress, single molecule assays using QDs will ultimately transition from proof-of-principles performed by specialists to general use by a broad biological and biophysical community.

Acknowledgments

We acknowledge NRL, the Office of Naval Research, Army Research Office, and DTRA for financial support.

References

[1] Deniz, A.A., T.A. Laurence, M. Dahan, et al., "Ratiometric single-molecule studies of freely diffusing biomolecules." *Annual Review of Physical Chemistry*, Vol. 52, No. 2001, pp. 233-253.

[2] Xie, X.S. and J.K. Trautman, "Optical Studies of Single Molecules at Room Temperature." *Annual Review of Physical Chemistry*, Vol. 49, No. 1998, pp. 441-480.

[3] Medintz, I.L., H.T. Uyeda, E.R. Goldman, et al., "Quantum dot bioconjugates for imaging, labelling and sensing." *Nature Materials*, Vol. 4, No. 6, 2005, pp. 435-446.

[4] Michalet, X., F.F. Pinaud, L.A. Bentolila, et al., "Quantum dots for live cells, in vivo imaging, and diagnostics." *Science*, Vol. 307, No. 5709, 2005, pp. 538-544.

[5] Jaiswal, J.K., H. Mattoussi, J.M. Mauro, et al., "Long-term multiple color imaging of live cells using quantum dot bioconjugates." *Nature Biotechnology*, Vol. 21, No. 1, 2003, pp. 47-51.

[6] Nirmal, M., B.O. Dabbousi, M.G. Bawendi, et al., "Fluorescence intermittency in single cadmium selenide nanocrystals." *Nature*, Vol. 383, No. 6603, 1996, pp. 802-804.

[7] Kuno, M., D.P. Fromm, H.F. Hamann, et al., "Nonexponential "blinking" kinetics of single CdSe quantum dots: A universal power law behavior." *Journal of Chemical Physics*, Vol. 112, No. 7, 2000, pp. 3117-3120.

[8] Kuno, M., D.P. Fromm, S.T. Johnson, et al., "Modeling distributed kinetics in isolated semiconductor quantum dots." *Physical Review Letters B*, Vol. 67, No. 2003, pp. 125304.

[9] Ho, Y.P., M.C. Kung, S. Yang, et al., "Multiplexed hybridization detection with multicolor colocalization of quantum dot nanoprobes." *Nano Letters*, Vol. 5, No. 9, 2005, pp. 1693-1697.

[10] Agrawal, A., C.Y. Zhang, T. Byassee, et al., "Counting single native biomolecules and intact viruses with color-coded nanoparticles." *Analytical Chemistry*, Vol. 78, No. 4, 2006, pp. 1061-1070.

[11] Crut, A., B. Geron-Landre, I. Bonnet, et al., "Detection of single DNA molecules by multicolor quantum-dot end-labeling." *Nucleic Acids Research*, Vol. 33, No. 11, 2005, pp.

[12] Edgar, R., M. McKinstry, J. Hwang, et al., "High-sensitivity bacterial detection using biotin-tagged phage and quantum-dot nanocomplexes." *Proceedings of the National Academy of Sciences of the United States of America*, Vol. 103, No. 13, 2006, pp. 4841-4845.

[13] Hahn, M.A., J.S. Tabb, and T.D. Krauss, "Detection of single bacterial pathogens with semiconductor quantum dots." *Analytical Chemistry*, Vol. 77, No. 15, 2005, pp. 4861-4869.

[14] Yao, J., D.R. Larson, H.D. Vishwasrao, et al., "Blinking and nonradiant dark fraction of water-soluble quantum dots in aqueous solution." *Proceedings of the National Academy of Sciences of the United States of America*, Vol. 102, No. 2005, pp. 14284-14289.

[15] Deniz, A.A., M. Dahan, J.R. Grunwell, et al., "Single-pair fluorescence resonance energy transfer on freely diffusing molecules: Observation of Förster distance dependence and subpopulations." *Proceedings of the National Academy of Sciences of the United States of America*, Vol. 96, No. 1999, pp. 3670-3675.

[16] Ha, T., T. Enderle, D.F. Ogletree, et al., "Probing the interaction between two single molecules: fluorescence resonance energy transfer between a single donor and a single acceptor." *Proceedings of the National Academy of Sciences of the United States of America*, Vol. 93, No. 1996, pp. 6264-6268.

[17] Clapp, A.R., I.L. Medintz, and H. Mattoussi, "Forster resonance energy transfer investigations using quantum-dot fluorophores." *Chemphyschem*, Vol. 7, No. 1, 2006, pp. 47-57.

[18] Clapp, A.R., I.L. Medintz, J.M. Mauro, et al., "Fluorescence resonance energy transfer between quantum dot donors and dye-labeled protein acceptors." *Journal of the American Chemical Society*, Vol. 126, No. 1, 2004, pp. 301-310.

[19] Sapsford, K.E., L. Berti, and I.L. Medintz, "Materials for fluorescence resonance energy transfer analysis: Beyond traditional donor-acceptor combinations." *Angewandte Chemie International Edition*, Vol. 45, No. 28, 2006, pp. 4562-4588.

[20] Medintz, I.L., A.R. Clapp, H. Mattoussi, et al., "Self-assembled nanoscale biosensors based on quantum dot FRET donors." *Nature Materials*, Vol. 2, No. 9, 2003, pp. 630-638.

[21] Medintz, I.L., A.R. Clapp, F.M. Brunel, et al., "Proteolytic activity monitored by fluorescence resonance energy transfer through quantum-dot-peptide conjugates." *Nature Materials*, Vol. 5, No. 7, 2006, pp. 581-589.

[22] Medintz, I.L., J.H. Konnert, A.R. Clapp, et al., "A fluorescence resonance energy transfer-derived structure of a quantum dot-protein bioconjugate nanoassembly." *Proceedings of the National Academy of Sciences of the United States of America*, Vol. 101, No. 26, 2004, pp. 9612-9617.

[23] Hohng, S. and T. Ha, "Single-molecule quantum-dot fluorescence resonance energy transfer." *Chemphyschem*, Vol. 6, No. 5, 2005, pp. 956-960.

[24] Pons, T., I.L. Medintz, X. Wang, et al., "Solution Phase Single Quantum Dot Fluorescence Resonance Energy Transfer." *Journal of the American Chemical Society*, Vol. 128, No. 47, 2006, pp. 15324-15331.

[25] Zhang, C.Y., H.C. Yeh, M.T. Kuroki, et al., "Single-quantum-dot-based DNA nanosensor." *Nature Materials*, Vol. 4, No. 11, 2005, pp. 826-831.

[26] Zhang, C.Y. and L.W. Johnson, "Quantum dot-based fluorescence resonance energy transfer with improved FRET efficiency in capillary flows." *Analytical Chemistry*, Vol. 78, No. 15, 2006, pp. 5532-5537.

[27] Zhang, C.Y. and L.W. Johnson, "Quantifying RNA-Peptide Interaction by Single-quantum Dot-Based Nanosensor: An Approach for Drug Screening." *Analytical Chemistry*, Vol. 79, No. 2007, pp. 7775-7781.

[28] Saxton, M. and K. Jacobson, "Single-Particle Tracking: Applications to Membrane Dynamics." *Annual Reviews - Biophysics and Biomolecular Structure*, Vol. 26, No. 1997, pp. 373.

[29] Ueda, M., Y. Sako, T. Tanaka, et al., "Single-Molecule Analysis of Chemotactic Signaling in Dictyostelium Cells." *Science*, Vol. 294, No. 2001, pp. 864.

[30] Mansson, A., M. Sundberg, M. Balaz, et al., "In vitro sliding of actin filaments labelled with single quantum dots." *Biochemical and Biophysical Research Communication*, Vol. 314, No. 2, 2004, pp. 529-534.

[31] Leduc, C., F. Ruhnow, J. Howard, et al., "Detection of fractional steps in cargo movement by the collective operation of kinesin-1 motors." *Proceedings of the National Academy of Sciences of the United States of America*, Vol. 104, No. 26, 2007, pp. 10847-10852.

[32] Seitz, A. and T. Surrey, "Processive movement of single kinesins on crowded microtubules visualized using quantum dots." *EMBO Journal*, Vol. 25, No. 2, 2006, pp. 267-277.

[33] Warshaw, D.M., G.G. Kennedy, S.S. Work, et al., "Differential Labeling of myosin V heads with quantum dots allows direct visualization of hand-over-hand processivity." *Biophysical Journal*, Vol. 88, No. 5, 2005, pp. L30-L32.

[34] Dahan, M., S. Levi, C. Luccardini, et al., "Diffusion dynamics of glycine receptors revealed by single-quantum dot tracking." *Science*, Vol. 302, No. 5644, 2003, pp. 442-445.

[35] Bats, C., L. Groc, and D. Choquet, "The interaction between stargazin and PSD-95 regulates AMPA receptor surface trafficking." *Neuron*, Vol. 53, No. 5, 2007, pp. 719-734.

[36] Bouzigues, C. and M. Dahan, "Transient directed motions of GABA(A) receptors in growth cones detected by a speed correlation index." *Biophysical Journal*, Vol. 92, No. 2, 2007, pp. 654-660.

[37] Bouzigues, C., M. Morel, A. Triller, et al., "Asymmetric redistribution of GABA receptors during GABA gradient sensing by nerve growth cones analyzed by single quantum dot imaging." *Proceedings of the National Academy of Sciences of the United States of America*, Vol. 104, No. 27, 2007, pp. 11251-11256.

[38] Charrier, C., M.V. Ehrensperger, M. Dahan, et al., "Cytoskeleton regulation of glycine receptor number at synapses and diffusion in the plasma membrane." *Journal of Neuroscience*, Vol. 26, No. 33, 2006, pp. 8502-8511.

[39] Ehrensperger, M.V., C. Hanus, C. Vannier, et al., "Multiple association states between glycine receptors and gephyrin identified by SPT analysis." *Biophysical Journal*, Vol. 92, No. 10, 2007, pp. 3706-3718.

[40] Chen, H.F., I. Titushkin, M. Stroscio, et al., "Altered membrane dynamics of quantum dot-conjugated integrins during osteogenic differentiation of human bone marrow derived progenitor cells." *Biophysical Journal*, Vol. 92, No. 4, 2007, pp. 1399-1408.

[41] Haggie, P.M., J.K. Kim, G.L. Lukacs, et al., "Tracking of quantum dot-labeled CFTR shows near immobilization by C-terminal PDZ interactions." *Molecular Biology of the Cell*, Vol. 17, No. 12, 2006, pp. 4937-4945.

[42] Lidke, D.S., P. Nagy, R. Heintzmann, et al., "Quantum dot ligands provide new insights into erbB/HER receptor-mediated signal transduction." *Nature Biotechnology*, Vol. 22, No. 2, 2004, pp. 198-203.

[43] Lidke, D.S., K.A. Lidke, B. Rieger, et al., "Reaching out for signals: filopodia sense EGF and respond by directed retrograde transport of activated receptors." *Journal of Cell Biology*, Vol. 170, No. 4, 2005, pp. 619–626.

[44] Rajan, S.S. and T.Q. Vu, "Quantum dots monitor TrkA receptor dynamics in the interior of neural PC12 cells." *Nano Letters*, Vol. 6, No. 9, 2006, pp. 2049-2059.

[45] Durisic, N., A.I. Bachir, D.L. Kolin, et al., "Detection and correction of blinking bias in image correlation transport measurements of quantum dot tagged macromolecules." *Biophysical Journal*, Vol. 93, No. 4, 2007, pp. 1338-1346.

[46] Brokmann, X., M.V. Ehrensperger, J.P. Hermier, et al., "Orientational imaging and tracking of single CdSe nanocrystals by defocused microscopy." *Chemical Physics Letters*, Vol. 406, No. 1-3, 2005, pp. 210-214.

[47] Lagerholm, B.C., L. Averett, G.E. Weinreb, et al., "Analysis method for measuring submicroscopic distances with blinking quantum dots." *Biophysical Journal*, Vol. 91, No. 8, 2006, pp. 3050-3060.

CHAPTER 7

Assessment of the Issues Related to the Toxicity of Quantum Dots

Françoise M. Winnik and Dusica Maysinger

7.1 Introduction

With the exciting possibilities offered by quantum dots (QDs) in clinical applications, the potential toxicity of QDs has become a serious concern. To date there is not sufficient information available in the literature or unanimous consent on whether or not QDs induce harmful effects when they are introduced into biological systems. However, in the past few years there has been a number of important investigations on the safety of QDs pointing out some key factors that may contribute to the harmful interactions of QDs with cells in vivo and in vitro. In view of their size, QDs belong to a class of materials known as *engineered nanomaterials* that are under investigation by regulatory agencies worldwide regarding hazard identification. Several reviews on the potential detrimental health effects of nanoparticles and on screening strategies have appeared recently and should be consulted by readers wishing to gain insights into the burgeoning field of nanotoxicity and its implications in engineering, research, and health management [1–5].

In his toxicologic review of QDs published in 2006, Hardman offers an excellent introduction to the complexity of the problem [6]. He stressed that the extent of cytotoxicity depends on a number of factors related not only to the physicochemical properties of the particles but also to the modalities of their use. A large section of a 2008 review by Lewinski et al. on the cytotoxicity of nanoparticles is devoted to semiconductor nanoparticles [7]. It provides a list of the experimental setups and results on CdSe and CdTe QDs reported from 2002 to 2007, including data on cell lines, conditions of exposures, assays employed, and surface characteristics of the QDs. This information is very useful, since cell type and cell status at the time of QD exposure critically influence the extent of QD-induced cell toxicity. All these biological variables together with the richness of QDs in terms of chemistry and breadth of applications have led to confusing and sometimes contradictory statements on QD-induced toxicity. Our objective in this review is to help the reader in identifying the risks involved with the use of QDs and in designing protocols that will eliminate undesirable side effects, or at least minimize them, within the context of a specific application. The review examines first the routes of exposure to QDs and the mechanisms of their cellular internalization. This section includes a brief description of common in vitro assays of cellular damage. Then, we expose the experimental evidence of cellular damage induced by QDs via four mechanistic pathways: (1) release of toxic metal ions; (2) release of capping material; (3) production of reactive oxygen species (ROS); and (4) genomic and epigenomic damage. A final section is devoted to the current status on QD bioaccumulation and clearance in vivo.

7.2 General Considerations

7.2.1 Routes of Exposure

Given that QDs show great promise as medical imaging agents, exposure resulting from administration to patients for medicinal purpose is of greatest concern, at least theoretically, since no QD product is currently approved for diagnostics or therapeutic purposes. A majority of the studies on the potential toxicity of QDs were designed such that they model this putative administrative route of exposure for humans, as will be described later. Nonetheless, it is important to assess incidental or accidental modes of exposure, such as those met in the workplace by researchers, engineers, or clinicians, who may be exposed to QDs by inhalation, through dermal contact, or by accidental ingestion. Most protocols currently in use for synthesis of QDs are solvent based and require handling of solutions. Little is known on the conditions under which QDs may form aerosols or whether they form aggregates in air. Guidelines to assess the risks of QD inhalation are provided by the large body of work on the health effects of exposure to airborne nanoparticles similar to QDs in term of their size (mineral dust particles, silicates, and so on) [1, 8, 9]. Topical exposure, either accidental or through cosmetic applications, provides another potential route of entry.

A study by confocal microscopy has revealed that QDs can penetrate the stratum corneum of intact porcine skin and localize within the epidermal and dermal layers after 8 to 24 hours of exposure [10]. The study encompassed QDs of different sizes and shapes (spherical 4.6 nm in diameter and ellipsoidal 12 nm × 6 nm) with neutral (PEG), anionic (COO^-), and cationic ($PEG\text{-}NH_2$) coatings. Localization of QDs in the epidermal layers was confirmed in all cases after a 24-hour exposure, but the kinetics of penetration depended on the QDs characteristics. Furthermore, the group showed that anionic and cationic QDs, but not neutral QDs, are internalized by epidermal keratinocytes (HEK cells) and localize in the cytoplasm and the nucleus [11, 12]. Intradermal (ID) injection of CdSe/ZnS core/shell nanoparticles coated with poly(ethylene glycol) (PEG) emitting at 621 nm with a diameter of 37 nm was performed into female SKH-1 hairless mice as a model system for determining tissue localization following intradermal infiltration [13]. The QDs remained as a deposit in skin and penetrated the surrounding viable subcutis. They were distributed to draining lymph node, to the liver, and to other organs.

Nanoparticle exposure through contaminated environmental media is also of concern, given the large range of possible applications, which may necessitate sizeable production volume of these nanoproducts. Most QD metals (e.g., Cd, Te, and Se) are known to be toxic to vertebrates at low concentration (ppm); thus, degradation of QDs upon storage in the dark or under photolytic conditions could have harmful environmental consequences. Unfortunately, little is known on the stability of QDs subjected to environmental transformations. Contaminations of the environment could occur via streams polluted with waste matter originating from manufacturing or clinical settings [14]. Proper procedures for the disposal of QD-containing waste should be established in order to minimize the risk of environmental contamination, as numerous studies described later have confirmed that many cell types are able to internalize QDs.

7.2.2 Mechanisms of Cellular Internalization of QDs

Different cellular uptake mechanisms may contribute to the internalization of QDs (Figure 7.1). The relevance of each pathway depends on the physicochemical properties of the QDs (e.g., size, surface charge, coating, ligands, and aggregation status) and on the exposed cell type. For cells from the immune system, such as macrophages, uptake of nanoparticles occurs via phagocytosis, a process through which particles are engulfed by the membrane receptors leading to the formation of phagosomes [15, 16]. The translocation mechanism available to all cells is endocytosis, a term that encompasses several distinct mechanisms and eventually leads to the formation of intracellular vesicles, the endosomes, which are led to various cell compartments [17, 18]. Nanoparticles that cannot be used by the cells are trafficked to acidic compartments (the lysosomes, pH ~ 5) or to the peroxisomes, which provide a highly oxidative environment favoring degradation of the particles [19]. Examples of specific endocytotic processes include pinocytosis, which involves the formation of macropinosomes that mature and form lysosomes. Clathrin-mediated endocytosis occurs at specific locations of the membrane known as clathrin-coated pits and yields intermediate vesicles, which are processed by early endosomes and late endosomes. Nonclathrin and noncaveolae-mediated endocytosis are also available to cells. For example, particles may be internalized via so-called lipid rafts. Internalization of nanoparticles by simple diffusion, a pas-

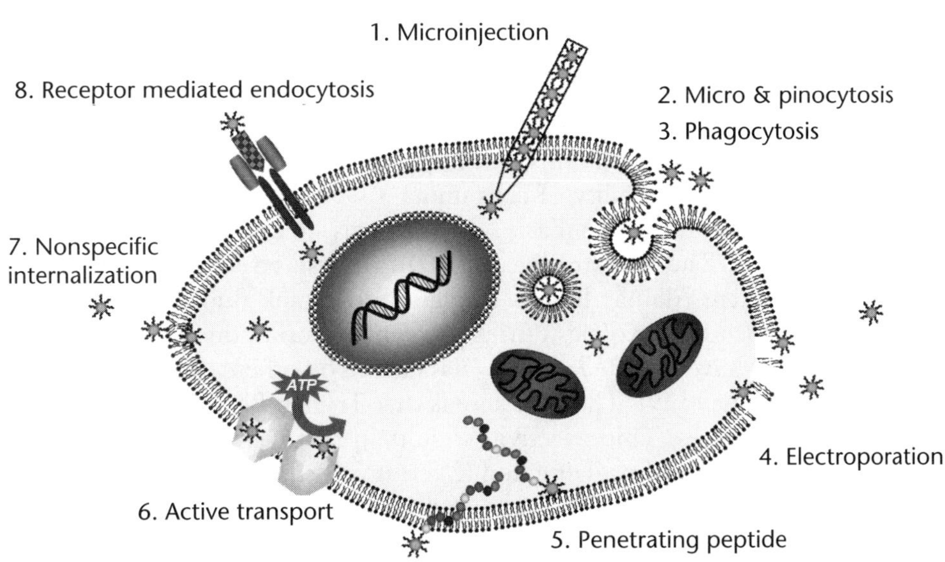

Figure 7.1 Cellular uptake mechanisms available for the internalization of quantum dots. (See Color Plate 14.)

sive process, may also account for nanoparticle entry into cells. Recently, an active transport of nonfunctionalized QDs was also reported [20].

Several or all of the internalization processes are available to nanoparticles as they come in contact with live cells [21]. The selection of the most probable mechanism of entry depends on factors such as (1) the physicochemical properties of the particles, in particular their size, shape, surface chemistry, and aggregation state; (2) the experimental conditions of the in vitro or in vivo assay, which will affect the nanoparticle indirectly via processes such as opsonization by serum components or modifications by proteins or lipids; and (3) the characteristics of the cell ("professional" phagocytes or not, normal versus "cancerous" cells, differentiation status). The interaction of a given nanoparticle with a cell and the final outcome of the exposure are dictated by these factors as a whole. To conduct mechanistic investigations on the cytotoxicity of nanoparticles, it is necessary to control as many parameters as possible in order to clarify the relation between the uptake mechanism and subsequent cellular distribution pattern of the particles and monitor which cellular pathways are triggered by internalized nanoparticles.

7.2.3 Detection of QD-Induced Cytotoxicity

The first in vivo studies aimed at demonstrating the exceptional imaging capabilities of QDs did not indicate marked cytotoxic effects [22]. Yet in vitro investigations provided evidence of cytotoxicity, raising the question of the relevance of in vitro tests in the context of QDs evaluation for in vivo applications. Nonetheless cell culture assays need to be conducted in order to minimize unnecessary in vivo experiments and to gain mechanistic information. In the following section, we describe briefly the assays commonly employed in studies addressing the question of QD cytotoxicity in order to help the reader to appreciate the limitations of each technique.

In a large number of studies, conclusions are drawn from colorimetric assays, such as the MTT viability assay, aimed at distinguishing between live and dead cells. In this test, a yellow dye, 3-(4,5-dimethylzol-2-yl)-2,5-diphenyl tetrazolium bromide (MTT), is converted into a dark blue formazan dye upon reaction with mitochondrial dehydrogenase enzymes [23, 24]. This conversion occurs only in live cells. Hence, the production of formazan, quantified by its absorbance at 492 nm, can be correlated to the viability of cells under a given set of conditions. The WST-1 and WST-8 tests function similarly, on the basis of different water-soluble formazan dyes [25, 26]. The Alamar Blue (or resazurin) test is a colorimetric assay in which the nonfluorescent Alamar Blue is converted to a pink fluorescent dye by NADP and FADH-dependent enzymes during oxygen consumption in healthy cells [27, 28]. A few studies have reported viability data based on other tests, such as the Trypan Blue exclusion assay [29]. The idea here is that Trypan Blue only enters cells with damaged membranes. This selectivity results in two cell populations: (1) stained cells that are either dead or dying and (2) clear cells that are alive with uncompromised membranes. This assay is widely used in biology due to its simplicity.

Viability assays yield no information on sublethal effects of QDs that may have implications in the longer timeframe or that may help in elucidating mechanistic pathways. A number of tests have been developed to assess such damages. For instance, the glutathione assay detects levels of glutathione (GSH) using Ellman's reagent (5,5'-dithio-bis-2-nitrobenzoic acid, DTNB), which reacts with thiol groups to produce yellow 5-thio-2-nitrobenzoic acid (TNB) and oxidized glutathione (GSSG) [30, 31]. The production of TNB is measured from the absorbance (405 or 412 nm), and these concentrations are correlated to the concentration of GSH in the sample. Peroxidation of membrane lipids is assessed by specific assays, such as the thiobarbituric (TBA) test, which detects the formation of a lipid-peroxidation byproduct known to form a fluorescent pink dye upon treatment with TBA (heat in acidic conditions) [32]. The fluorescent dye BODIPY-581/591 C_{11} is a lipid dye that inserts into lipid membranes. It allows the quantification of oxidized versus nonoxidized lipids, using the ratio of green to red fluorescence intensity, which scales with the ratio of oxidized to nonoxidized lipids. The lactate dehydrogenase (LDH) release assay, another measure of membrane integrity, is a colorimetric assay involving the conversion of a tetrazolium salt into a formazan, quantified by its absorbance at 490 nm [33, 34]. The extent of LDH enzyme release into the cellular environment is proportional to the number of cells with compromised membranes. QD exposure-triggered inflammation can be tested via the production of pro-inflammatory cytokines detected by enzyme-linked immunosorbant assays (ELISA). The most commonly measured markers of inflammation are cytokines, such as interleukins (e.g., IL-1Beta, IL-6), and tumor necrosis factors (e.g., TNF-alpha). ELISA assays are generally sensitive, fast, and easily performed in laboratories without need for expensive and sophisticated equipment.

A useful method to assess the occurrence of DNA damage on QD-treated cells uses flow cytometry of cells stained with propidium iodide or Annexin V [35, 36]. Propidium iodide only enters cells with leaky membranes and the dye becomes strongly fluorescent upon binding to DNA. The emission intensity is a measure of the extent of damaged plasma membrane (i.e., the more extensive the damage, the more dye will get into the cell nuclei and the stronger the fluorescence intensity). Flow cytometry provides reliable information on different populations of cells exposed to injurious agents. However this technique does not reveal any information on possible morphological changes in the nucleus and other organelles. Transmission electron microscopy is the most reliable technique to detect such changes. However, this technique is time consuming. It can only provide information on a relatively limited number of cells at one time, and it is not practical for determining the dynamics of a deterioration process. The Comet assay or single cell gel electrophoresis (SCGE) assay is a rapid, sensitive, and relatively simple method to detect DNA damage at the level of individual cells [37]. In the original procedure cell lysis and subsequent electrophoresis were done under neutral conditions, and staining was done with acridine orange [38]. The image obtained resembles a comet with a distinct head comprising of intact DNA and a tail consisting of damaged or fragmented DNA. A more versatile alkaline method was developed later to measure low levels of strand breaks with high sensitivity [39]. This assay is semiquantitative, and interpretation of different types of tails is sometimes difficult. High-throughput assays, such as the GeneChip assay (Affymetrix) provide fast and effective means of profiling changes in gene expression upon treatment of cells with nanoparticles, including QDs.

There is no question that the most reliable information on cytotoxicity is obtained by combining several different techniques. A considerably larger palette of approaches must be applied if the questions are directed toward revealing a particular type of cell death or degeneration. Subtle cellular damage, which could eventually lead to long-term impairment, can only be revealed by functional assays (e.g., electrophysiological assessments of channel functions; release of neurotransmitters or hormones, histone acetylation, post-translational modification, methylation, and phosphorylation) coupled with real-time live cell imaging. Description of these assays is beyond the scope of this chapter.

7.3 Mechanisms of Quantum Dots Cytotoxicity

There is a general consensus that QD-induced cellular impairment and eventual cell death can involve the following events: (1) the release of the highly toxic heavy metals (Cd, Te, Se); (2) the desorption of the organic capping layer; (3) the formation of reactive oxygen species (ROS) and the cascade of events triggered by ROS; and (4) epigenetic and genetic changes involving histone modifications and DNA cleavage.

7.3.1 Release of Toxic Metal Ions

Cadmium, selenium, and tellurium, the core components of the most widely used QDs, are known to cause acute and chronic toxic effects in humans. A great deal of toxicological data is available on cadmium and selenium, which are of serious environmental concern. They are known to accumulate in vertebrates, with a biologic half-life in humans of 15 to 20 years (in the case of cadmium) [40]. Cadmium can be retained in all organs [41], and it has been shown to cross the blood brain barrier and induce neurological damage [42, 43]. The liver and kidney are the main target organs of cadmium toxicity [44], which involves, among other factors, interference with antioxidant enzymes [45], alterations in thiol proteins [46], inhibition of energy metabolism [47], generation of ROS and lipid peroxidation [48], and alteration in DNA structure [49]. Less is known on the toxicity of tellurium, although it was shown almost 20 years ago that this metal can induce significant damage in the peripheral nervous system [50].

Several groups have demonstrated that the amount of free Cd^{2+} in solutions of QDs prior to their addition to cells correlates with the cytotoxicity in vitro [51,52]. The free Cd^{2+} concentration, determined by techniques such as inductively coupled, plasma optical emission spectroscopy (ICP/EOS), in a 0.25 mg/mL solution of QDs ranged from 6 ppm (~ 50 μM) for nontoxic CdSe/ZnS QDs to as much as 126 ppm (~ 1.05×10^3 μM) for the highly toxic CdSe QDs [53]. The latter value is within the range of Cd^{2+} levels known to induce significant decrease in cell viability (100 to 400 μM) [54]. Derfus et al. demonstrated that the level of Cd^{2+} contaminating solutions of CdSe QDs depends on the type of coating and on storage conditions, such as exposure to light and air [53]. Their work suggests that Cd^{2+} generation results from the gradual erosion of the nanoparticle outer surface.

More recent work indicates that a ZnS outer layer provides the CdSe core with a robust, mostly defect-free coating of enhanced resistance against degradation in oxidative media. For instance, CdSe/ZnS QDs were shown to be nontoxic and did not interfere with the liver-specific functions of primary hepatocytes after exposure to low concentrations (< 0.25 mg/mL) and relatively short periods of time (< 1 hr) [53, 55, 56, 57]. Various ZnS-protected QDs have been used in a large number of in vivo and in vitro studies during which QD-induced cytotoxicity was not observed within the imaging time period [51, 58, 59]. These studies and others suggest that one key requirement is to protect the core with an outer layer that withstands aggressions from oxidative, acidic, or basic environments, and to verify that there is no trace of Cd or Se release during storage, upon irradiation, and upon contact with the biological media. Most studies suggest that this criterion is met by QDs covered with a zinc sulfide or cadmium sulfide (ZnS or CdS) outer layer synthesized according to the core-shell model, a number of which are currently commercially available. Silica-coated CdSe or CdSe/ZnS particles, which also present this robust core-shell morphology, were shown to be nontoxic in various types of cells—HepG2 (human liver carcinoma), NIH 3T3 (mouse embryonic fibroblasts), and COS-7 (monkey kidney fibroblasts) based on the Alamar Blue viability assay [60]. In these studies, the silica outer surface was hydrophilic due to the presence of PEG chains or amine groups originating from the aminopropylsilane used during the synthesis of the silica shell. Leaking of Cd^{2+} from silica-coated particles is believed to be precluded, although the absence of free Cd^{2+} in cells treated with SiO_2-coated QDs has not been demonstrated experimentally.

Cadmium telluride-QDs also induce cytotoxic effects in vitro and in vivo. Their toxicity was ascribed in part to the presence of free Cd^{2+} in a study of Cho et al., who tested exposure of human breast cancer cells (MCF-7) to CdTe QDs with no protective coating other than an adsorbed layer of hydrophilic ligands, such as mercaptopropionic acid (MPA) or cysteamine (Cys) [61]. They measured the intracellular concentration of Cd^{2+} in MCF-7 cells incubated for 24 hours with various QDs (10 μg/mL) using a Cd-specific cellular assay (Measure-iT). This study revealed that there is no linear correlation between the *intracellular* Cd^{2+} concentration measured in QD-exposed cells and the percent loss of metabolic activity (MTT assay) of the same cells treated with the same QDs under the same conditions. For example, MPA-coated CdTe QDs were significantly more toxic than Cys-coated CdTe QDs, yet the intracellular Cd^{2+} concentration was significantly lower in MPA-CdTe treated cells, compared to Cys-CdTe treated cells. Cho et al. also reported that CdSe/ZnS QDs were nontoxic to MCF-7 cells under the same conditions and that the intracellular Cd^{2+} concentration in cells treated with CdSe/ZnS QDs was not detectable within the sensitivity limits of the assay.

Kirchner et al. pointed out that the concentration of Cd^{2+} ions released from unprotected CdSe particles should scale with the concentration of Cd atoms on the surface of the CdSe core, a value that can be estimated from the size and concentration of the CdSe particles (i.e., a 1-nM solution of CdSe particles with 100 surface Cd-atoms has a surface Cd concentration of 100 nM) [51]. Using this indicator of Cd^{2+} concentration as a means to compare the cytotoxic effect of various CdSe QDs on several cell lines (NRK fibroblasts, MDA-MB-435S breast cancer cells, CHO cells, and RBL cells), these authors concluded that there is no correlation between the Cd^{2+} surface concentration and the viability of cells exposed to QDs in serum free medium [51]. This study corroborates the findings of Cho et al. indicating that the toxicity of QDs (CdTe or CdSe) cannot be accounted solely by the inherent toxicity of released Cd^{2+}.

7.3.2 Effects of Capping Materials on Cytotoxicity

The standard protocol for QD synthesis involves first the formation of semiconductor crystals in an organic solvent, and second exchange of the lipophilic ligand, usually trioctylphosphine oxide (TOPO), with a hydrophilic ligand, yielding water-soluble QDs. Since TOPO is a cytotoxic compound, it is important to ensure its complete removal during the exchange step [62]. The chemical structure of the lipophilic ligand needs to be selected with a view on its toxicity, since it has been speculated that exposure to acidic or oxidative intracellular environments or competitive adsorption of cellular components may trigger its desorption and intracellular release. The toxicity of several standard low molecular weight ligands was tested in the absence of QDs [62]. Some compounds, such as thioglycerol, were shown to be innocuous to cells; others turned out to be harmful. For example, mercaptoundecanoic acid (MUA) induced DNA damage at 50 μg/mL, and at concentrations > 100 μg/mL proved to be toxic in human lymphoblastoid WTK1 cells. Cysteamine, another commonly used capping agent, was found to be weakly genotoxic after a 12h treatment. These materials, whether inadvertently present in the QD solution or desorbed from the QDs in vitro or in vivo, can contribute to the overall cytotoxicity of QDs [63].

Several groups have demonstrated that the replacement of low molecular weight ligands by a biocompatible hydrophilic polymer can alleviate the harmful effects of QDs. Thus, PEG chains [51] or PEG-grafted polymers [60] yield water-dispersible, stable, and generally nontoxic QDs. However, PEGylation increases substantially the hydrodynamic volume of the QDs and lessens their cellular uptake, compared to QDs with less bulky hydrophilic capping. These trends were observed in a study of CdSe/Si-PEG QDs, which presented no toxic effects in NRK fibroblasts up to a concentration of 30 μM, as determined from the ratio of adherent cells after and before QD exposure. However, cellular uptake of the PEGylated QDs was greatly reduced compared to the corresponding non-PEGylated QDs that had cytotoxic effects [51]. A recent study by Ryman-Rasmussen et al. provides useful information on the toxicity of various commercial PEG-coated CdSe/ZnS toward skin cells, primary neonatal human epidermal keratinocytes (NHEK) [12]. The QDs carried neutral PEG chains, amine-terminated-PEG, or COOH terminated PEG-chains. They were shown to localize in the cytoplasm and the nucleus of NHEK cells. The three types of QDs were nontoxic, as determined by the MTT assay, when used in low concentration (2 nM). Exposure to higher concentrations of QDs (10 nM) revealed that the amine- and carboxylic acid-functionalized QDs were toxic and triggered pro-inflammatory cytokine release, whereas QDs coated with neutral PEG remained harmless. Further experiments correlated the coating-dependent cytotoxicity of QDs to the mechanism of their interactions with the cells [11].

Entrapment of CdSe QDs into poly(D-L)lactide nanoparticles stabilized by surfactants (overall hydrodynamic diameter of the composite particles: 160 to 260 nm) was reported as yet another means to insulate the QD core from the cellular environment [65]. The QD-containing particles, when coated with neutral or negatively charged surfactants, were shown to be nontoxic toward HepG2 cells, as assessed by the MTT test. Similar particles stabilized with a cationic surfactant (cetyltrimethyl ammonium bromide) proved to be toxic to the cells. This study highlights some of the problems related to the use of polymer-coated QDs, namely, increased size, and introduction of materials, other than the metal core, which may be inherently toxic.

7.3.3 Effects of QD Size on Cytotoxicity

A comparison of the toxicity of QDs with identical, or at least similar, composition and surface coating but different in size or hydrodynamic volume points to the rather general trend that smaller QDs are more cytotoxic than larger ones. Kirchner et al. tested the toxicity of different size CdSe QDs in several cell lines and attributed this trend to the higher surface-to-volume ratio of small nanoparticles compared to larger ones (or higher Cd^{2+} surface concentration per mol or weight of QD) [51]. Lovric et al. also noted that green CdTe QDs (diameter ~2.2–3 nm) were significantly more toxic than red ones (~5.2–6 nm), with identical surface covering as assessed by the MTT assay [66]. Moreover, they observed that the red QDs localize primarily in the cell cytoplasm and do not enter in the nucleus, whereas the smaller green QDs are found within the nucleus, where damage of the DNA can occur. Similar trends were reported also during an in vitro study of the interactions of green (~2 nm), yellow (~4 nm), and red (~6 nm) CdTe QDs in human hepatoma cells (HepG2) in concentrations up to 100 μM treated for 48h [67]. The viability of cells was assessed by the MTT assay and reported as IC_{50} values or concentration of QD causing a 50 percent reduction in viability. The IC_{50} values were 3.0, 4.8, and 19.1 μM for the green, yellow, and red QDs, respectively. Note that the researcher carried out in parallel an in vivo trial, exposing the same QDs to Sprague-Dawley rats [67]. The animals experienced a temporary decrease in locomotion immediately upon injection and some weight loss. However, after a 4-hr treatment, there was no noticeable damage to the specific organs.

Most of cytotoxicity data from QD exposure in vitro relate loss of viability and other cellular impairments to the concentration of the QD solution added to system investigated. This concentration is a good estimate of the extracellular QD concentration prior to internalization. If the QD size, coating, and concentration are such that the nanoparticles are readily endocytosed by the cells employed, then one may assume that the intracellular concentration will be equal, or similar, to the initial concentration, given sufficient time for internalization to occur. However, this may not be the case at all, since there is great variability in QD internalization, as revealed by numerous studies. These considerations motivated Chang et al. to evaluate the toxicity of a set of CdSe/CdS QDs (core/shell structure) toward a human breast cancer cell line (SK-BR-3) on the basis on the *intracellular* QD concentration, rather than the initial QD concentration added to cells [64]. The QDs were either coated with a thin polymeric shell bearing carboxylates or PEGylated with PEG chains (MW 750 or 6000). Cell viability was assessed by the live/dead assay. Cytotoxicity was shown to be (1) concentration dependent—the higher the dose, the higher the cell death—a trend reported in many previous studies and (2) surface dependent—the "bare" carboxylated QDs caused the largest decrease in cell viability for a given initial concentration. However, the intracellular QD concentration, after a 4-hr incubation at 37 degrees C, differed greatly for the three types of QDs: the intracellular concentration of uncoated QDs was approximately five times higher than that of the PEGylated QDs. A plot of the fraction of cell death versus intracellular QD concentration indicated no significant difference between viability data obtained for the three types of QDs, although initial concentration/toxicity studies revealed different cytotoxicities for each surface-modified QD (Figure 7.2). Hence, the study suggests that the apparent improved biocompatibility of some QDs arises from a reduced cellular uptake of QDs and is not a good indicator of the intrinsic toxicity level of the QDs.

The generality of this observation remains to be confirmed. Nonetheless it points to the importance of assessing the toxicity of QDs on the basis of their intracellular concentration, a protocol rarely followed in the past. Special experimental care needs to be taken in order to ensure the reliability of the intracellular QD concentration determination. Several protocols have been reported and usually involve several steps [68, 69]: (a) removal of excess extracellular QDs by washing the cells; (b) determination of cell number; and (c) measurement of the sample luminescence (from QDs) using appropriate controls and calibration curves. Some authors recommend subjecting the cells to an alkali treatment (2-hr incubation in 0.1M NaOH) prior to luminescence measurement in order to destroy the cell and all the organelles. Cellular residues are then removed by centrifugation prior to fluorometric quantification.

7.3.4 Effects of Reactive Oxygen Species on Cytotoxicity

7.3.4.1 Oxidative Stress

The generation of ROS upon exposure of cells to nanoparticles is currently considered to be one of the major contributors to their toxicity [2, 4]. Alteration of the

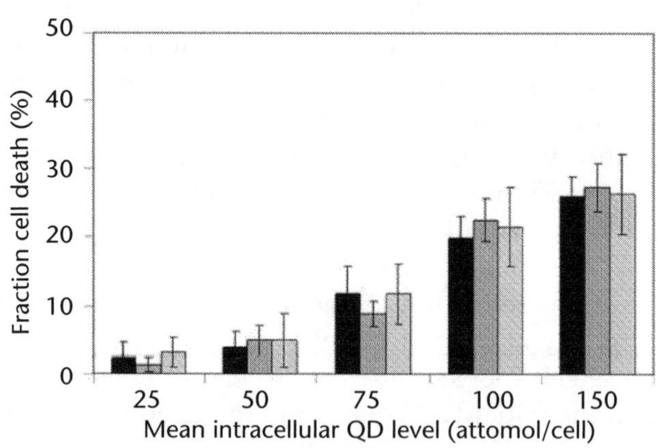

Figure 7.2 Cytotoxicity evaluation based on the same number of intracellular QDs for non PEG-substituted, 750- and 6000-Mw PEG-substituted QDs (black, dark gray, and light gray, respectively) on SK-BR-3 cells ($n = 4$). QDs were taken up into cells by endocytosis during a 4-h incubation, and intracellular levels were quantified by photoluminescence measurements. Cytotoxicity was determined using a commercial live/dead assay. Reproduced from [68] with permission from Wiley-VCH.

steady-state balance between oxidant and antioxidant agents in the cell causes what is known as oxidative stress, which disrupts normal physiological processes sufficiently to inhibit proliferation, induce differentiation [70], and, eventually, lead to cell death [71]. There are many different types of cell death, and it is commonly believed that QDs lead not only to apoptosis, but also to necrosis and cell death with autophagy [72]. Several modes for the activation of cellular signaling cascades by ROS have been identified and discussed in detail [73]. Cellular response depends on the severity of the oxidative stress, cell type, expression of antioxidant enzymes, microenvironment, and many other factors including other possible stressors present together with QDs. At its lowest level, oxidative stress induces the generation of antioxidants and the synthesis of detoxification enzymes [74]. At higher levels, this protective response is overtaken by inflammation initiated through activation of proinflammatory signaling cascades. It is well documented that certain types of QDs cause cytokine release and the release of proapoptotic factors [11]. Programmed cell death can be initiated either extrinsically or intrinsically. A well-characterized extrinsically initiated program involves the signal transduction cascade starting with the Fas (CD95) receptor, which is a prototypical "death receptor" [75]. Activation of the Fas receptor eventually leads to caspase activation and cell death [76]. Downstream signaling of Fas can also induce activation of lipases and pro-apoptotic transcription factors such as p53, which then potentiate apoptosis [77].

Various assays have been developed to detect and quantify the cellular responses at each level of oxidative stress. Parameters assessed include increased expression of antioxidant enzymes and cytokines, upregulation of "death receptors" such as Fas, or cell membrane damage, including lipid peroxidation. ROS themselves can be detected by electron spin resonance spectroscopy [78], an approach that tends to be cumbersome with tissues or cells, or via in vitro assays using a variety of fluorescent dyes [79, 80]. Dichlorodihydrofluorescein diacetate is often used in preliminary screening since it detects nearly all ROS [81, 82]. Other dyes are much more specific to individual types of free radicals. Two ROS species often implicated in the oxidative stress induced by nanoparticles are superoxide and singlet oxygen, which can be detected by dihydroethidium and singlet oxygen green sensor, respectively.

Imaging by confocal fluorescence microscopy of cells stained with organelle-specific dyes is a powerful tool to assess signature morphological damages inflicted by ROS on cell organelles, such as the mitochondria (e.g., visualized with MitoTracker Deep Red), lysosomes (e.g., LysoTracker DND 99), the nucleus (e.g., DAPI and Draq5), and lipid droplets (e.g., Oil Red O). Cells damaged upon treatment with CdTe QDs (2–3 nm, green positively charged) are visualized by this technique, as presented in Figure 7.3, together with micrographs of normal cells obtained under the same conditions [83]. By comparing the micrographs recorded for normal cells and cells subjected to oxidative stress, one notices that in injured cells the nuclei are deformed and is chromatin condensed, the mitochondria are swollen and often localized in the perinuclear region; the lysosomes are swollen, and the number of lipid droplets is increased.

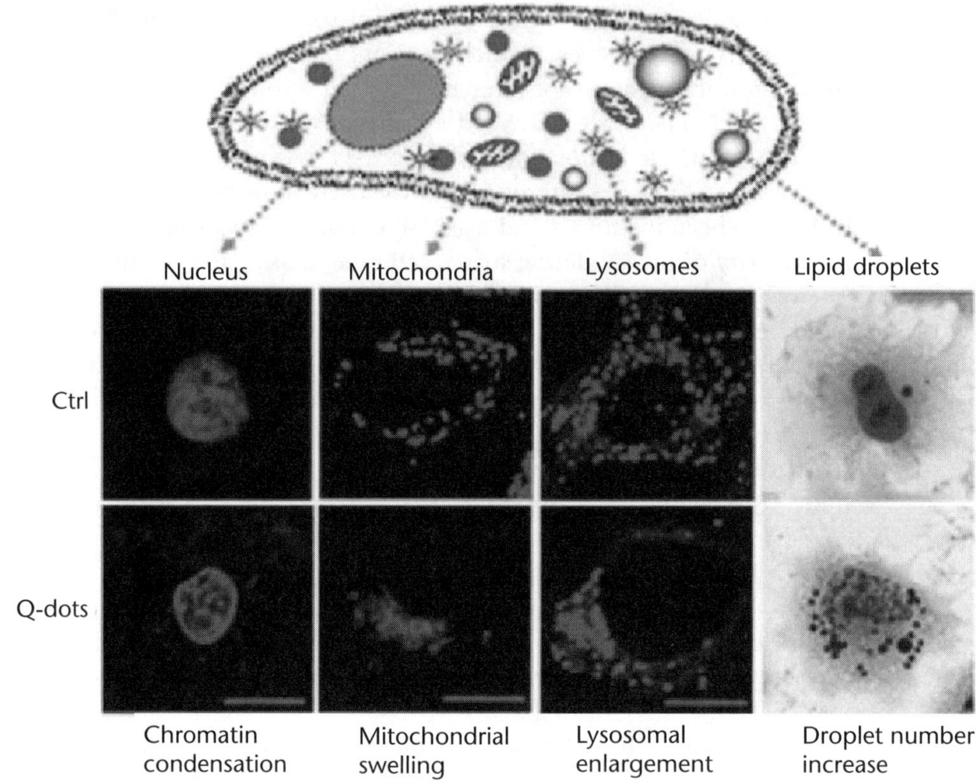

Figure 7.3 Organelle states and functions under normal conditions and under oxidative stress; Top: schematic representation of the cellular compartments observed. Top row: organelles under normal conditions. Bottom row: changes in organelles exposed to quantum dots for 24 hours. Column 1: nuclei are deformed and often have condensed chromatin. Column 2: mitochondria are swollen and often localized in the perinuclear region. Column 3: lysosomes are swollen in Q-dot treated cells. Column 4: lipid droplets are more abundant and enlarged in CdTe Q-dot (10 mg mL^{-1}) treated cells than in the untreated controls. Cells were stained with Draq5 (0.5 mM, nucleus), MitoTracker deep red (0.5 mM, mitochondria); LysoTracker DND 99 (0.5 mM, lysosomes) and oil red O (1 mM, lipid droplets). Reproduced from [83] by permission of the Royal Society of Chemistry. (See Color Plate 15.)

7.3.4.2 Mechanisms of QD-Induced Oxidative Stress

While several studies, described later, point to the involvement of ROS generation as one factor contributing to the toxicity of QDs, the exact mechanism by which QDs cause ROS formation is not yet fully understood. Enhanced ROS generation may occur by direct reaction of the QDs with molecular oxygen present in biological fluids or via physical interaction with cellular structures involved in the catalysis of biological reduction/oxidation (redox) processes. Specific mechanisms that have been suggested include the following: (a) light-induced energy transfer, in the presence of a photosensitizer, leading to the formation of singlet oxygen ($^1O_2$) [61, 84]. The generation of $^1O_2$ upon irradiation of QDs has been shown to occur, but it is generally not an efficient process, except in the case of QD-photosensitizer conjugates, such as those investigated for applications in photodynamic therapy [85–87]. (b) Photoexcitation to generate free electrons and subsequent electron transfer to oxygen yielding superoxide (O_2^-), which disproportionates spontaneously or upon enzymatic catalysis to produce hydrogen peroxide. Hydrogen peroxide can be fully reduced to water by peroxidases or else partially reduced in the presence of redox active transition metal ions in their reduced form, such as Fe^{2+} or Cu^+ (Fenton reaction), resulting in the production of hydroxyl radicals, which are potent initiators of radical chain reactions with diverse biomolecules. In this context, it is useful to recall the results of Ipe et al. [78], who performed a study of free radical generation in aqueous solution by photoirradiation of CdS, CdSe, and CdSe/ZnS QDs coated with mercaptopropionic acid. The study confirmed that QDs are able to produce free of radicals upon UV irradiation, but the type and quantity of radical formed depend on the QD composition. While CdS QDs have sufficient redox power to generate both hydroxyl and superoxide radicals, CdSe QDs exclusively generate hydroxyl radicals. Importantly, irradiation of CdSe/ZnS core/shell QDs did not produce free radicals under the conditions used.

7.3.4.3 Oxidative Stress and Free Cd2+

The situation is somewhat complicated by the fact that ROS generation can be induced also by Cd^{2+} ions present inadvertently or leaked out of the QDs. A number of authors have reported this mechanism to account for the toxicity of Cd^{2+} added as soluble salt (not as QD) while investigating its effect on different cell types [88–90]. Often ROS formation is detected in the early stages of Cd^{2+}-induced toxicity. Lipid peroxidation has also been associated to ROS produced from Cd^{2+}, rather than by direct Cd^{2+} involvement. All the parameters studied (ROS formation, mitochondrial potential dysfunction, and so on) were found to be lower in the presence of serum than in its absence, implying a serum protection against oxidative stress [48]. The protection is believed to be mediated by sequestration of cadmium by thiol groups of serum proteins, which decreases the effective concentration of Cd^{2+} and consequently reduces the damage caused by Cd^{2+}. It is worthwhile to remember here that several researchers have noted a similar protective effect of serum against QD-inflicted damages.

7.3.4.4 Experimental Evidence

In an early study, Lovric et al. [66], who examined the interactions of CdTe QDs capped with small ligands on rat pheochromocytoma (PC12) cells, noted that QDs coated with MPA or cysteamine were cytotoxic at concentrations of 10 μg/mL. Cell death was characterized by chromatin condensation and membrane blebbing, commonly detected in cells undergoing apoptotic cell death. Based on the morphological changes of cells upon exposure to QDs, the authors proposed that cell death was caused by the generation of ROS and that, consequently, the outcome of exposure may be altered by treating the cells with agents known to protect cells under oxidative stress, such as N-acetylcysteine (NAC). Indeed, addition of NAC to cells exposed to CdTe QDs significantly enhanced cell survival. Such a remarkable protective effect by NAC is not only due to its antioxidant effect via interaction with thiol groups but also due to several other mechanisms including its role as a glutathione precursor, as a transcription regulator for genes involved in cellular homeostasis, and as a cell survival promoter via inhibition of apoptotic signal transduction pathways.

The generation of ROS was shown to take place also in QD-exposed human neuroblastoma cells [91]. For example IMR-32 cells, treated with mercaptoacetic acid (MPA) coated CdSe QDs underwent severe biochemical changes ascribed to the generation of ROS detected in vitro by the 2',7'-dichlorofluorescein diacetate fluorescence assay. In contrast, none of these changes were observed when IMR-32 cells were treated with CdSe/ZnS core-shell QDs, confirming previous reports on the protective effect of the ZnS shell. Damages inflicted by CdSe QDs were alleviated by pretreatment of the cells with ROS scavengers, such as NAC or α-tocopherol. Information on the apoptotic signal pwathways was gathered from a battery of cellular assays that revealed activation of the protein kinase c-Jun-N-terminal kinase (JNK) and of caspase-9 and caspase-3, but not caspase-8, decrease of the mitochondrial membrane potential, and mitochondrial release of cytochrome c. Moreover, CdSe QDs were shown to inhibit survival-related signaling events, such as the expression of the Ras and Raf-1 proteins, and to decrease activation of the extracellular signal regulated kinase (ERK).

The effects caused to another human neuroblastoma cell line, SH-SY5Y, by exposure to CdTe QDs were assessed by Choi et al. [92], who confirmed the role of oxidative stress in cell death based on the results of experiments that combined biochemical assessment of cellular mechanisms and chemical modification of the QD surface layer. Various cellular responses were identified by treating SH-SY5Y cells with either NAC-conjugated, NAC-capped, or cysteamine-capped CdTe QDs. The NAC-modified QDs led to reduced cell death, decreased Fas expression, decreased mitochondrial membrane lipid peroxidation, and less extensive perturbation of the mitochondrial membrane potential, compared to cysteamine-capped QDs. The authors noted also that cellular uptake was reduced for NAC-modified QDs, compared to cysteamine-QDs. These studies illustrate the fact that even if the surface of the QDs is modified with molecules endowed of antioxidant therapeutic properties, it is not possible to completely compensate for the lack of stable capping (e.g., by ZnS). An additional reason for the partial but not full protection of cells exposed to the uncapped CdTe QDs is that the most effective concentrations of NAC are within the millimolar range (2–5 mM) which is unattainable with the number of NAC molecules associated with surfaces of low nanomolar QD concentrations. This notion was confirmed by treating the cells concomitantly with unbound and QD-bound NAC to achieve millimolar concentrations. This treatment provided full protection from QD-induced toxicity.

In summary, CdSe and CdTe QDs are prone to disturb cellular ROS equilibria to various extents depending on the type and redox status of the cell or organelle in contact with the QDs. This characteristic of uncapped CdSe and CdTe QDs is a limitation for their in vitro or in vivo long-term applications. In contrast, little evidence has been reported so far indicating that core-shell type QDs, such as CdSe/ZnS QDs, induce detectable levels of oxidative stress in the cellular environment.

7.3.5 Effects of QDs on Genomic DNA

Some nanoparticles, such as titanium dioxide, fullerenes, or diesel exhaust particles, have been shown to elicit nuclear DNA damage [3], which could have major long-term physiological and pathological implications for cells, tissues, and organisms. On the single cell level, such particle-induced injury may have three major consequences: (1) induction and fixation of mutations; (2) induction of DNA cell cycle arrest; and (3) activation of signal transduction pathways that promote apoptosis [93]. Damages are thought to occur either by direct interaction of the nanoparticles with DNA or via ROS originating from cell exposure to nanoparticles. In the case of QDs, evidence of damage to DNA by direct interaction is scarce. Green and Howman reported some DNA damage upon treatment with biotin-conjugated CdSe/ZnS QDs in the dark and under UV irradiation [94]. The experiments were conducted with solutions of supercoiled double stranded DNA, which is highly sensitive to free radicals. Damage occurred immediately upon contact of DNA with QDs. However, the authors of this study observed that ~70 percent of the DNA was adsorbed irreversibly on the QDs and hence unavailable for analysis. The DNA nicking detected was attributed to the photo- or dark-generation of free radicals in QD solutions. DNA damage was reported also by Liang et al. [95], who studied the interactions of MAA-capped CdSe QDs with calf thymus DNA. In this case, however, damage was noted only if the DNA/QD solution was subjected to UV irradiation. It was also attributed to the generation of free radicals and ROS. Control experiments confirmed that the damage was not caused by free Cd^{2+} ions.

It is difficult to transpose these experimental results to the situation encountered in the cellular environments. However, since there is evidence that QDs can penetrate the cell nucleus and that they can generate ROS intracellularly, there is a need to assess the long-term effects of QD exposure on the genomic and epigenetic levels. This aspect of the cytotoxicity of QDs is largely unexplored at this time, but several research groups have initiated studies probing this issue. T. Zhang et al. [96] performed a high throughput gene expression analysis to assess genotoxic effects in two cell types, a human skin cell line (HSF-42) and lung fibroblasts (IMR-90), exposed to low (2 nM) and high (> 20 nM) doses of core-shell CdSe/ZnS QDs covered with a PEG-silane outer layer. The two cell lines were selected as representative of situations corresponding to dermal exposure or inhalation. The QD inner core had a diameter of ~ 3 nm and the entire nanoparticle was 8 to 10 nm in diameter. The gene expression assay failed to reveal any significant difference in the phenotypic response of either cell line to high or low doses on QDs in the short term. Twenty to 30 percent of the genes were affected and a reduced expression of genes involved in M-phase exit was observed, together with an increased expression of genes involved in vesicle transport and cell protection. Such changes could be deleterious in the long run. There was no evidence for altered expression of any genes involved in Cd and Se toxicity, confirming that a combination of ZnS shell(s) and silylation is effective in preventing leakage of Cd^{2+} from the QDs inner core. Using various colorimetric assays, Zhang et al. confirmed by standard methodologies that the PEG-Si-CdSe/ZnS QDs used in the high-throughput assay do not affect cell proliferation significantly. A very modest increase in both necrosis and apoptosis was noted for cells treated with high (10 nM) or low (2 nM) concentration of QDs.

Imaging by confocal fluorescence microscopy of HSF-42 cells after a 48-hour exposure to the QDs revealed that QDs had been internalized. They were localized in the cytoplasm and the perinuclear region, but were unable to cross the nuclear membrane. The authors conclude that the ZnS/Si-PEG-shielded QDs have minimal impact on cells and on its genomic content, making them suitable for imaging of cellular compartments, except for the nucleus, which they cannot enter.

Other types of QDs, however, are able to penetrate the cell nucleus via mechanisms that are not yet fully understood. Treatment of cells with such QDs has an increased probability to induce DNA damage. Nabiev et al. [20] demonstrated that small QDs (2–3 nm in diameter) enter the nucleus via nuclear pore complexes and specifically target histones in the nuclei and nucleoli. Recalling that histones play an important role in the normal cell cycle and in tumor growth, the authors speculate that QDs may have a different "tropism" for histones at some stages of the cell cycle. The study was carried out with CdTe QDs capped with thioglycolic acid (d = 2.1 and 3.4 nm) as well as CdSe/ZnS QDs solubilized with cysteine (d = 3.8 nm) and commercial CdSe/ZnS 605 nm QDs. Cells assessed were of various types: blood monocyte-derived primary macrophages, human THP-1 monocytes, transformed epithelial cell lines (HCT-116 and AGS), and vascular endothelial HUVEC cells. It is important to observe that the QDs had no cytotoxic effects over the 72-hr incubation period during which the assays were performed. Nabiev et al. pointed out, however, that the specific intracellular and intranuclear accumulation of unfunctionalized QDs may produce unknown delayed effects in the long term, adding that given the fast nuclear localization of QDs exposed to epithelial cells and macrophages, it seems important to implement strict environmental control of nanoparticles.

A study by Choi et al. [97] aimed at assessing the long-term effects of exposure to QDs provides strong evidence that small CdTe QDs coated with mercaptopropionic acid are able to trigger genotoxic and epigenetic changes in human breast cancer cells (MCF-7). Fluorescence microscopy imaging together with TEM confirmed that the CdTe/MPA QDs were internalized by the cells and translocated in the nucleus, where they induced chromatin condensation and reorganization, as well as overall nuclear shrinking in the case of a high-dose (10 μg/mL) 24-hr exposure. These macroscopic changes were traced to hypoacetylation of histone 3, suggesting reduced gene transcription. RT-PCR amplification studies indicated that the mRNA levels of two genes involved in preventing cell death (*cIAP*-1 and *Hsp70*) were significantly reduced in QD-treated cells and that *GPx* (glutathione peroxidase) mRNA expression was completely suppressed upon QD treatment. Other effects were noted to occur simultaneously, in particular upregulation of proapoptotic genes (*Bax*, *Puma*, and *Noxa*), as well as a dramatic increase in phosphorylated p53 protein levels in the nucleus, cytosol, and mitochondria. The authors speculate that it may be possible that, despite the global hypoacetylation observed after QD treatment, local p53 recruitment brings about local hyperacetylation to allow for increased mRNA production. The authors suggest that changes in the cell epigenome may be triggered by QD-generated ROS and by free Cd^{2+} released by the QDs, two phenomena that have been associated previously to CdTe QDs. A schematic representation of the overall changes that occur upon exposure of MCF-7 cells to minute amounts of intracellular CdTe QDs is given in Figure 7.4. Information on the effects of QDs on the epigenome, such as histone modification and DNA methylation, is scarce. The study by Choi et al., who employed poorly protected CdTe QDs prone to degradation, shows that, aside from genotoxic effects, nanoparticles may cause more subtle epigenetic changes, which need to be examined thoroughly in particular when medical applications are to be considered.

The long-term effects of QDs and their impact on cell differentiation have been evaluated also from the viewpoint of their impact on stem cell growth, differentiation, and functions. Hsieh et al. [98] monitored human bone marrow mesenchymal stem cells (hBMSC) exposed to CdSe/ZnS QDs in the presence of lipofectamine.

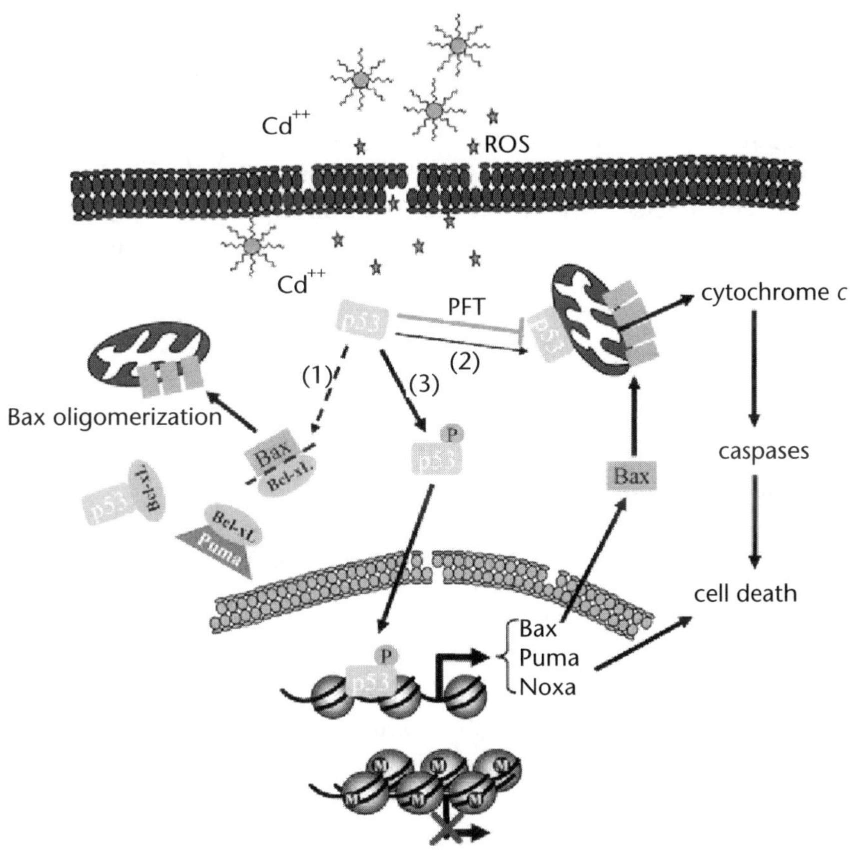

Figure 7.4 Schematic representation of the changes induced by QDs at the cellular epigenic and genomic levels. QDs release reactive oxygen species (ROS)and free cadmium ions extra- and intracellularly, triggering changes in the epigenome through chromatin condensation and histone hypoacetylation. QDs induce increased protein levels and activation of the transcription factor p53 resulting in: 1 cytosolic p53 directly activating Bax by freeing it from its binding proteins and facilitating the mitochondrial accumulation of Bax; 2. p53 proteins can mistranslocate to the mitochondria, leading to membrane permeabilization and consequential cell death. Pifithrin-á (PFT), a specific inhibitor of p53, can prevent this mistranslocation, and thereby can partially prevent QD-induced cell death; 3 activated (phosphorylated) p53 induces the transcription of proapoptotic genes, including Bax, Puma, and Noxa. Bax proteins accumulate and oligomerize at the mitochondrial membrane, forming pores and releasing cytochrome c, leading to cell death. Puma facilitates Bax mitochondrial accumulation by occupying Bax-binding proteins (i.e., Bcl-xL), freeing cytosolic Ba. Reproduced from [97] with permission from Springer Science and Business Media. (See Color Plate 16.)

They assessed other methods of QDs internalization, such as the presence of calcium phosphate or of the HIV-derived Tat peptides, which were not effective in mediating the transport of QDs through the cell membrane. The internalized QDs localized in endosome-like structures. They had no damaging effect on cell proliferation, and the cell cycle distribution was not disturbed. Hsieh et al. also carried out RT-PCR on treated cells and noticed that the expression of two osteogenic markers, osteopontin and osteocalcin, was inhibited significantly. They concluded that exposure to CdSe/ZnS QDs prevents the full response of hBMSCs in the induction of osteogenic differentiation. The authors observed that the effect took place independently of the QD size, although no data was provided. Another study by the same group suggests that QD labeling of hBMSCs also inhibits the elaboration of chondrogenic matrix [99].

In contrast, Shah et al. [100] did not observe any QD-induced damaging effects in the course of a study of primary BMSCs exposed to CdSe/ZnS (λ_{em} 600 ± 10 nm) conjugated to a peptide (CGGGRGD). The conjugated QDs, which had a tendency to aggregate, were internalized by the cells but did not translocate in the nucleus. QD-treated cells were able to proliferate for extended periods (up to 28 days) with no sign of adverse effect. Moreover, multilineage differentiation of the BMSCs into osteoblasts, chondrocytes, and adipocytes occurred, yielding QD-labeled differentiated cells. The successful outcome of cell differentiation was verified by matrix biosynthesis markers. Possible QD-inflicted damage to the DNA was not assessed and therefore cannot be entirely ruled out.

7.4 Bioaccumulation and Clearance of QDs

The palette of QDs currently available for in vitro studies of cellular mechanisms is quite staggering. As described in the preceding sections, a number of design rules have emerged to guide the elaboration of QDs able to perform a specific imaging task without affecting the cell functions significantly, at least in the short term. In vitro studies have answered in part some of the key biological questions related to QD uptake, subcellular distribution, and functional consequences. The next step is to introduce QDs in animals and eventually into the human body for live, real-time imaging. Early in vivo imaging experiments with QDs gave no indication of acute toxicity over the experiment time period (up to 24 hrs) [22]. These experiments demonstrated the power of QDs to image various tissues and to allow the precise imaging of tumors and the simultaneous identification of different populations of cells.

However, early in vivo studies suggested also that QDs may be systemically distributed in rodent animals and accumulate in various organs. Ballou et al. [101] assessed the effect of the size and surface coating of QDs on their biodistribution. This study indicated that QDs accumulate and can be detected in the lymph nodes, bone marrow, liver, and spleen up to four months after injection. In addition, Ballou's experiments demonstrated that the organs and tissues in which QDs tend to accumulate depend on the size and surface charge of the QDs. A recent study suggests that QDs with appropriate organic coating are retained in injected animals (mice) for more than two years, with minimal toxicity as assessed by pathological examination [102]. Akerman et al. [22] investigated the in vivo fate of CdSe/ZnS

QDs coated with lung- and tumor-targeting peptides injected (intravenously) in mice. The QDs were shown to accumulate, not only in the targeted organs, but also in the liver and spleen, regardless of the peptide conjugated to the QDs.

In these studies, the strong QD emission was exploited for detection and qualitative measure of QD concentration. This approach is not suitable for accurate assessment of QD concentrations, given the impact of environmental variability on the intensity of QD emission. Studies by Ballou et al. and Akerman et al. were the first reports of the exceptional potential of QDs in experimental biology and medicine and of the possible pitfalls of nanoparticle-based medical imaging techniques.

Recently, a few research groups have carried out quantitative pharmacokinetic analyses in which the QD concentrations were determined from Cd concentration in various organs obtained by inductively coupled plasma atomic emission spectroscopy (ICP-AES) or inductively coupled plasma mass spectroscopy (ICP-MS). This analytical technique yields accurate quantitative values, unlike measurements relying on the light emitting properties of QDs. Gopee et al. [99] have evaluated the biodistribution of intradermally injected QDs (CdSe/ZnS PEG coated, diameter = 37 nm, emission at 621 nm) in mice. The QDs migrated rapidly from the injection site to regional lymph nodes. Quantification of the QDs 24 hrs after dosing revealed that residual QDs remained at the injection site, but there was also a significant accumulation in the liver, regional draining lymph nodes, kidneys, spleen, and hepatic lymph nodes.

Fischer et al. [104] performed a pharmacokinetic study in Sprague-Dawley rats (intravenous injection) with two samples of CdSe/ZnS QDs (core size = 5.5 nm) coated either with mercaptoundecanoic acid with lysine crosslinking (total hydrodynamic diameter = 25 nm) or with bovine serum albumin (BSA, total hydrodynamic diameter (HD) = 80 nm). The plasma half-life was longer for the smaller QDs (58 ± 17 min versus 39 ± 3 min or clearances of 0.59 ± 0.16 mL min^{-1} kg^{-1} versus 1.23 ± 0.22 mL min^{-1} kg^{-1}). Negligible clearance in the urine or feces was observed for both QD samples over a period of up to 10 days after injection, leading the authors to conclude that the QDs are sequestered and not excreted. The liver took up most of the QD dose (99 percent of the BSA-coated QDs and 40 percent of the smaller QDs after 90 min), and, in the liver, the QDs were localized in vesicles within the Kupffer cells. Small amounts of both types of QDs were localized in the spleen, kidney, and bone marrow with some level of selectivity depending on the coating of the QDs. The authors carried out experiments aimed at detecting the presence of free cadmium in spleen and liver tissues, but they were unable to detect any Cd that might have leaked from the QDs.

Yang et al. [105] monitored the pharmacokinetics of commercial QD705 CdTe/ZnS coated with methoxy-PEG-5000, diameter ~13 nm) after a single intravenous injection in mice. The QDs had a plasma half-life of 18.5 hrs. After a period of 24 hrs post injection, high levels of QDs were detected in the liver, spleen, and kidney. Complete QD mass balance studies were carried 1 day and 28 days after dosing. High levels of QDs persisted in the liver, spleen, and kidney. Over time, the liver uptake appeared to increase relative to the QD content in all other organs (Figure 7.5). About 50 percent of the QD mass was retained in the carcass, mainly distributed in large masses of muscle, skin, and bone. No excretion occurred over 28 days, except for minute amounts of QDs (accounting for 0.01 to 0.04 percent of

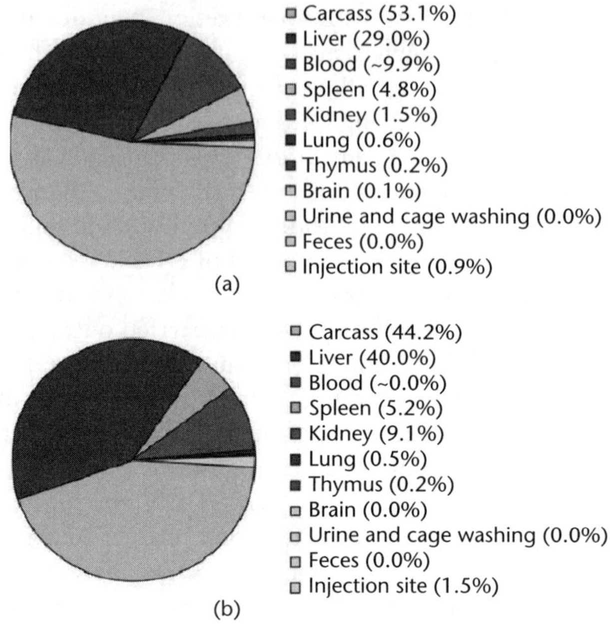

Figure 7.5 Mass balance studies of an intravenous dose of QD705 injected in ICR mice; (a) 24 hours after injection, and (b) 28 days after injection. Reproduced from [105] with permission from *Environmental Health Perspectives*.

the total dose) found in the urine. Tissue localizations, judged from imaging by fluorescence microscopy of the red QD emission, were mainly in the linings of hepatic sinusoids, renal vessels, and glomerular vasculature in the kidneys.

The accumulation of QDs may cause renal and hepatic toxicity in the long term, even if they remain intact and do not erode and exude free cadmium ions. The retention of metal particles in various organs can also interfere with subsequent medical tests, such as radiological tests by X-ray imaging or magnetic resonance imaging. Thus, for nanoparticles such as QDs, which do not and should not degrade in vivo, body clearance needs to be one of the required design parameters for clinical applications. This criterion is related to the size of the nanoparticles, since glomerular filtration in the kidneys, controlled by the effective renal pore size, is a sensitive function of the hydrodynamic particle size. The liver is designed specifically to capture and eliminate particles 10 to 20 nm in size. Particles that remain intact in the liver can be excreted via the bile and the feces. However transport of intact particles from the liver to bile is very slow, which accounts for the significant long-term accumulation of QDs in the liver as observed in most in vivo imaging experiments.

Long-term problems related to persistent retention of QDs in the liver and kidneys can be avoided by using QDs able to be cleared rapidly from the body via renal filtration. Based on the assumption that the renal filtration threshold of QDs is a function of the hydrodynamic diameter of the nanoparticles, H.-S Choi et al. [106] carried out a pharmacokinetic study of QDs with different hydrodynamic diameters but identical compositions and surface properties. They employed cysteine-coated CdSe/ZnS QDs ranging in hydrodynamic diameter from 4.4 nm to 8.7 nm by increasing the core size while keeping the same organic coating. The authors carefully selected an organic coating able to withstand the adsorption of serum proteins, in order to prevent undesirable size increase of the QDs upon injection. Particles were labeled with a chelated form of the γ-ray emitting isotope ^{99m}Tc. Radioscintigraphic images were recorded to monitor the distribution and clearance of QDs upon intravenous injection into CD mice. Four hours after injection with QDs of hydrodynamic diameter 4.36 nm, the dominant signal was in the bladder, whereas QDs of hydrodynamic diameter 8.65 nm exhibited a higher uptake in the liver, lung, and spleen. By measuring the radiographic intensity in urine (excreted and preexcreted) and in the entire carcass (less the bladder and urethra), H.-S Choi et al. obtained a relationship between hydrodynamic diameter, renal clearance, and total body retention (Figure 7.6). Results from these studies suggest that the upper limit of hydrodynamic diameter for total nanoparticle renal QD clearance (after 4 hrs) is approximately 5.5 nm. The authors conclude that larger particles are most likely not promising imaging tools for clinical applications.

7.5 Outlook

In view of their size and composition, QDs may impact physiological functions and exert toxic effects that cannot be ignored. However, there is no conclusive evidence that QD-induced effects will cause major problems to human health or to the environment. In this review, we have assessed the risks associated with the use of QDs as imaging agents in medical diagnostics, as well as those associated with inadvertent contact with QDs by inhalation, dermal exposure, or ingestion. We considered factors susceptible to trigger toxic effects and means to minimize them. The core/shell QDs of the current generation are very robust against surface erosion and leaching of toxic metal ions or coating materials, a severe concern associated with the use of the first generation QDs. However, the bioaccumulation/clearance issue needs to be addressed in detail, since QDs are potential inducers of oxidative stress upon cell internalization. This property of QDs needs to be fully understood on the

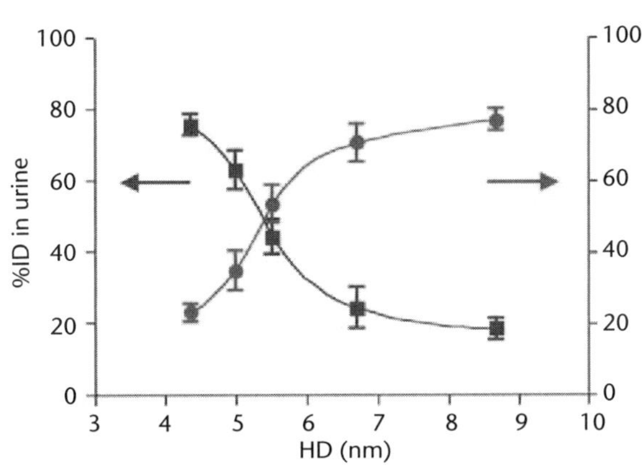

Figure 7.6 Urine excretion and carcass retention of ^{99m}TC-labeled QDs after intravenous injection into CD1-mice as a function of the hydrodynamic diameter of the QDs. Reproduced from [106] with permission from *Nature Biotechnology*.

nongenomic, genomic, and epigenomic levels. Even small, hardly detectable amounts of QDs can cause epigenetic changes, which remain programmed long after the initial signal has been removed. We are still far from solving the numerous problems related to the unknown fate of cells and tissues exposed to QDs for long time periods in intracellular concentrations so low that they cannot be determined accurately by currently available techniques. This issue can only be addressed by employing a combination of techniques, such as high throughput gene expression analysis, proteomics, lipidomics, metabolomics, and expertise in cell biology, physics, chemistry, and environmental science.

Acknowledgments

FMW acknowledges financial support from the Global Center of Excellence (G-COE) program "Education and Research Center for Emergence of New Molecular Chemistry" in the form of a G-COE invited Professorship in the Tokyo Institute of Technology, Tokyo, Japan. The authors gratefully acknowledge the help of Mr. A. Moquin and Ms. A. Choi for editorial assistance.

References

[1] Oberdörster, G., E. Oberdörster, E., and J. Oberdörster, J., "Nanotoxicology: An Emerging Discipline Evolving from Studies of Ultrafine Particles" *Environment. Health Persp.*, Vol. 113 (7), 2005, pp. 823–839.

[2] Oberdörster, G., A. Maynard, K. Donaldson, et al., "Principles for characterizing the potential human health effects from exposure to nanomaterials: elements of a screening strategy" *Particle and Fibre Toxicology*, 2005, 2 (8), pp. 1–35.

[3] Unfried, K., C. Albrecht, L.-O. Klotz, et al., "Cellular Responses to Nanoparticles: Target Structures and Mechanisms" *Nanotoxicology*, Vol. 1, No. 1, 2007, 1 (1) pp. 52–71.

[4] Nel, A., T. Xia, and L. Mädler, et al., "Toxic Potential of Materials at the Nanolevel" *Science*, Vol. 311 (5761), 2006, pp. 622–627.

[5] Fischer, H.C., and W.C.W. Chan, "Nanotoxicity: The Growing Need for in vivo Study" *Current Opinion Biotechnol.*, Vol. 18 (6), 2007, pp. 565–571.

[6] Hardman, R., "A Toxicologic Review of Quantum Dots: Toxicity Depends on Physicochemical and Environmental Factors" *Environmental Health Perspectives*, Vol. 114 (2), 2006, pp. 165–172.

[7] Lewinski, N., V. Colvin, and R. Drezek, "Cytotoxicity of Nanoparticles" *Small*, Vol. 4 (1), 2008, pp. 26–49.

[8] Donaldson, K., D. Brown, A. Clouter, et al., "The Pulmonary Toxicology of Ultrafine Particles" *J. Aerosol Med.*, Vol. 15 (2), 2002, pp. 213–220.

[9] Bermudez, E., J.B. Mangum, B.A. Wong, et al., "Pulmonary Responses of Mice, Rats, and Hamsters to Subchronic Inhalation of Ultrafine Titanium Dioxide Particles" *Toxicol. Sci.*, Vol. 77, 2004, pp. 347–357.

[10] Ryman-Rasmussen, J. P., J.E. Riviere, and N.A. Monteiro-Riviere, "Penetration of Intact Skin by Quantum Dots with Diverse Physicochemical Properties" *Toxicol. Sci.*, Vol. 91 (1), 2006, pp. 159–165.

[11] Ryman-Rasmussen, J. P., J.E. Riviere, and N.A. Monteiro-Riviere, "Surface Coatings Determine Cytotoxicity and Irritation Potential of Quantum Dot Nanoparticles in Epidermal Keratinocytes" *J. Invest. Dermatol.*, Vol. 127, 2007, pp. 143–153.

[12] Ryman-Rasmussen, J. P., J.E. Riviere, and N.A. Monteiro-Riviere, "Variables Influencing Interactions of Untargeted Quantum Dot Nanoparticles with Skin Cells and Identification of Biochemical Modulators" *Nano Letters*, Vol. 7 (5), 2007, pp. 1344–1348.

[13] Gopee, N.V., D.W. Roberts, P. Webb, et al., "Migration of Intradermally Injected Quantum Dots to Sentinel Organs in Mice" *Toxicol. Sci.*, Vol. 98 (1), 2007, pp. 249–257.

[14] Gagne, F., J. Auclair, P. Turcotte, et al., "Ecotoxicity of CdTe Quantum Dots to Freshwater Mussels: Impacts on Immune System, Oxidative Stress, and Genotoxicity" *Aquatic Toxicol.*, Vol. 86, 2008, pp. 333–340.

[15] Aderem, A., and D.M. Underhill, "Mechanisms of Phagocytosis in Macrophages" *Annu. Rev. Immunol.*, Vol. 17, 1999, pp. 593–623.

[16] Scott, C.C., R.J. Botelho, and S. Grinstein, "Phagosome maturation: A few Bugs in the System" *J. Membrane Biol.*, Vol. 193, 2003, pp. 137–152.

[17] Gruenberg, J., "The Endocytic Pathway: A Mosaic of Domains" *Nat. Rev. Mol. Cell Biol.*, Vol. 2, 2001, pp. 721–730.

[18] Mukherjee, S., R.N. Ghosh, and F.R. Maxfield, "Endocytosis" *Physiol. Rev.*, Vol. 77, 1997, pp. 759–803.

[19] Alberts, B., D. Bray, J. Lewis, et al., *Molecular Biology of the Cell*; New York, NY: 3rd ed., Garland Publishing, 1994.

[20] Nabiev, I., S. Mitchell, A. Davies, et al., "Nonfunctionalized Nanocrystals Can Exploit a Cell's Active Transport Machinery Delivering them to Specific Nuclear and Cytoplasmic Compartments" *Nano Letters*, Vol. 7, 2007, pp. 3452–3461.

[21] Maysinger, D., J. L. A. Eisenberg, et al., "Fate of Micelles and Quantum Dots in Cells" *Eur. J. Pharm. Biopharm.*, Vol.65 (3), 2006, pp. 270–281.

[22] Akerman, M., W.C. Chan, P. Laakkonen, et al., "Nanocrystal Targeting in vivo" *PNAS*, Vol. 99, 2002, pp. 12617–12621.

[23] Carmicheal, J., W.G. DeGraaf, A.F. Gazdar, et al., "Evaluation of a Tetrazolium-Based, Semi-Automated Colorimetric Assay: Assessment of Chemosensitivity Testing" *Cancer Res.*, Vol. 47, 1987, pp. 936–942.

[24] Mossman, T., "Rapid Colorimetric Assay for Cellular Growth and Survival: Application to Proliferation and Cytotoxicity Assays" *J. Immunol. Methods*, Vol. 65, 1983, pp. 55–63.

[25] Scudiero, D., R.H. Shoemaker, K.D. Paull, et al., "Evaluation of a Soluble Tetrazolium/Formazan Assay for Cell Growth and Drug Sensitivity in Culture Using Human and Other Cell Lines" *Cancer Res.*, Vol. 48, 1988, pp. 4827–4833.

[26] Roehm, N.W., G.H. Rodgers, S.M. Hatfield, et al., "An Improved Colorimetric Assay for Cell Proliferation and Viability Utilizing the Tetrazolium Salt XTT" *J. Immunol. Methods*, Vol. 142, 1991, pp. 257–265.

[27] Ahmed, S.A., R.M. Gogal Jr., and J.E. Walsh, "A New Rapid and Simple Non-Radioactive Assay to Monitor and Determine the Proliferation of Lymphocytes: An Alternative to [3H]Thymidine Incorporation Assay" *J. Immunol. Methods*, Vol. 170 (2), 1994, pp. 211–224.

[28] Nociari, M.M., A. Shalev, P. Benias, and C. Russo, "A Novel One-Step, Highly Sensitive Fluorometric Assay to Evaluate Cell-Mediated Cytotoxicity" *J. Immunol Methods*, Vol. 213 (2), 1998, pp. 157–167.

[29] Freshney, R.I., *Culture of Animal Cells: A Manual of Basic Technique*, New York, NY: Alan R. Liss, Inc., 1987, p. 117.

[30] Akerboom, T.P., and H. Sies, "Assay of Glutathione, Glutathione Disulfide, and Glutathione Mixed Disulfides in Biological Samples" *Methods Enzymol.*, Vol. 77, 1981, pp. 373–382.

[31] Ji, L.L., and R. Fu, "Responses of Glutathione System and Antioxidant Enzymes to Exhaustive Exercise and Hydroperoxide" *J. Appl. Physiol.*, Vol. 72, 1992, pp. 549–554.

[32] Free Radical Biology and Aging Program, *Methods in Biological Oxidative Stress*,Oklahoma Medical Research Foundation, Oklahoma City, OK, 2003, pp. 57–65

[33] Chen, J., G.C. Douglas, T.L. Thirkill, et al., "Effect of Bromodichloromethane on Chorionic Gonadotrophin Secretion by Human Placental Trophoblast Cultures" Toxicol. Sci., Vol. 76, 2003, pp. 75–82.

[34] Hernandez, J.M., M.H.T. Bui, K.-R. Han, et al., "Novel Kidney Cancer Immunotherapy Based on the Granulocyte-Macrophage Colony-Stimulating Factor and Carbonic Anhydrase IX Fusion Gene" Clin. Cancer Res., Vol. 9, 2003, pp. 1906–1916.

[35 Kuypers, F.A., R.A. Lewis, M. Hua, et al., "Detection of Altered Membrane Phospholipid Asymmetry in Subpopulations of Human Red Blood Cells Using Fluorescently Labeled Annexin V" *Blood*, Vol. 87, 1996, pp. 1179–1187.

[36] Koopman, G., C.P. Reutelingsperger, G.A. Kuijten, et al., "Annexin V for Flow Cytometric Detection of Phosphatidylserine Expression on B Cells Undergoing Apoptosis" *Blood*, Vol. 84, 1994, pp. 1415–1420.

[37] Santos, S.J., N.P. Singh, and A.T. Natarajan, "Fluorescence in Situ Hybridization with Comets" *Exp. Cell Res.*, Vol. 232, 1997, pp. 407–411.

[38] Ostling, O., and K.J. Johanson, "Microelectrophoretic Study of Radiation-Induced DNA Damage in Individual Mammalian Cells" *Biochem. Biophys. Res. Commun.*, Vol. 123, 1984, pp. 291–298.

[39] Collins, A. R., "Comet Assay for DNA Damage and Repair: Principles, Applications and Limitations" *Mol. Biotechnol.*, Vol. 26, 2004, pp. 249–261.

[40] Goyer, R.A., "Mechanisms of Lead and Cadmium Nephrotoxicity" *Toxicol. Lett.*, Vol. 46, 1989, pp. 153–162.

[41] Robards, K., and P. Worsfold, "Cadmium: Toxicology and Analysis" *Analyst.*, Vol. 116, 1991, pp. 549–568.

[42] Gabbiani, G., D. Baic, and C. Deziel, "Toxicity of Cadmium for the CNS" *Exp. Neurol.*, Vol. 18, 1967, pp. 154–160.

[43] Hart, R.P., C.S. Rose, and R.M. Hamer, "Neuropsychological Effects of Occupational Exposure to Cadmium" *J. Clin. Exp. Neuropsychol.*, Vol. 11, 1989, pp. 933–943.

[44] Goering, P.L., B.R. Fischer, and C.L. Kish, "Stress Protein Synthesis Induced in Rat Liver by Cadmium Precedes Hepatotoxicity" *Toxicol. Appl. Pharmacol.*, Vol. 122, 1993, pp. 139–148.

[45] Hussain, T., G.S. Shukla, and S.V. Shandra, "Effects of Cadmium on Superoxide Dismutase and Lipid Peroxidation in Liver and Kidney of Growing Rats: In vivo and in vitro Studies" *Pharmacol. Toxicol.*, Vol. 60, 1987, pp. 355–359.

[46] Belyaeva, E.A., and S.M. Korotkov, "Mechanism of Primary Cd2+-Induced Rat Liver Mitochondria Dysfunction: Discrete Modes of Cd2+ Action on Calcium and Thiol-Dependent Domains" *Toxicol Appl. Pharmacol.*, Vol. 192, 2003, pp. 56–68.

[47] Mueller, L., "Consequences of Cadmium Toxicity in Rat Hepatocytes: Mitochondrial Dysfunction and Lipid Peroxidation" *Toxicology*, Vol. 40 (3), 1986, pp. 285–295.

[48] Lopez, E., C. Arce, M.J. Oset-Gasque, et al., "Cadmium Induces Reactive Oxygen Species Generation and Lipid Peroxidation in Cortical Neurons in Culture" *Free Radical Biol. Med.*, Vol. 40 (6), 2006, pp. 940–951.

[49] Coogan, T.P., R.M. Bare, and M.P. Waalkes, "Cadmium-Induced DNA Strand Damage in Cultured Liver Cells: Reduction of Cadmium Genotoxicity Following Zinc Pretreatment" *Toxicol. Appl. Pharmacol.*, Vol. 113, 1992, pp. 227–233.

[50] Toews, A.D., S.Y. Lee, B. Popko, and P. Morell, "Tellurium-Induced Neuropathy: A Model for Reversible Reductions in Myelin Protein Gene Expression" *J. Neurosci. Res.*, Vol. 26 (4), 1990, pp. 501–507.

[51] Kirchner, C., T. Liedl, S. Kudera, et al., "Cytotoxicity of Colloidal CdSe and CdSe/ZnS Nanoparticles" *Nano Lett.*, Vol. 5 (2), 2005, pp. 331–338.

[52] Kirchner, C., A. Munoz Javier, A.S. Susha, et al., "Cytotoxicity of Nanoparticle-Loaded Polymer Capsules" *Talanta*, Vol. 67, 2005, pp. 486–491.

[53] Derfus, A.M., W.C.W. Chan, and S.N. Bhatia, "Probing the Cytotoxicity of Semiconductor Quantum Dots" *Nano Lett.*, Vol. 4, 2004, pp. 11–18.

[54] Limaye, D.A., and Z.A. Shaikh, "Cytotoxicity of Cadmium and Characteristics of its Transport in Cardiomyocytes" *Toxicol. Appl. Pharmacol.*, 154 (1), 1999, pp. 59–66.

[55] Dubertret, B., P. Skourides, D. J.Norris, et al., "In-Vivo Imaging of Quantum Dots Encapsulated in Phospholipid Micelles" *Science*, 2002, Vol. 298, pp 1759–1762.

[56] Voura, E. B., J. K. Jaiswal, H. Mattoussi, et al. "Tracking Metastatic Tumor Cell Extravasation with Quantum Dot Nanocrystals and Fluorescence Emission-Scanning Microscopy" *Nature Med.* 2004, Vol 10, pp 993–998.

[57] Delehanty, J. B., I. L. Medintz, T. Pons, et al. "Self-Assembled Quantum Dot-Peptide Bioconjugates for Selective Intracellular Delivery," *Bioconjugate Chem.* 2006, Vol 17, pp 920–927.

[58] Seleverstov, O., O. Zabirnyk, M. Zscharnack, et al., "Quantum Dots for Human Mesenchymal Stem Cells Labeling: A Size-Dependent Autophagy Activation" *Nano Lett.*, 6, 2006, pp. 2826–2832.

[59] Chan, W.-H., N.-H. Shiao, and P.-Z. Lu, "CdSe Quantum Dots Induce Apoptosis in Human Neuroblastoma Cells via Mitochondrial-Dependent Pathways and Inhibition of Survival Signals" *Toxicol. Lett.*, Vol. 167, 2006, pp. 191–200.

[60] Selvan, S.T., T.T. Tan, and J.Y. Ying, "Robust, Non-Cytotoxic, Silica-Coated CdSe Quantum Dots with Efficient Photoluminescence" *Adv. Mater.*, Vol. 17 (13), 2005, pp. 1620–1625.

[61] Cho, S.J., D. Maysinger, M. Jain, et al., "Long-Term Exposure to CdTe Quantum Dots Causes Functional Impairments in Live Cells" *Langmuir*, Vol. 23 (4), 2007, pp. 1974–1980.

[62] Hoshino, A., K. Fujioka, T. Oku, et al., "Physicochemical Properties and Cellular Toxicity of Nanocrystal Quantum Dots Depend on Their Surface Modification" *Nano Lett.*, Vol. 4, 2004, pp. 2163–2169.

[63] Ballou, B., "Quantum Dot Surfaces for Use in vivo and in vitro" *Curr. Top. Dev. Biol.*, Vol. 70, 2005, pp. 103–120.

[64] Duan, H., and S. Nie, "Cell-Penetrating Quantum Dots Based on Multivalent and Endosome-Disrupting Surface Coatings" *J. Am. Chem. Soc.*, Vol. 129 (11), 2007, pp. 3333–3339.

[65] Guo, G., W. Liu, J. Liang, et al., "Probing the Cytotoxicity of CdSe Quantum Dots with Surface Modification" *Mater. Lett.*, Vol. 61 (8-9), 2007, pp. 1641–1644.

[66] Lovriæ, J., S.J. Cho, F.M. Winnik, and D. Maysinger, "Unmodified Cadmium Telluride Quantum Dots Induce Reactive Oxygen Species Formation Leading to Multiple Organelle Damage and Cell Death" *Chem. Biol.*, Vol. 12, 2005, pp. 1227–1234.

[67] Zhang, Y.B.J., W. Chen, J. Zhang, et al., "In vitro and in vivo Toxicity of CdTe Nanoparticles" *Nanosci. Nanotech.*, Vol. 7 (2), 2007, pp. 497–503.

[68] Chang, E., et al., "Evaluation of Quantum Dot Cytotoxicity Based on Intracellular Uptake" *Small*, Vol. 2 (12), 2006, pp. 1412–1417.

[69] Ma, D., Z.J. Jakubek, and B. Simard, "A New Approach towards Controlled Synthesis of Multifunctional Core-Shell Nano-Architectures: Luminescent and Superparamagnetic" *J. Nanosci. Nanotechnol.*, Vol. 6 (12), 2006, pp. 3677–3684.

[70] Noble, M., M. Mayer-Pröschel, and C. Pröschel, "Redox Regulation of Precursor Cell Function: Insights and Paradoxes" *Antioxid. Redox. Signal*, Vol. 7 (11-12), 2005, pp. 1456-1467.

[71] Finkel, T., and N.J. Holbrook, "Oxidants, Oxidative Stress and the Biology of Ageing" *Nature*, Vol. 408 (6809), 2000, pp. 239–247.

[72] Kroemer, G., and M. Jaattela, "Lysosomes and Autophagy in Cell Death Control" *Nat. Rev. Cancer*, Vol. 5, 2005, 886–897.

[73] Halliwell, B., and J. Gutteridge, *Free Radicals in Biology and Medicine*, Oxford, UK: Oxford Univ. Press, 1999.

[74] Xiao, G.G., M. Wang, N. Li, et al., "Use of Proteomics to Demonstrate a Hierarchical Oxidative Stress Response to Diesel Exhaust Particle Chemicals in a Macrophage Cell Line" *J. Biol. Chem.*, Vol. 278, 2003, pp. 50781–50790.

[75] Ju, S.-T., D.J. Panka, H. Cui, et al., "Fas(CD95)/FasL Interactions Required for Programmed Cell Death after T-cell Activation" *Nature*, Vol. 373 (6513), 1995, pp. 444–448.

[76] Thorburn, A., "Death Receptor-Induced Cell Killing" *Cell Signal.*, Vol. 16 (2), pp. 139-144.

[77] Wallach, D., E.E. Varfolomeev, N.L. Malinin, et al., "Tumor Necrosis Factor Receptor and Fas Signaling Mechanisms" *Annu. Rev. Immunol.*, Vol. 17, 1999, pp. 331–367.

[78] Ipe, B.I., M. Lehnig, and C.M. Niemeyer, "On the Generation of Free Radical Species from Quantum Dots" *Small*, Vol. 1 (7), 2005, pp. 706–709.

[79] Bohne, C., K. Faulhaber, B. Giese, et al., "Studies on the Mechanism of the Photo-Induced DNA Damage in the Presence of Acridizinium Salts-Involvement of Singlet Oxygen and an Unusual Source for Hydroxyl Radicals" *J. Am. Chem. Soc.*, Vol. 127, 2005, 76–85.

[80] Iida, Y., K. Yasui, T. Tuziuti, et al., "Ultrasonic Cavitation in Microspace" *Chem. Comm.*, 2004, pp. 2280–2281.

[81] Tsuchiya, M., M. Suematsu, and H. Suzuchi, "In vivo Visualization of Oxygen Radical-Dependent Photo Emission" *Methods Enzymol.*, Vol. 233, 1994, pp. 128–140.

[82] Bonini, M.G., C. Rota, A. Tomasi, and R.P. Mason, "The Oxidation of 2',7'-Dichlorofluorescin to Reactive Oxygen Species: A Self-Fulfilling Prophesy?" *Free Radical Biol. Med.*, Vol. 40 (6), 2006, pp. 968–975.

[83] Maysinger, D., "Nanoparticles and Cells: Good Companions and Doomed Partnerships" *Org. Biomol. Chem.*, Vol. 5, 2007, pp. 2335–2342.

[84] Klotz, L.O., "Oxidant-Induced Signaling: Effects of Peroxynitrite and Singlet Oxygen" *Biol. Chem.*, Vol. 383, 2002, pp. 443–456.

[85] Samia, A.C.S., C. Burda, and X. Chen, "Semiconductor Quantum Dots for Photodynamic Therapy" *JACS*, Vol. 125, 2003, pp. 15736–15737.

[86] Shi, L., B. Hernandez, and M. Selke, "Singlet Oxygen Generation from Water-Soluble Quantum Dot-Organic Dye Nanocomposites" *J. Am. Chem. S*, Vol. 128, 2006, pp. 6278–6279.oc.

[87] Tsay, J.M., M. Trzoss, L. Shi, et al., "Singlet Oxygen Production by Peptide-Coated Quantum Dot-Photosensitizer Conjugates" *J. Am. Chem. Soc.*, Vol. 129, 2007, pp. 6865–6871.

[88] Yang, C.-F., H.M. Shen, Y. Shen, et al., "Cadmium-Induced Oxidative Cellular Damage in Human Fetal Lung Fibroblasts (MRC-5 Cells)" *Environ. Health Perspect.*, Vol. 105,1997, pp. 712–716.

[89] Koizumi, T., H. Shirakura, H. Kumagai, et al., "Mechanism of Cadmium-Induced Cytotoxicity in Rat Hepatocytes: Cadmium-Induced Active Oxygen-Related Permeability Changes of the Plasma Membrane" *Toxicology*, Vol. 114, 1996, pp. 125–134.

[90] Hassoun, E.A., and S.J. Stohs, "Cadmium-Induced Production of Superoxide Anion and Nitric Oxide, DNA Single Strand Breaks and Lactate Dehydrogenase Leakage in J774A.1 Cell Cultures" *Toxicology*, Vol. 112 (3), 1996, pp. 219–226.

[91] Chan, W.-H., N.H. Shiao, and P.Z. Lu, "CdSe Quantum Dots Induce Apoptosis in Human Neuroblastoma Cells via Mitochondrial-Dependent Pathways and Inhibition of Survival Signals" *Toxicol. Lett.*, Vol. 167 (3), 2006, pp. 191–200.

[92] Choi, A.O., S.J. Cho, J. Desbarats, et al., "Quantum Dot-Induced Cell Death Involves Fas Upregulation and Lipid Peroxidation in Human Neuroblastoma Cells" *J. Nanobiotechnol.*, Vol. 5 (1), 2007, pp. 1–13.

[93] Schins, R.P.F., and T.K. Hei, *Genotoxic Effects of Particles* in: *Particle Toxicology*, Boca Raton: CRC Press and Francis Group, 2006, pp. 285–298.

[94] Green, M., and E. Howman, "Semiconductor Quantum Dots and Free Radical Induced DNA Nicking" *Chem. Comm.*, 2005, pp. 121–123.

[95] Liang, J., Z. He, S. Zhang, et al., "Study on DNA Damage Induced by CdSe Quantum Dots Using Nucleic Acid Molecular "Light Switches" as Probe" *Talanta*, Vol. 71 (4), 2007, pp. 1675–1678.

[96] Zhang, T., J.L. Stilwell, D. Gerion, et al., "Cellular Effect of High Doses of Silica-Coated Quantum Dot Profiled with High Throughput Gene Expression Analysis and High Content Cellomics Measurements" *Nano Lett.*, Vol. 6 (4), 2006, pp. 800–808.

[97] Choi, A.O., S.E. Brown, M. Szyf, and D. Maysinger, "Quantum Dot Induced Epigenetic and Genotoxic Changes in Human Breast Cancer Cells" *J. Mol. Med.*, Vol. 86 (3), 2008, pp. 291–302.

[98] Hsieh, S.-C., F.-F. Wang, C.-S. Lin, et al., "The Inhibition of Osteogenesis with Human Bone Marrow Mesenchymal Stem Cells by CdSe/ZnS Quantum Dot Labels" *Biomaterials*, Vol. 27 (8), 2006, pp. 1656–1664.

[99] Hsieh, S.-C., F.-F. Wang, S.-C. Hung, et al., "The Internalized CdSe/ZnS Quantum Dots Impair the Chondrogenesis of Bone Marrow Mesenchymal Stem Cells" *J. Biomed. Mat. Res. part B*, Vol. 79, 2006, pp. 95–101.

[100] Shah, B.S., P.A. Clark, E.K. Moioli, et al., "Labeling of Mesenchymal Stem Cells by Bioconjugated Quantum Dots" *Nano Lett.*, Vol. 7 (10), 2007, pp. 3071–3079.

[101] Ballou, B., B.C. Langerholm, L.A. Ernst, et al., "Noninvasive Imaging of Quantum Dots in Mice" *Bioconjugate Chem.*, Vol. 15, 2004, pp. 79–86.

[102] Ballou, B., L.A. Ernst, S. Andreko, et al., "Sentinel Lymph Node Imaging Using Quantum Dots in Mouse Tumor Models" *Bioconjugate Chem.*, Vol. 18 (2), 2007, pp. 389–395.

[103] Gopee, N.V., D.W. Roberts, P. Webb, et al., "Migration of Intradermally Injected Quantum Dots to Sentinel Organs in Mice" *Toxicol. Sci.*, Vol. 98 (1), 2007, pp. 249–257.

[104] Fischer, H.C., L. Liu, K.S. Pang, and W.C.W. Chan, "Pharmacokinetics of Nanoscale Quantum Dots: In vivo Distribution, Sequestration, and Clearance in the Rat" *Adv. Funct. Mat.*, Vol. 16 (10), 2006, pp. 1299–1305.

[105] Yang, R.S.H., L.W. Chang, J.-P. Wu, et al., "Persistent Tissue Kinetics and Redistribution of Nanoparticles, Quantum Dot 705, in Mice: ICP-MS Quantitative Assessment" *Environm. Health Perspectives*, Vol. 115, 2007, pp. 1339–1343.

[106] Choi, H.S., W. Liu, P. Misra, et al., "Renal Clearance of Quantum Dots" *Nature Biotech.*, Vol. 25 (10), 2007, pp. 1165–1170.

CHAPTER 8

Chemical and Biological Sensing Based on Gold Nanoparticles

Chang-Cheng You, Sarit S. Agasti, Myoung-Hwan Park, and Vincent M. Rotello

8.1 Introduction

Chemical and biological sensing plays a significant role in medical, forensic, agricultural, and environmental sciences [1]. The prompt and accurate sensing of diseases and harmful agents will give significant improvement in various fields such as healthcare, food safety, and environmental monitoring. In general, sensor systems consist of a recognition component for target binding and a transduction element for signaling the binding event. There are multiple criteria for the creation of efficient sensors, including response time, signal-to-noise characteristics, sensitivity, and selectivity. Thus, sensing technology has been concerned with both developments of the recognition process and understanding of the transduction mechanism through the use of new materials. Similarly, the miniaturization of a sensor often increases its signal-to-noise ratio, facilitating the signal transduction [2]. To this end, nanomaterials are particularly interesting in creating novel chemical and biological sensors due to unique physicochemical properties that are absent in macro-scaled materials [3].

Gold nanoparticles (AuNPs) are stable materials that can be readily fabricated through either chemical reduction of gold salts or physical treatment of bulk gold. AuNPs possess unique optical and electronic properties due to the large surface-to-volume ratio with high density, and they show excellent biocompatibility with varied ligands [4]. The optoelectronic properties of AuNPs depend on their size and shape, as well as upon the surrounding chemical environment. As shown in Figure 8.1, the binding event may change the physicochemical properties of AuNPs such as surface plasmon resonance, conductivity, and redox behavior, leading to detectable signals. In this regard, AuNPs behave as signal transducers. On the other hand, AuNPs provide an adaptable platform for multiple functionalization with either small organic ligands or large biomacromolecules. The resultant functionalized AuNPs offer opportunities in the selective binding and sensing of organic as well as biological targets [5–7].

In this chapter, we have organized our discussion on the basis of the transduction mechanisms that have been used with these sensors, including absorption, quenching, conductivity, redox, and density. Within these sections, we will

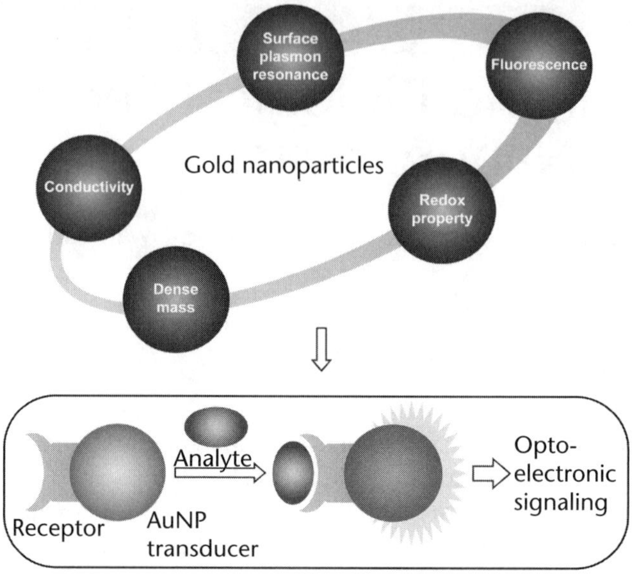

Figure 8.1 Physical properties of AuNPs and the schematic depiction of an AuNP-based sensor.

focus on the recent research activities involving the use of AuNPs in the detection of a variety of target analytes including metal ions, volatile molecules, organic compounds, oligonucleotides, and proteins.

8.2 Synthesis of Gold Nanoparticles

The synthesis of colloidal gold dates back to Faraday, who obtained gold hydrosols by the reduction of an aqueous solution of chloroaurate using phosphorus dissolved in carbon disulfide in 1857 [8]. During the past few decades, many efforts have been devoted to the preparation of AuNPs with control over their size, shape, stability, solubility, and surface functionality. Both “top-down” (e.g., physical manipulation) and “bottom-up” (e.g., chemical transformation) methods have been successfully developed. AuNPs with varying core sizes can be prepared by the chemical reduction of gold salts in the presence of appropriate stabilizing agents that provide the necessary barrier to particle coalescence. Some common synthetic methods of core-shell AuNPs are summarized in Table 8.1. It should be noted that the terms *colloid* and *cluster* are often used interchangeably; the former generally refers to particles with diameters larger than 10 nm, while the latter refers to smaller particles.

Turkevich et al. developed a simple synthetic method of gold colloids in 1951 by the treatment of hydrogen tetrachloroaurate with citric acid in boiling water [18]. In this approach, citric acid acts as both reducing and stabilizing agent. Frens’s group further refined this method and manipulated the core sizes by changing the feed ratio of gold salt to sodium citrate [19]. This protocol is usually used to prepare spherical AuNPs in diameters of 10 to 20 nm, though larger AuNPs (e.g., 100 nm) can also be prepared.

Triphenylphosphine has been used as the capping agent to prepare small gold clusters. Monodisperse AuNPs in diameters of 1–2 nm are obtained by reduction of

Table 8.1 Synthetic Methods and Capping Agents for AuNPs of Diverse Core Size

Core Size (d)	*Synthetic Methods*	*Capping Agents*	*References*
1–2 nm	Reduction of $AuCl(PPh_3)$ with diborane or sodium borohydride	Phosphine	[9–11]
1.5–5 nm	Biphasic reduction of $HAuCl_4$ by sodium borohydride in the presence of thiol capping agents	Alkanethiol	[12–14]
5–8 nm	Reduction of $HAuCl_4$ by sodium borohydride in the presence of TOAB	Quaternary ammonium salt (TOAB)	[15]
8–20 nm	Reduction of $HAuCl_4$ by oleyl amine in water under heating	Oleyl amine	[16, 17]
10–40 nm	Reduction of $HAuCl_4$ with sodium citrate in water	Citrate	[18–20]

$AuCl(PPh_3)$ with diborane [9] or sodium borohydride [11]. Particularly, particles of formula $Au_{55}(PPh_3)_{12}Cl_6$ (or $Au_{101}(PPh_3)_{21}Cl_5$) [11] constitute the predominant fraction of the products. These small AuNPs have found interesting applications in molecular devices [10, 21]. Kinetic studies have revealed that phosphine-capped AuNPs undergo rapid exchange of capping ligand phosphine with dissociated phosphine [22].

In 1990s, a breakthrough in the AuNP synthesis was achieved, involving the transfer of hydrogen tetrachloroaurate from aqueous phase to toluene phase by the surfactant tetraoctylammonium bromide (TOAB) and the subsequent reduction by sodium borohydride in the presence of alkanethiols to generate nanoparticles that are soluble in organic solvents [12]. This synthetic approach, known as Brust-Schiffrin method, leads to relatively monodisperse AuNPs protected by thiol ligands with controlled diameters ranging from 1.5 to 5 nm. The nanoparticle size can be readily varied by the various reaction conditions, including gold-to-thiol ratio, reduction rate, and reaction temperature [14]. Thiol-protected AuNPs possess superior stability to most of the other AuNPs due to the synergistic effect of strong thiol-gold interactions and van der Waals interactions of the ligands. Nanoparticles of this kind can be thoroughly dried and redispersed in solution without any aggregation. Monophasic reduction of gold salts by sodium borohydride in the presence of thiols has also been developed [23, 24], through which water-soluble AuNPs could be prepared in a single step. In the biphasic reduction protocol, the absence of thiol ligands can lead to slightly larger nanoparticles stabilized by quaternary ammonium, which show considerable stability in solution and serve as excellent precursors for other functionalized nanoparticles [15].

Various reducing/capping agents, such as amino acid [25], oleyl amine [16], aliphatic and aromatic amines [26, 27], and hyperbranched polyethylenimine [28] have been used to reduce gold salts into nanoparticles with various core sizes and dispersities. The size and shape of AuNPs can be further manipulated by physicochemical treatments including light-irradiation and thermolysis [13, 31]. For example, conventional ripening [29, 30] and digestive ripening [32, 33] treatments have been conducted to increase and decrease the nanoparticle size, with the concurrent decrease in polydispersity. UV and laser irradiation provides another powerful approach to improve the nanoparticle quality [34, 35]. The capping agents listed in Table 8.1 are generally lacking in chemical functionality, thus restricting their applications in sensing. One efficient approach for the nanoparticle functionalization is the place-exchange process introduced by Murray et al. [36]. Initially, the thiol ligands are anchored on the nanoparticle surface, and then they're replaced by the presence of external thiol ligands [37]. The loading of functional ligands can be controlled by modulating the reaction time and/or the amount of incoming ligands. Mixed monolayer-protected gold clusters can be obtained by place-exchange reactions using a mixture of two or more ligands as the incoming agents. The thiol ligands on gold surface possess a certain level of mobility, and consequently they can undergo reposition on the surface to optimize interaction with analytes [38], as well as slowly hop between nanoparticles [39].

Labile capping agents such as citrate [40], triphenylphosphine [41], and dimethylaminopyridine [42] can be displaced by thiols under mild reaction conditions with no residual capping agent. Citrate-stabilized AuNPs are important precursors for large functionalized colloidal ensembles such as those carrying oligonucleotide [43], protein, or antibody functionalities [44]. However, the chemisorption of thiol ligands onto the citrate-stabilized nanoparticles can cause irreversible aggregation [45]. In this case, the addition of nonionic surfactant such as Tween 20 can prevent aggregation during the place-exchange [46].

8.3 Physical Properties of Gold Nanoparticles

AuNPs possess unique size- and shape-dependent optical and electronic properties. Solutions of spherical AuNPs exhibit a diverse range of colors including brown, red, and violet as the core size increases from 1 to 100 nm. Generally, AuNPs show an intense absorption peak from 500 to 550 nm [47], referred to as *surface plasmon band*, which arises from the collective oscillation of the conduction electrons due to the resonant excitation by the incident photons (Figure 8.2). This surface plasmon band is absent in both small nanoparticles ($d < 2$ nm) and bulk materials. Mie theoretically interpreted the surface plasmon resonance (SPR) phenomena in 1908 [48], and his theory has been extensively correlated with the experimental results [49, 50]. The SPR is sensitive not only to nanoparticle size, but also to the surrounding environment such as ligand, solvent, and temperature. Particularly, the SPR frequency is dependent on the proximity to other nanoparticles. Thus, under nanoparticle aggregation, the surface plasmon band shows significant red-shifting (to ca. 650 nm) and broadening, and the solution displays a red-to-blue color change due to the interparticle plasmon coupling [51]. This phenomenon constitutes the cornerstone for their application in colorimetric sensing, which will be discussed in detail in the following sections.

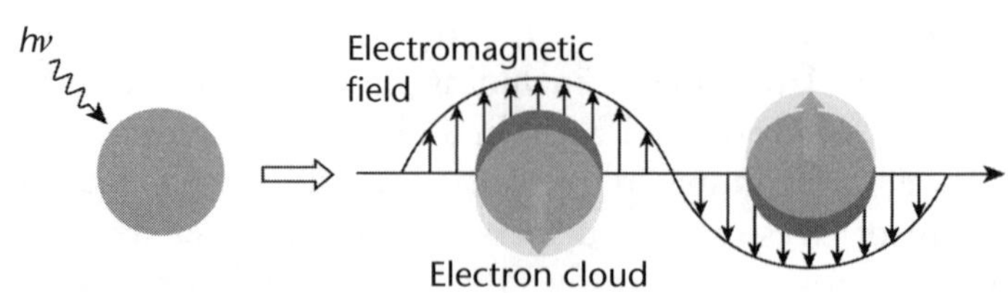

Figure 8.2 Schematic representation of the oscillation of conduction electrons across the nanoparticle in the electromagnetic field of the incident light.

Generally, it is not easy to determine AuNP concentrations. As the molar extinction coefficient of colloidal gold (520 nm) is ~4000 M^{-1} cm^{-1} per gold atom [52], the nanoparticle concentration can then be roughly estimated based on the number of gold atoms. The extinction coefficients of AuNPs with different sizes and capping ligands have also been measured experimentally [53]. A linear relationship is observed between logarithms of molar extinction coefficient (ε) and core diameter (*d*), essentially irrespective of the ligands and solvents:

$$\ln \varepsilon = k \ln d + c \tag{8.1}$$

where $k = 3.32$ and $c = 10.8$ ($\lambda = 506$ nm). The nanoparticle concentrations can be readily deduced from Beer-Lambert Law once the nanoparticle size is known (from TEM). For example, it is estimated that the AuNP of 20-nm diameter has a molar extinction coefficient of 1×10^9 M^{-1} cm^{-1} from (8.1). This value is at least three orders higher than that of common organic dyes ($10^4 - 10^6$ M^{-1} cm^{-1}), indicating that AuNPs may serve as excellent light collectors [54].

Not only can AuNPs show photoluminescence under certain conditions [55, 56], but they can also enhance fluorescence at appropriate fluorophore-to-metal distances on solid substrates [57], based on the superb quenching ability of AuNPs to proximal fluorophores. This effect could be explained by the reflected far-field radiation from the fluorophore back on itself, which depends on the distance from the metal surface. The lifetime of fluorophore was decreased when the reflected field amplitude was increased, whereas it was increased when the field was opposed. Fluorescence resonance energy transfer (FRET) is an important deactivation pathway for the excited fluorophores in case of a good overlap between the donor's emission spectrum and the gold surface plasmon band [58, 59]. Both radiative and nonradiative decay rates of fluorescent molecules are distinctly affected, indicating highly efficient fluorescence quenching with small (1-nm) nanoparticles. Photoinduced electron transfer (PET) can also quench fluorophores in the vicinity of AuNPs, where the nanoparticles act as electron acceptors [5]. The electron transfer process can be modulated by charging/discharging the gold core, providing an interesting opportunity for sensor fabrication [60].

In contrast to bulk metals, a band gap exists between the valence and the conduction bands of small metal nanoparticles. Therefore, small metal nanoparticles display size-dependent quantization effects, leading to the discrete electron-transition energy levels. For example, 15 redox states have been observed for hexanethiol-capped AuNPs (Au_{147}, $r = 0.81$ nm) at room temperature [61], indicating that AuNPs are multivalent redox species with molecule-like redox properties [62]. The quantized capacitance charging behavior of AuNPs is distinctly affected by applied electrolyte ions, external ligands, and magnetic fields, expanding their utility in electronic devices and electrochemical labels [21].

8.4 Colorimetric Sensing

The clustering of AuNPs of appropriate sizes ($d > 3.5$ nm) results in interparticle surface plasmon coupling [63], resulting in a color change from red to blue. These color changes can be easily observed by the naked eye at nanomolar concentrations. Therefore, AuNPs have been intensely used in the colorimetric sensing of diverse substances ranging from simple metal ions and small molecules to complex polynucleotides and proteins [3].

8.4.1 Colorimetric Detection of Metal Ions and Anions

The colorimetric detection of metal ions using AuNPs requires the incorporation of chelating agents onto the nanoparticle surface (Figure 8.3). AuNPs carrying 15-crown-5 moieties have been fabricated to detect potassium ions, which are physiologically important [64], through a red-to-blue color change. The concentration ranges of K^+ detection are from μM to mM, depending upon the concentrations of colloid gold. Attractively, this sensor system is still viable in the presence of a large amount of interferential Na^+. This system, extended to the detection of Na^+, has been achieved by the incorporation of 12-crown-4 onto the AuNPs [65]. Similarly, phenanthroline-functionalized 4-nm AuNPs and lactose-functionalized 16-nm AuNPs have been constructed, respectively, to detect Li^+ and Ca^{2+} with little interference from other metal ions [66, 67].

Heavy metal ions such as Pb^{2+}, Cd^{2+}, and Hg^{2+} are quite toxic. Hupp et al. have reported a simple metal ion sensing system based on 11-mercaptoundecanoic acid (MUA)-functionalized 13 nm AuNPs [68]. In their design, the surface carboxylates act as metal ion receptors and the nanoparticle aggregation is driven by heavy-metal ion chelation. The presence of Pb^{2+}, Cd^{2+}, or Hg^{2+} (= 400 μM) causes nanoparticle aggregation, whereas Zn^{2+} exhibits no response. Fine control of the buffer composite can significantly improve the selectivity and sensitivity of this system [69]. Mixed monolayer-protected AuNPs carrying both carboxylate and 15-crown-5 functionalities provide a colorimetric sensor for Pb^{2+}, where Pb^{2+} ions disrupt the initially hydrogen-bonded assemblies [70]. Cysteine and peptide-functionalized AuNPs have been fabricated and used to detect Cu^{2+} and Hg^{2+}, respectively [71, 72]. These sensing systems are able to detect the target analytes at submicromolar concentrations. Recently, Mirkin et al. reported a detection limit of 100 nM with DNA-functionalized AuNPs [73].

In general, selectivity and sensitivity are very important in ionic sensing. Liu and Lu have devised a highly selective lead biosensors using DNAzyme-directed assembly of AuNPs [74–76]. DNAzymes are catalytically active DNA molecules and show metal-dependent activities. In the sensor design, a Pb^{2+}-specific DNAzyme was chosen as the target recognition element and DNA-functionalized AuNPs as the signal transducer. The DNAzyme consists of an enzyme strand and a substrate strand, and

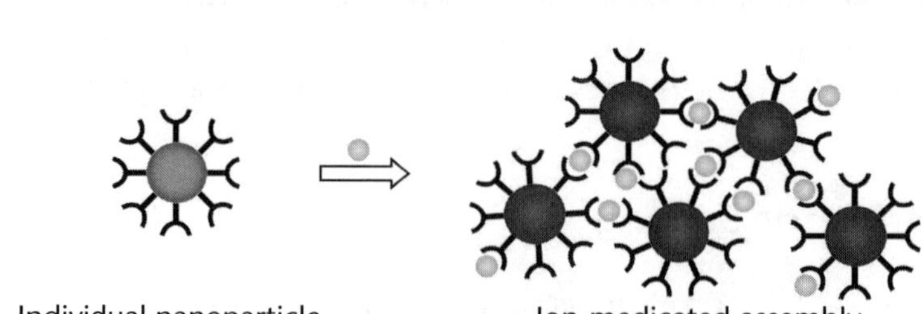

Figure 8.3 Schematic illustration of metal ion-induced nanoparticle aggregation.

both ends are extended with bases that are complementary to the DNA anchored on AuNPs. The DNAzyme and the DNA-functionalized AuNPs initially form blue-colored assemblies through Watson-Crick base pairing [77, 78]. In the presence of Pb^{2+}, the DNAzyme is activated and cleaves the substrate strand to disassemble the AuNPs, resulting in a blue-to-red color change. In addition, the sensor is available for detecting Pb^{2+} of 100 nM, while other divalent metal ions such as Ca^{2+}, Co^{2+}, Ni^{2+}, and Cd^{2+} show only background blue color. Further investigation indicated that it's very important to arrange AuNPs' assemblies in the disassembly process, because "head-to-tail" manner might result in a large steric hindrance that could disfavor the assembly, comparing with the "tail-to-tail" alignment [79]. Thus, optimization of the AuNP alignment in the assemblies allows a fast detection of Pb^{2+} (< 10 min) at ambient temperature [76, 79]. This approach has also been extended to the detection of adenosine by using AuNPs functionalized with an adenosine-specific aptazyme [80].

In comparison with metal ions, the colorimetric detection of anions using AuNPs is still limited mainly due to the lack of appropriate anion receptors. Kubo et al. have attached isothiouronium groups onto AuNPs and then explored their colorimetric sensing of oxoanions in aqueous methanol solution [81]. The presence of Cl^- does not affect the absorption properties of the nanoparticle, whereas oxanions such as AcO^-, HPO_4^{2-}, and malonate induce color changes. Particularly, ditopic malonate causes the big color change from red to blue due to the significant AuNP aggregation. Thioglucose-coated AuNPs have been used to sense fluoride anions in water [82]. Although other anions such as Cl^-, Br^-, I^-, AcO^-, and NO_3^- show only a little color change, the relatively narrow concentration range (20 ~ 40 mM) for F^- detection restricts the practical application of this system.

8.4.2 Colorimetric Detection of Biomaterials

In solution-based colorimetric detection, it is critical to introduce appropriate receptors onto AuNPs such that aggregation or disaggregation can be triggered by target complexations. However, this recognition is not readily achieved for the small organic molecule sensing, as the small organic analytes cannot serve as the bridging agents for nanoparticle assembly in most cases. On the basis of a competitive colorimetric assay, Geddes et al. have demonstrated glucose sensing by using assemblies of concanavalin A (Con A) and dextran-functionalized AuNPs [83, 84]. Con A is a multivalent protein (four sugar binding sites at pH 7), which allows dextran-coated nanoparticles to cross-link, affording assemblies with broadened and red-shifted SPR. When glucose is present, it competitively interacts with Con A, releasing the individual dextran-coated AuNPs. This process can be readily monitored by either conventional UV/Vis spectrometry [83] or wavelength-ratiometric resonance light scattering [84]. Significantly, the dynamic range for glucose sensing can be modulated by various factors such as dextran length, particle size, and the loading amount of dextran or Con A. A glucose dynamic sensing range of 1–40 mM has been achieved, and it can potentially be used to diagnose the blood glucose level in healthy people (3–8 mM) and in diabetics (2–40 mM).

Incorporation of AuNPs into the polymer matrix of molecularly imprinted polymers (MIPs) provides SPR-based molecular sensors. For example,

MUA-AuNPs have been immobilized into a MIP gel placed between two glass slides to serve as a colorimetric adrenaline sensor [85]. The initially shrunken MIP gel in the absence of adrenaline affords the close proximity of AuNPs. The selective binding of target analytes, however, causes a blue-shift in the SPR band of the immobilized AuNPs due to the swelling of the MIP gel. This AuNP-MIP system selectively detects adrenaline with a dynamic range from 5 μM to 2 mM.

Aptamers are single-stranded oligonucleic acid-based binding molecules that can bind a great variety of targets with high affinity and specificity [86]. For example, Lu and coworkers have designed an effective cocaine sensor using a cocaine aptamer-mediated AuNP assembly [87]. As illustrated in Figure 8.4, the sensor consists of two kinds of single-stranded (ss) DNA-modified AuNPs and a linker DNA molecule that carries cocaine aptamer. The linker molecule pairs respectively with two ssDNA-functionalized AuNPs to generate blue aggregates where a part of cocaine aptamer takes part in the DNA hybridization. When cocaine is present in the system, the aptamer changes its structure to bind cocaine, resulting in the disassembly of the aggregates with a concomitant blue-to-red color change whose rate depends upon the cocaine concentration (50 to 500 μM). This sensing approach is of general significance in the sensor design, as any aptamer of choice can potentially be grafted into this system [87]. Interestingly, the use of a mixture of different aptamers provides smart materials for responding to the combination of analytes [88]. Recently, both adenosine and cocaine aptamer-linked nanoparticle aggregates have been immobilized onto a lateral flow device, allowing a more sensitive "dipstick" test that can be performed in complex sample matrices such as human blood serum [89].

DNA-meditated AuNP assembly was first described by Mirkin et al. in 1996 [77]. Since then, the oligonucleotide-directed AuNP aggregation has been extensively used in the colorimetric detection of oligonucleotides [78, 90–97] and fabrication of structured assemblies [98]. Generally, two ssDNA-modified AuNPs are used for the detection of oligonucleotides, where the base sequences are respectively complementary to both ends of the target oligonucleotides. Therefore, the presence of target oligonucleotides causes the AuNP aggregation accompanied with a color change. The intense absorptivity of AuNPs coupled with the strong and highly specific base-pairing of DNA molecules enables the ultrasensitive detection of oligonuceotides in a quantitative manner. When large AuNPs (e.g., 50 nm or 100 nm) are employed, the detection limit was subpicomolar without the assistance of

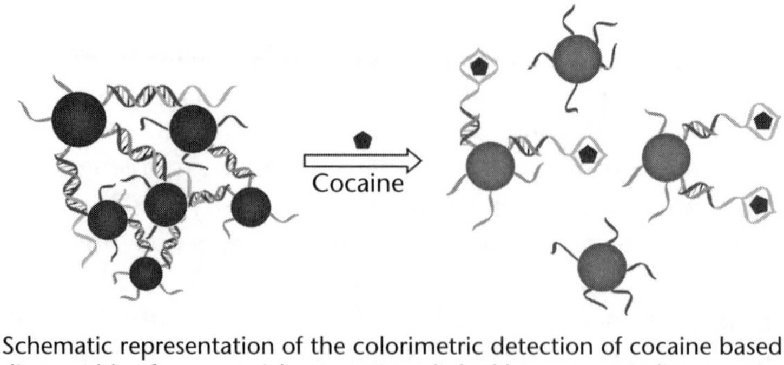

Figure 8.4 Schematic representation of the colorimetric detection of cocaine based on the target-induced disassembly of nanoparticle aggregates linked by corresponding aptamers.

polymerase chain reaction (PCR) [91]. Interestingly, citrate-stabilized AuNPs can distinguish ssDNA and dsDNA at the level of 100 fmol based on simple electrostatic interactions [99], such as single-base-pair mismatches.

The oligonucleotide-directed AuNP assembly has important applications in the colorimetric screening of DNA binders [100] and triplex DNA binders [101]. In the latter case, the assay is composed of two sets of noncomplementary AuNPs and a free strand of DNA that can form triplexes with those on the nanoparticles with no aggregation at room temperature due to the low stability of the triplex structure (Figure 8.5). However, the appropriate triplex DNA binders can stabilize the complexes, inducing the aggregation of AuNPs. The simplicity of this approach makes it more convenient than other methods such as competitive dialysis, mass spectroscopy, and electrophoresis, thus being suitable in high-throughput screening of potential triplex binders from large combinatorial libraries [101].

Protein detection and identification is important in medical diagnostics, proteomics, and antibioterrorism. Ligand-modified AuNPs provide a promising scaffold for colorimetric detection of proteins. For example, agglutinin, a bivalent lectin that can specifically recognize β-D-galactose, induces the aggregation of galactose-functionalized AuNPs based on the lectin concentration, allowing the quantitative detection of the protein [102]. Significantly, the sensitivity of this system is appreciably high enough to detect the lectin concentration of 1 ppm, comparable to that of immunological assay methods such as ELISA [102]. Protein-directed glyconanoparticle assembly has been used to detect protein-protein interactions. Interestingly, Chen et al. used the assemblies Con A and mannose-modified AuNPs to identify the binding partners for Con A, since the protein-protein interactions disrupt the initial nanoparticle-protein assemblies, affording both quantitative results [103]. Recently, the controlled aggregation of glyconanoparticles has been harnessed to attain colorimetric detection of cholera toxin [104]. By using the high binding affinity between biotin and avidin, biotin-functionalized AuNPs have been deposited on glass substrates, with colorimetric changes upon streptavidin binding with nanoparticle size-dependent sensitivity [105, 106].

Aptamers rival antibodies in terms of binding ability. AuNPs carrying an aptamer that is specific to platelet-derived growth factors (PDGFs) have been

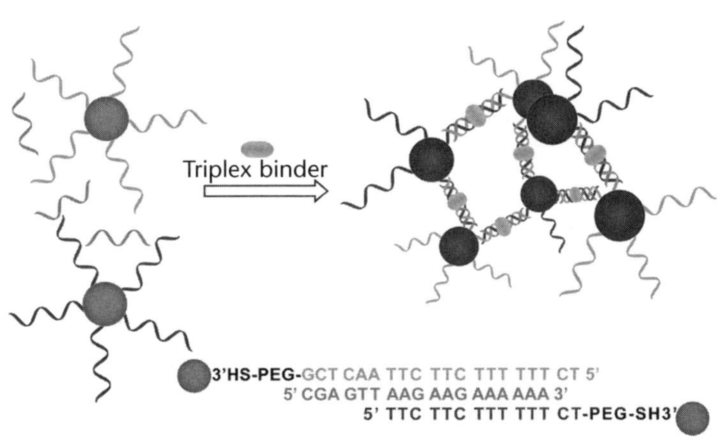

Figure 8.5 Schematic depiction of the screening of DNA triplex binder using DNA-directed AuNP assembly.

exploited to detect PDGFs by monitoring the changes in color and extinction of the AuNPs as a consequence of aggregation [107]. Noteworthy, this assembly of aptamer-AuNP-PDGF could also be used to detect PDGF receptors through a competitive binding mechanism. Recently, Dong's group reported a much simpler aptamer-based colorimetric sensing system by thrombin-binding aptamers [108]. The aptamers fold into a structure of G-quadruplex/duplex in the presence of thrombin due to the aptamer-protein recognition, losing their protecting function. The AuNP aggregates are formed accordingly with a detection limit of 0.83 nM for thrombin.

Willner et al. have achieved thrombin sensing using thrombin aptamer-modified glass surface [109]. The functionalized glass substrate was treated with thrombin targets and aptamer-functionalized AuNPs successively, leading to a "sandwich" complex. The immobilized AuNPs are further enlarged in a growth solution containing $HAuCl_4$, CTAB, and NADH [110], which initiates the SPR coupling interaction of adjacent nanoparticles with a sensitivity limit of 2 nM.

Dithiols have long been used as cross-linkers in the assembly of AuNPs [111]. In case of dithiol-functionalized peptides as bridging agents, the AuNP assemblies provide a powerful platform for colorimetric detection of proteases [112]. In a representative study, Scrimin and coworkers designed two C- and N-terminal cysteinyl derivatives of peptide substrates that are specific to thrombin and lethal factor, respectively [113]. First, the peptides were treated with the analytes, and then they were incubated with citrate-stabilized 12-nm AuNPs. In the absence of target proteases, the intact peptides induce nanoparticle aggregations, showing a red-to-blue color change, while the protease-cleaved peptides do not bring any color change with the sensitivity in the low nanomolar range. Stevens et al. further simplified this two-stage approach by using AuNPs functionalized with Fmoc-protected peptides (substrate of thermolysin) with a cysteine anchor. The π-π stacking interactions between Fmoc groups led to an assembled state of AuNPs, which can be directly subjected to protein sensing. Once thermolysin is present, the peptide ligands are digested and AuNPs are dispersed in the solution along with a blue-to-red color change. This system has achieved an impressive sensitivity of 90 zg mL^{-1} (less than 380 molecules) [114]. Based on the enzymatic cleavage of DNA molecules, real-time colorimetric screening methods for endonuclease activity and inhibition have been developed by using DNA-mediated AuNP assemblies [115]. Similarly, the principle of enzyme-triggered AuNP assembly/disassembly has been employed to detect kinase [116] and phosphatases [117, 118], along with the screening of their activity. It has also been demonstrated that AuNPs can act as a colorimetric sensor for protein conformational changes [119].

8.5 Fluorescence Sensing

As it has been demonstrated earlier, AuNPs can be treated as nonmolecular chromophores with high molar extinction coefficients. Their exceptional quenching ability makes them excellent energy acceptors in the FRET assays [58, 120]. Poly-pyridyl complex $[Ru(bpy)^3]^{3+}$ is a well-known fluorophore, which is effectively quenched by anionic tiopronin-coated AuNPs [121]. The electrostatic interaction-driven complexes can be dissociated by addition of electrolytes such as K^+, Bu_4N^+, and Ca^{2+} salts. The fluorescence quenching and recovery follow Stern-Volmer relations, thus showing promising exploitation in the detection of these ions [121]. By employing the same principle, Rhodamine B-adsorbed AuNPs have been used in the turn-on fluorescence sensing of Hg^{2+} [122]. By optimizing the AuNP surface functionality and the chelating agent in the sample solution, the selectivity of this system for Hg^{2+} is 50-fold over other metal ions (e.g., Pb^{2+}, Cd^{2+}, Co^{2+}) with a detection limit of 2.0 ppb. Similarly, Nile red-adsorbed AuNPs show the selective detection of aminothiols [123], whereas Zhu, Li, and collaborators have fabricated bispyridyl perylene bridged AuNPs as Cu^{2+} sensors [124]. The fluorescence of perylene is quenched by AuNPs, while Cu^{2+} ions release the dye from the aggregate by stronger pyridine-Cu^{2+} coordination, regenerating the fluorescence. Significantly, this system can also be used in the colorimetric sensing of Cu^{2+} as the ion recognition involves the aggregation and disaggregation of AuNPs. Recently, lanthanum complexes of bipyridine-functionalized AuNPs have been used as phosphorescent sensors for alkaline earth metal ions and transition metal ions [125].

AuNP-based molecular beacons have been designed to provide fluorescence sensing of DNA [126]. As shown in Figure 8.6, the dye molecules within the initial closed hairpin structure are in close proximity to the AuNPs, resulting in effective fluorescence quenching through FRET. The hybridization of target DNA opens up the hairpin structure, increasing the donor-acceptor distance and providing a significant increase in fluorescence. In comparison with common molecular quenchers, this AuNP-based molecular beacon exhibits a sensitivity enhanced up to 100-fold with significantly improved detection of a single mismatch. Similarly, Nie et al. reported that oligonucleotide-functionalized AuNPs with fluorophore-terminus spontaneously assemble into a constrained arch-like conformation with close donor-acceptor distance, which responds to target ssDNA by a hybridization-induced strand stretching and consequent fluorescence light-up [127]. The distance-dependent FRET also provides a powerful way for the detection of DNA cleavage [128].

As with organic fluorescent dyes, the emission of semiconductor quantum dots can be effectively quenched by AuNPs in the appropriate vicinity. Melvin et al. have designed a fluorescent competitive assay for DNA detection using QDs and AuNPs as the FRET donor-acceptor couple [129]. In their protocol, the CdSe QDs linked to a short DNA strand are hybridized with a complementary DNA strand linked to an AuNP, leading to quenched assemblies due to the surface contact between QDs and AuNPs. When unlabelled complementary oligonucleotides are present, the AuNP-DNA is displaced from the QD-DNA, regenerating the QD fluorescence.

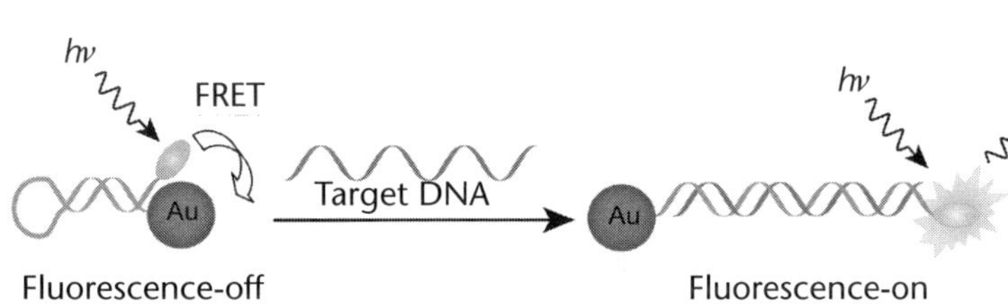

Figure 8.6 Schematic drawings of the conformational changes of the dye-oligonucleotide-AuNP conjugates before and after hybridization with the target DNA.

Kim, Oh, and coworkers have fabricated an inhibition assay of proteins on the basis of FRET between QDs and AuNPs [130]. The streptavidin-functionalized QDs specifically interact with biotinylated AuNPs to afford quenched assemblies through a QD-to-AuNP FRET process (Figure 8.7). This system has been exploited to the target avidin, which releases the biotinylated AuNPs from QDs through a competitive binding and regenerates the photoluminescence of QDs with a detection limit of 10 nM coupled with a dynamic range up to 2 μM. This study provides a generic tactic for designing protein sensors. For example, the assembly of dextran-functionalized QDs and Con A–coated AuNPs are available for the detection of glycoproteins in the protein sensing through specific protein-ligand interactions [131].

On the basis of fluorescent indicator-displacement assay coupled with "chemical nose" approach, Rotello and collaborators have devised a sensor array consisting of six cationic AuNPs and one anionic poly(*p*-phenyleneethynylene) (PPE) polymer, which can properly identify seven common proteins [132]. The initially quenched polymer-AuNP complexes are disrupted by protein analytes through competitive binding, resulting in fluorescence restoration, as shown in Figure 8.8(a). Because the protein-nanoparticle interactions are determined by their respective structural features such as charged, hydrophobic, hydrophilic, and hydrogen-bonding sites [133, 134], the diverse particle-protein affinities generate a distinguished fluorescence response pattern for individual proteins (Figure 8.8(b)). Linear discrimination analysis (LDA) has been used to differentiate the response patterns in high accuracy. Protein samples with both unknown identity and concentration have been subjected to the detection with the sensor array. With the training matrix (7 proteins $\times$ 6 sensors $\times$ 6 replicates) as the standard, an identification accuracy of 94.2 percent was obtained on the basis of 52 samples, and the protein concentrations were generally determined within $\pm$5 percent error.

8.6 Electrical and Electrochemical Sensing

Attributes such as the roughening of the conductive sensing interface, the catalytic properties, and the conductivity properties of AuNPs make them excellent candi-

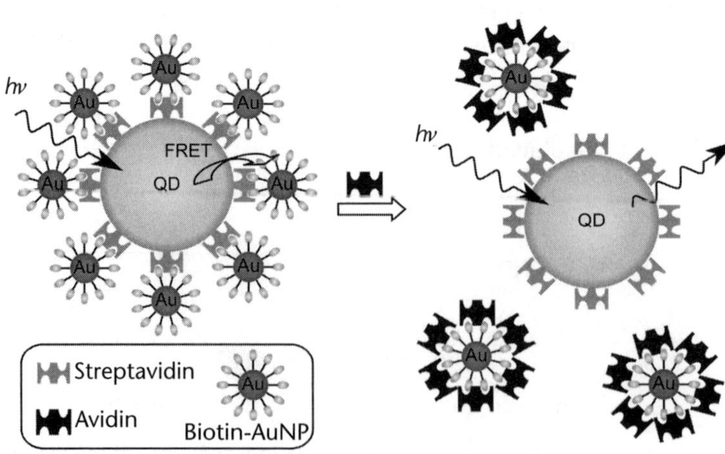

Figure 8.7 Competitive inhibition assay for the detection of avidin by using QD-AuNP couple.

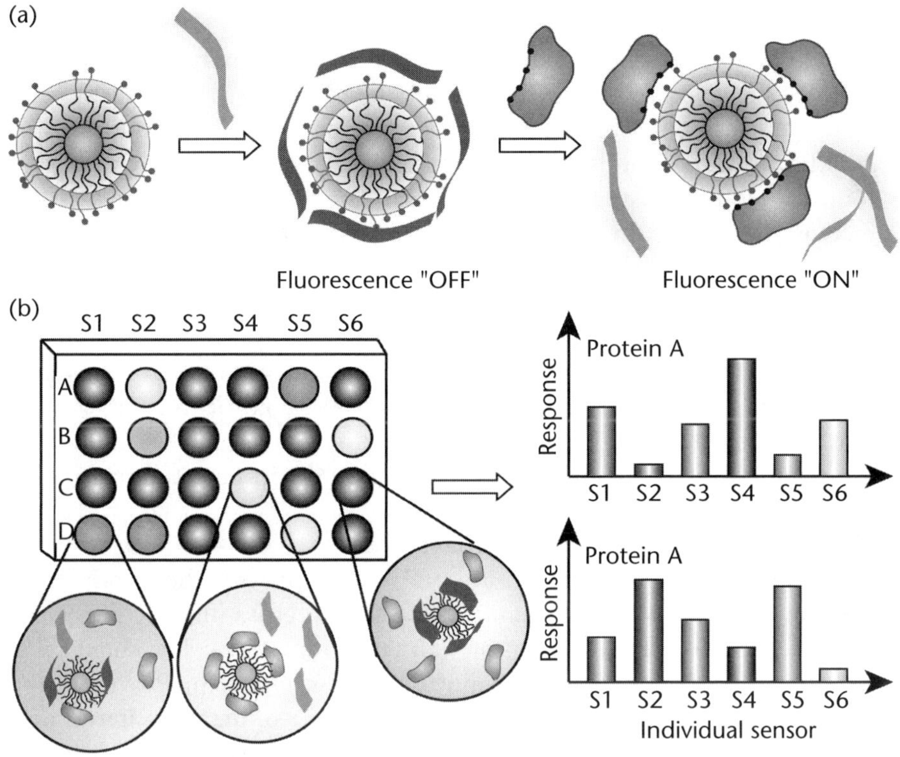

Figure 8.8 Schematic illustration of "chemical nose" sensor array based on AuNP-fluorescent polymer conjugates: (a) The competitive binding between protein and quenched polymer-AuNP complexes leads to the fluorescence light-up. (b) The combination of an array of sensors generates fingerprint response patterns for individual proteins.

dates for electroanalytical applications [135]. The assembly of multilayered AuNPs onto electrodes significantly enhances electrode surface area, enabling the highly sensitive electrochemical detection of redox analytes [136]. On the other hand, the analyte or redox partners on a roughened electrode have more freedom in orientation to facilitate the electron transfer through the conducting pathways provided by AuNPs. Particularly, the AuNP-decorated electrode displays high electrocatalytic activity in comparison with bulk electrodes. For example, AuNP-electrodes are able to discriminate the voltammetric signals of dopamine, ascorbate, and uric acid [137, 138].

Chemiresistors are solid-state devices that exhibit electrical resistance changes upon interaction with chemical species. The electronic conductivities of self-assembled films of monolayer-protected AuNPs can be varied by particle size, interparticle separation, ligand properties, and chemical environments [139]. These materials have been widely used to build chemiresistors for vapor sensing during the past decade [135]. Recently, Wohltjen and Snow have fabricated a sensor by deposition of a thin film of octanethiol-coated AuNPs ($d \sim 2$ nm) onto an interdigitated microelectrode [140]. This sensor shows a large and rapid decrease in the conductance upon exposure to toluene and tetrachloroethylene, with a detection limit of ca. 1 ppm. The increase of the resistance indicates that the film swelling dominates the vapor sensing, leading to an increase of the interparticle distances. Once the coated ligands of AuNPs are replaced by those bearing polar functional groups, the resultant chemiresistors are more sensitive to polar analytes [141].

Vossmeyer et al. have systematically investigated the sensing system with vapor of toluene and tetrachloroethylene from films formed by dodecylamine-stabilized AuNPs and α,ω-dithiols with different chain lengths (C_6, C_9, C_{12}, C_{16}) [142]. It was found that the resistance responses at a given concentration of toluene analyte increase exponentially with increasing number of methylene units. This effect has been attributed to the augmentation of sorption sites along with increasing the ligand length. Zhong and coworkers have tested the cofactors influencing the performance of sensor arrays constructed from AuNP films and interdigitated microelectrodes, proving the correlation between the vapor-response sensitivity and the interparticle spacing properties [143, 144]. Significantly, it was demonstrated that a compromised balance between the interparticle chain-chain cohesive interdigitation and the film-vapor interaction determines the relative change of the electrical resistance.

AuNP-dendrimer composites have likewise been used in vapor sensing [145]. In these layer-by-layer self-assemblies, the AuNPs provide the film material with electric conductivity, while the dendrimers serve to cross-link the particles and to provide sites for the selective sorption of analyte molecules. The chemical selectivity of the films is predominantly determined by the solubility properties of the dendrimer component. In an early study, an interesting bioconjugate material has been fabricated by the in situ reduction of gold salts to nanoparticles by spider silk [146]. The spider-silk fiber displays environmentally dependent expansion/contraction that consequently changes the conductivity of the adhesive nanoparticles. This material distinguishes the polarity of alcohol vapors (from methanol to butanol) by distinct conductivity changes and shows excellent cycling efficiency for exposure to methanol vapor.

The combination of the electroactivity of AuNPs and the complexation features of macrocyclic compounds lead to attractive sensory materials. In a series of studies [147–150], Willner and coworkers have demonstrated an attractive concept to realize three-dimensional electrode surfaces, where citrate-stabilized AuNPs and oligocationic cyclophanes or molecular squares were alternately deposited onto a 3-aminopropyltriethoxysilane-modified indium-doped tin oxide (ITO) conductive glass (Figure 8.9). In these systems, the AuNPs provide conductive surfaces, while the macrocycles serve as "molecular glues" that associate with π-donor substrates such as hydroquinone in their cavities. The molecular recognition increases the local concentration of substrates at the electrode surface, facilitating the detection of targets at low concentration (e.g., 1 μM of hydroquinone) where the bare ITO electrode describes no electrical response [151]. The sensitivity of this system can be readily tuned by adjusting the number of the assembled layers, as the electrical response of the analytes are proportional to the number of layers [147]. The preconcentration of substrates can be determined by controlling the binding affinity between macrocycles and analytes, providing selectivity. For example, the multilayered electrodes built up from AuNPs and cyclobis(paraquat-*p*-phenylene) cyclophane respond to hydroquninone, whereas the electrodes consisting of multilayers of AuNPs and the enlarged cyclophane cyclobis(paraquat- *p*biphenylene) respond only

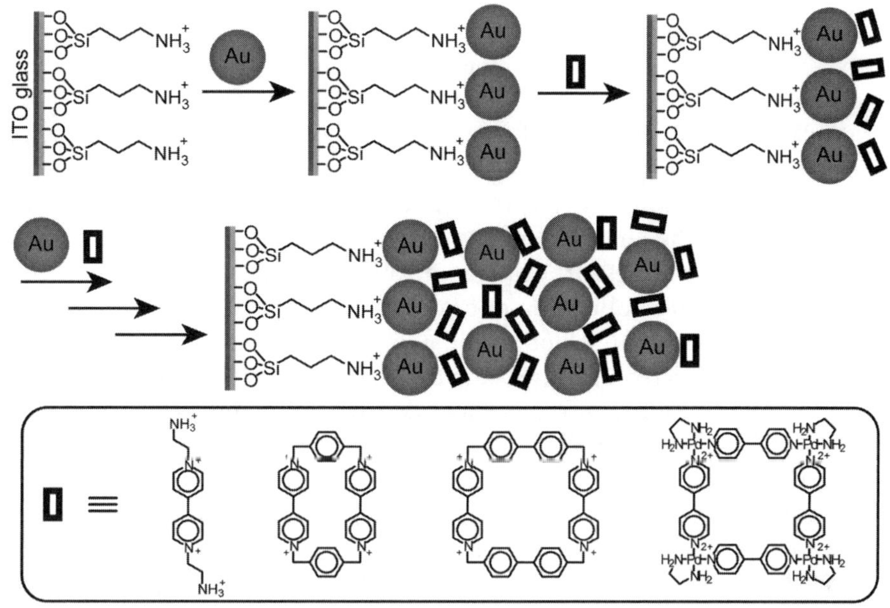

Figure 8.9 Electroactive multilayers formed by the self-assembly of anionic AuNPs and bipyridinium-based oligocations.

to dihydroxymethyl ferrocene [149]. Sensing studies on anionic π-donor analytes such as 3,4-dihydroxyphenylacetic acid confirm that the preconcentration of analytes at the conductive support originates from the specific π donor-acceptor interactions rather than nonspecific electrostatic interactions [148].

In most cases, the electrochemical sensors can only be used to detect redox-active analytes due to their voltammetric nature. To allow the analysis of nonredox-active compounds, Willner et al. have deposited a film composed of polyethyleneimine, AuNPs, and cyclobis(paraquat-*p*-phenylene) on the Al_2O_3 insulating layer of an ion-sensitive field-effect transistor to serve as a sensing interface [152]. This device is able to sense any charged analytes that are bound to the cyclophane, irrespective of their redox activity. With adrenaline as a model compound, it was demonstrated that the analysis could be accomplished by measuring either the source-drain current or the gate-source voltage. Significantly, the sensing device is reusable (at least 100 cycles) with high stability. Recently, AuNP-based microelectronic devices have been fabricated to detect H_2S where the adsorption of H_2S molecules onto the nanoparticles drastically changes the hopping behavior of electrons through the particles and consequently the current-voltage profile [153].

Although bulk Au metal is chemically inert, AuNPs have proven to be catalysts for many reactions. These materials feature extraordinary catalytic activity due to their large surface-to-volume ratio and interface-dominated properties [4, 154]. Therefore, AuNP-modified electrodes hold great promises in the electrocatalytic detection of organic and biological molecules [137, 155–157]. As an example, Jena and Raj have demonstrated the electrocatalytic sensing of glucose by using an AuNP-coated gold electrode [156]. The AuNPs are self-assembled on a three-dimensional silicate network anchored on an electrode followed by enlargement with hydroxylamine. The enzyme-free amperometric response of this system increases linearly with the glucose concentration with a detection limit of 50 nM.

While the integration of enzymes and electrodes would lead to highly selective electrical biosensors, the direct immobilization of redox enzymes onto the electrodes generally results in low sensitivity due to the lack of mutual electrical communication between the enzyme and the electrode. AuNPs and redox enzymes have been codeposited on the electrodes to improve such electrical communication [158–161]; likewise, the immobilization of enzymes onto AuNPs can often increase their turnover rates [162, 163], which would potentially reinforce the detection sensitivity. To facilitate the electron transfer between the enzyme active sites and the electrode support, Willner and coworkers have constructed a bioelectrocatalytic system with highly efficient electrical contacting of glucose oxidase (GOx) with electrode support by the reconstitution of apo-glucose oxidase (apo-GOx) on a 1.4-nm gold nanoparticle that was functionalized with the cofactor flavin adenine dinucleotide (FAD) (Figure 8.10) [164]. The nanoparticle-reconstituted enzyme electrodes exhibited extremely efficient electrical communication with the electrode, with electron-transfer turnover rate of ca. 5000 s^{-1} sevenfold higher than the electron-transfer rate constant of native GOx.

AuNP-based electrochemical detection of DNA has been developed as an alternative to optical approaches [165]. In this route, the DNA recognition events are transduced into electrical or electrochemical signals by using AuNPs as mediators. For example, Mirkin et al. have fabricated a DNA array detection method in which the binding of oligonucleotide-functionalized AuNPs leads to conductivity changes associated with target binding events [166]. First, short capture oligonucleotides were immobilized on the SiO_2 surface between two electrodes, and then the target DNA and AuNPs functionalized with oligonucleotides were added successively for hybridization. Finally, the enlargement of metal nanoparticles was conducted to

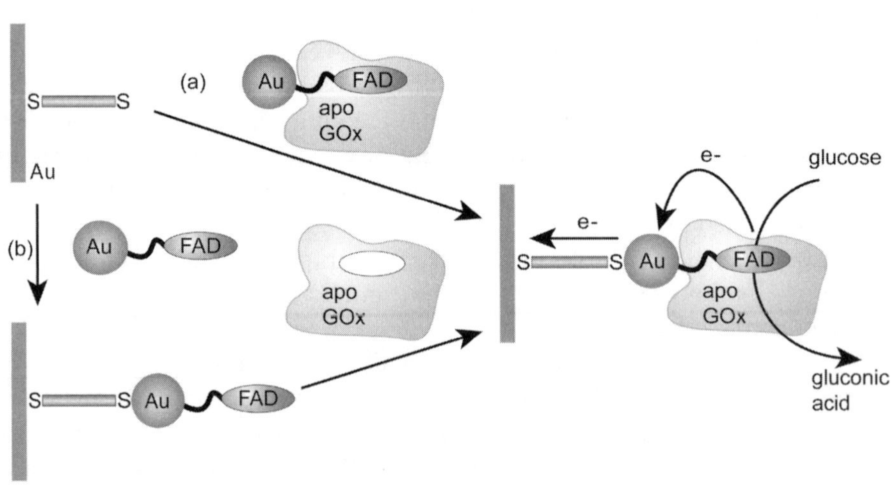

Figure 8.10 Fabrication of GOx electrode by the reconstitution of apo-GOx on a FAD-functionalized AuNP: (a) The adsorption of AuNP-reconstituted apo-GOx to a dithiol monolayer assembled on a gold electrode, and (b) the adsorption of FAD-AuNPs to a dithiol monolayer assembled on a gold electrode followed by the reconstitution of apo-GOx on the functional nanoparticles. Both routes afforded almost identical monolayers.

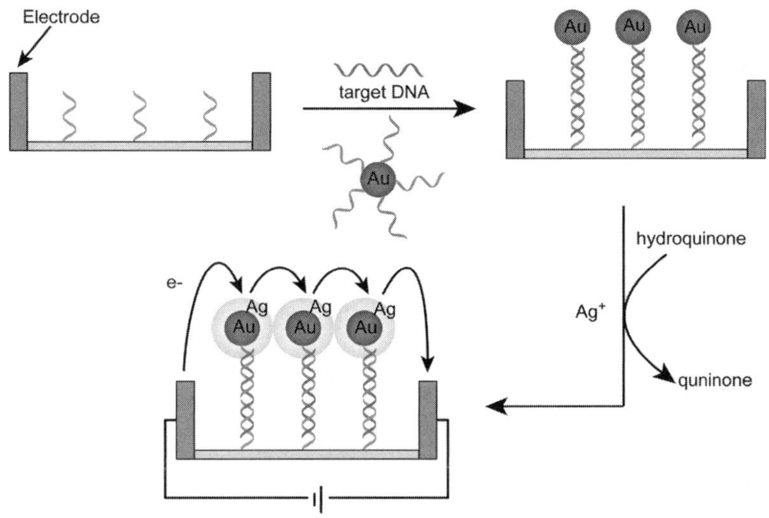

Figure 8.11 Electrical detection of DNA based on the "sandwich" hybridization with DNA-functionalized AuNPs followed by silver deposition.

enhance the conductivity by deposition of silver onto AuNPs (Figure 8.11). Using this method, the target DNA has been detected at concentrations as low as 500 femtomolar with a point mutation selectivity factor of ~100,000:1 [166].

The redox properties of AuNPs further enable their applications as electrochemical labels in oligonucleotide detection. In a representative study, Ozsoz et al. have shown that the treatment of a target DNA-modified electrode with complementary probes conjugated to AuNPs resulted in the appearance of a gold oxide wave at +1.2V, showing the detection limit as low as 0.78 fmol with the assistance of PCR amplification [167]. So far, several amplification tactics that are readily accessible have been developed, involving the nanoparticle enhancement by silver deposition [168] and the incorporation of electrochemically active groups onto AuNPs [169, 170]. As an example, ferrocene-capped AuNP/streptavidin conjugates were attached to a biotinylated DNA detection probe of a "sandwich" DNA complex on the electrode, showing good selectivity and reproducibility with a detection limit of 2 pM, in spite of its simplicity [169, 171]. Similarly, Fan et al. described a sandwich detection system involving hybridization with AuNP-labeled reporter probe DNA and subsequent treatment with $[Ru(NH_3)_6]^{3+}$ complexes [172]. The quantitative adsorption of $[Ru(NH_3)_6]^{3+}$ to the surface-confined capture probe DNA via electrostatic interactions resulted in amplified electrochemical signals under chronocoulometric interrogation. The DNA sensor could detect as low as femtomolar (zeptomoles) DNA targets and exhibit excellent selectivity against even a single base mismatch. More recently, Willner et al. reported a novel amplified electrochemical detection of DNA through the aggregation of AuNPs on electrodes and the intercalation of methylene blue into the DNA-crosslinked structure [173]. In this system, the methylene blue units act as a specific electrochemical indicator for the double-stranded DNA formation, while the AuNP assemblies facilitate the electrical contact of the intercalated methylene blue with the electrodes. Therefore, this approach exhibits a detection limit of 0.1 pM for a 27-mer DNA.

AuNP-based immunoassays have been employed in the protein sensing by monitoring either the conductivity changes or the electrochemical signaling. A conductivity immunoassay system designed by Velev and Kaler involved the adsorption of proteins between antibodies immobilized in an electrode gap and a secondary AuNP-tagged antibody followed by AuNPs that are enlarged and fused together by a metastable solution of silver salts, which via nucleation deposits a silver layer on top of the gold (this is called *silver enhancement*) [174]. Conductive paths were formed across interdigitated electrodes, leading to a measurable conductivity changes. This assay has achieved ultrasensitive detection of human IgG at 0.2 pM. Likewise, Limoges et al. devised a highly electrochemical immunoassay by using AuNP-labeled antibodies [175]. As illustrated in Figure 8.12, the AuNP-labeled antibody forms sandwich complexes with the goat IgG target and the immobilized antibody. After removal of the unbound labeled antibody, AuNPs were dissolved in an acidic bromine-bromide solution to release gold ions, which are quantitatively determined at a disposable carbon-based screen-printed electrode (SPE) by anodic stripping voltammetry (ASV). With 18 ± 5 nm AuNPs as the label, a detection limit of 3 pM was obtained through this protocol benefiting from the sensitive ASV determination of Au(III) at a SPE (5 nM) and the large number of atoms in AuNPs (1.7×10^5 gold atoms in a 18 nm AuNP). In an early study, a new strategy based on cyclic accumulation of AuNPs has been developed for determination of human IgG by ASV [176]. In this protocol, the probe antibody in the sandwich complexes is labeled with dethiobiotin and advidin-AuNPs, which are introduced for further complexation. The alternative treatment of the system with biotin solution and avidin-AuNPs could realize cyclic accumulation of AuNPs. The detection limit of this method reaches as low as 0.1 ng mL^{-1} human IgG.

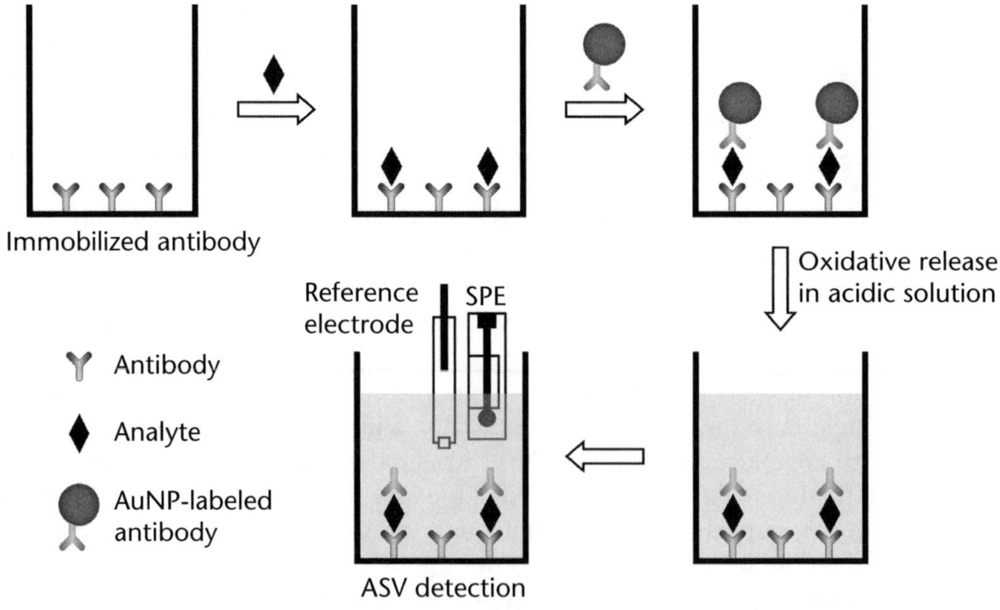

Figure 8.12 Schematic representation of the sandwich electrochemical immunoassay with an AuNP label.

8.7 Surface Enhanced Raman Scattering-Based Sensing

Raman scattering is the inelastic scattering of incident photons, which is sensitive to different vibrational modes and consequently provides the fingerprint of the target molecules. The cross-section of Raman scattering is about 10 to 15 orders smaller than that of fluorescence, which severely restricts the direct application of this technique. It has been demonstrated that when a molecule is adsorbed on rough metal surfaces, its Raman scattering may be significantly enhanced by up to 15 orders of magnitude, enabling single molecule detection [177]. This surface-enhanced Raman scattering (SERS) has been attributed to a local electromagnetic field enhancement induced by a plasmon resonance of optically active nanoparticles [178, 179]. The field enhancement is dependent on the nanoparticle size, shape, orientation, and aggregation.

AuNP-based SERS has been successfully exploited in biological sensing. In a representative study, Mirkin et al. used AuNP probes labeled with oligonucleotides and Raman-active dyes to achieve multiplexed detection of oligonucleotide targets [180]. Through a sandwich assay approach followed by silver enhancement, SERS signals are detected exclusively from the Raman dyes immobilized on the particles, showing a detection limit of 20 fM. Specifically, this method is able to discriminate single nucleotide polymorphisms relating to six different viruses, benefiting from the specificity of complementary probe sequences as well as the fingerprint of the Raman dyes. Recently, nonfluorescent Raman tags have been incorporated into DNA-functionalized 30-nm AuNP probes for the SERS detection of DNA [181]. In this system, the intensity of Raman signal of the probes could be controlled by the surface coverage of the Raman tags on the particles, indicating a simultaneous identification of up to eight probes in a mixture and a detection limit of ca. 100 nM without further metal enhancement.

AuNPs functionalized with either protein ligands or antibodies and Raman dyes have been developed to detect the protein-small molecule and protein-protein interactions [182]. However, this approach required further silver enhancement to get appropriate SERS when 13-nm AuNPs were used. Lipert, Porter, and coworkers have coated 30-nm AuNPs with a monolayer of an intrinsically strong Raman scatter (5-thiol-2-nitrobenzoate) followed by a layer of covalently linked antibodies for SERS detection [183]. This design not only minimizes the separation between label and particle surface but also maximizes the number of labels on each particle, so that the sensitivity can be drastically enhanced. This immunoassay system has been exploited in the detection of free prostate-specific antigen (PSA) through a sandwich assay format based on monoclonal antibodies. Detection limits of ~1 pg mL^{-1} in human serum and ~ 4 pg mL^{-1} in bovine serum albumin have been achieved with a spectrometer readout time of 60s. In addition, Nie et al. reported biocompatible and nontoxic AuNPs for in vivo tumor targeting and detection based on pegylated AuNPs and SERS [184]. These particles were >200 times brighter than near-infrared-emitting quantum dots and allowed spectroscopic detection of small tumors (0.03 cm^3) at a penetration depth of 1–2 cm.

8.8 Gold Nanoparticle-Amplified SPR Sensing

The excitation of planar noble metal film by light leads to SPR, which is dependent on the refractive index of layers present in the interfacial region. This phenomenon has been extensively exploited in chemical and biological sensing, and some sensors have been commercialized [185]. SPR sensors exhibit higher sensitivity for large analyte molecules because their effect on the refractive index is proportionally greater. Accordingly, the introduction of AuNPs onto the sensing surface provides an effective way to enhance this effect attributing to their high mass coupled with the high dielectric constant of AuNPs and the electromagnetic coupling between AuNPs and the metal film [186]. By way of example, a MIP gel with embedded AuNPs has been prepared on a gold film-coated chip [187]. Not only can the swelling of MIPs by binding of analytes lead to the significant changes in dielectric constant near the gold substrate surface, it can also increase the distance between the AuNPs within the polymer and the substrate surface, drastically enhancing the degree of SPR angle shift. By using this method, dopamine could be detected at as low as nanomolar concentrations [187], as compared to the micromolar sensitivity of colorimetric methods [85].

The specific base pairing in nucleotide interactions facilitates the highly selective sensing of oligoncucleotides. The sensitivity of oligonucleotide detection can be drastically improved by using AuNP-amplified SPR [188, 189]. Keating et al. have designed a sandwich approach where a monolayer of 12-mer oligonucleotides were first immobilized onto a gold substrate and the target DNA and AuNPs carrying complementary DNA molecules were combined successively [188]. The AuNP-tagged surface shows a greater than 10-fold increase in angle shift, corresponding to a more than 1,000-fold improvement in sensitivity for the target DNA compared with the nonamplified assay. As a consequence, a ~10 pM limit of quantification was achieved for a 24-mer DNA. The nonspecific adsorption of AuNPs onto the surface may attenuate the SPR signal enhancement. It has been shown that a dextran layer between the gold film and the immobilized DNA molecules effectively reduces the nonspecific adsorption, leading to an extremely sensitive detection of a 39-mer DNA at femtomolar level [190]. The real-time multicolor DNA detection has been achieved by using ssDNA-modified AuNPs and micropatterned chemoresponsive diffraction gratings interrogated simultaneously at multiple laser wavelengths [191].

Highly specific antibody-antigen recognition holds great promise in selective protein sensing [192]. Natan et al. devised the first AuNP-enhanced SPR immunosensing system by using either antigen- or antibody-functionalized AuNPs as signal amplifier [193]. In a typical sandwich immunoassay, the gold film is first coated with γ-chain-specific monoclonal goat antihuman immunoglobulin G (α-h-IgG(γ)). Subsequently, the addition of h-IgG and the second free antibody leads only a small plasmon angle shift. While the second free antibody is replaced by an electrostatic conjugate between 10-nm-diameter AuNP and α-h-IgG(Fc), the plasmon angle shift drastically increases by 28 times compared with the unamplified assay. Picomolar detection of h-IgG has been realized using such particle enhancement. Recently, both competitive and sandwich immunoassays have been developed to quantify human tissue inhibitor of metalloproteinases-2 on the basis of AuNP-enhanced SPR [194].

8.9 Quartz Crystal Microbalance-Based Sensing

Quartz crystal microbalance (QCM) (i.e., a piezoelectric microbalance) measures mass changes on a quartz crystal resonator in gas phase or in aqueous solution by following the respective frequency changes. This technique has been widely used in the sensing of various targets ranging from volatile molecules to microorganisms due to its high sensitivity, economic effectiveness, and convenient operation [195]. The integration of AuNPs into QCM-based sensing systems is of great interest mainly due to their two appealing attributes. First, nanoparticles possess large surface area and surface-to-volume ratio. Accordingly, AuNPs and AuNP-dendrimer acting as sorptive materials have been used for applications in vapor sensing [196–198]. Based on the relatively heavy mass of AuNPs and the direct response of QCM related to surface mass changes, the use of nanoparticles as "mass enhancers" provides a powerful approach for promoting detection sensitivity by amplifying frequency changes [199].

Efforts have been focused on the detection of oligonucleotides using QCM sensors with the assistance of AuNPs. Generally, the experimental setup involves the immobilization of thiol-terminated ssDNA onto the gold-coated QCM, followed by hybridization with target oligonucleotides. It was demonstrated that the introduction of a layer of AuNPs between the gold film and the immobilized ssDNA significantly improves the detection capacity of the system as a consequence of the large surface of AuNPs [200]. On the other hand, sandwich approaches can drastically improve the detection limit, where one end of target oligonucleotides hybridizes with the immobilized ssDNA molecules (recognition elements) while the other end hybridizes with ssDNA-modified AuNPs (signal amplifier) [201–205]. Particularly, multivalent ssDNA-modified AuNPs are able to further hybridize with AuNPs functionalized with complementary ssDNA and provide the dendritic amplification effect [202]. Catalyzed deposition of gold onto the amplifier AuNPs has also been conducted to improve the sensitivity of the QCM approach, and a detection limit of ca. 1 fM has been attained [206]. However, it should be noted that nonspecific adsorption of AuNPs to the gold film of QCM needs to be avoided in the amplification process, as it will lead to an overestimate of signal enhancement [207]. Recently, a microcantilever-based DNA sensor has been designed as an analogy to QCM [208]. In comparison with QCM, the sensor element is 100 times smaller, enabling the construction of a high-density senor array for multiplexed detection. On the basis of the sandwich approach coupled with AuNP-amplification, a detection limit of 23 pM has been achieved on a microcantilever for sensing a 30-mer DNA [208].

Detection of streptavidin on a QCM has been reported using AuNPs as a signal amplification probe [209]. In the experimental setup, biotinylated BSA was first immobilized on the gold surface of the QCM electrode and the combination of strepatvidin induced small frequency changes of the piezoelectric crystal. The further treatment of the resulting interface with biotin-functionalized AuNP enhanced the sensing signal with an additional frequency change two times higher, resulting in a wide detection window from 1 ng mL^{-1} to 10 μg mL^{-1}.

8.10 Gold Nanoparticle-Based Bio-Barcode Assay

Mirkin's group has developed an AuNP-based bio-barcode assay to amplify the target molecules with highly multiplexed and ultrasensitive detection of proteins and nucleic acids. In order to prove this concept, the bio-barcode assay was first employed to analyze PSA, which is a biomarker protein for prostate and breast cancer [210]. As shown in Figure 8.13(a), a magnetic microparticle carrying antibodies that specifically bind PSA was first used to capture the protein. Subsequently, a 30-nm AuNP that was functionalized with barcode DNA and antibodies unique to the protein target was combined to sandwich the protein between magnetic and gold particles. Magnetic separation of this assembly followed by thermal dehybridization of double-stranded DNA on AuNPs yielded the ssDNA-functionalized AuNPs and free barcode nucleic acids. The free barcode DNA was analyzed directly by using chip-based sandwich hybridization with ss-DNA functionalized AuNP probes, followed by silver amplification, leading to a detection limit of 30 aM. When PCR amplification on the barcode DNA was conducted, an unprecedented sensitivity of 3

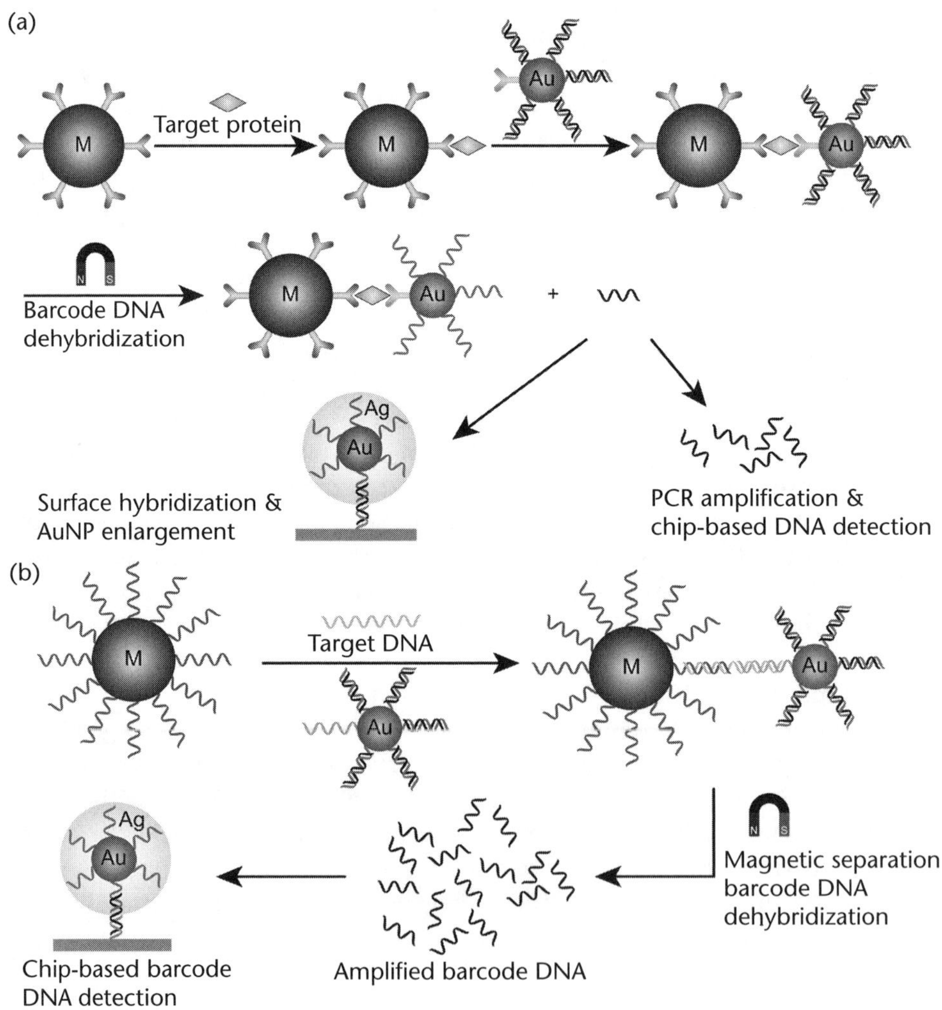

Figure 8.13 AuNP-based bio-barcode assay of (a) proteins and (b) DNA.

attomolar was obtained [210]. The feasibility of this bio-barcode approach has also been verified by the detection of amyloid-β-derived diffusible ligands, a soluble pathogenic Alzheimer's disease marker, in the cerebrospinal fluid [211]. Interestingly, this approach has proven to be able to achieve multiplexed detection of protein cancer markers by using a mixture of different biobarcoded AuNP probes [212]. During the detection process, the released barcode DNA molecules can be specifically immobilized onto a DNA functionalized surface, followed by hybridization with ssDNA-AuNP and silver amplification. Therefore, the barcode oligonucleotides can be scanometrically identified.

To simplify the signal readout, fluorophore-tagged biobarcoded AuNPs have been used in protein detection [213]. As the released barcode DNA is fluorescent, it can be readily quantified by measuring the fluorescence intensity. With PSA as the model protein, a detection limit of 300 aM was obtained without other amplification. Nam and Groves et al. developed a colorimetric bio-barcode assay for protein detection [214, 215]. In their approach, the released barcode nucleotides serve as a bridging agent of two ssDNA-functionalized barcode-capture AuNPs. The barcode-directed AuNP aggregation leads to a red-to-blue color change. Through this method, cytokine has been detected at 30 aM, which far higher than that of conventional colorimetric detection.

Ultrasensitive detection of DNA has also been developed through the principle of biobarcode amplification [216, 217]. As illustrated in Figure 8.13(b), the antibodies in the protein detection system are replaced by specific ssDNA. Consequently, the target DNA can hybridize with both the magnetic particle probes and the biobarcoded AuNP probes to form sandwich assemblies. The magnetic separation followed by thermal dehybridization releases the free barcode nucleotides for analysis. Using scanometric detection, this method has led to a 500-zeptomolar sensitivity, which is comparable to many PCR-based approaches without the need for enzymatic amplification [216]. Multiplexed DNA detection is also feasible using a mixture of different biobarcoded nanoparticle probes [217].

8.11 Concluding Remarks

AuNPs present a versatile scaffold for the creation of chemical and biological sensors. First, the particles provide an adaptable platform for the incorporation of various functionalities ranging from small organic ligands to large biomacromolecules, allowing the binding of target molecules with appropriate affinity and selectivity. Additionally, the physical, optical, and electronic attributes of AuNPs can be utilized to recognize the transduction of the binding events. Thus, functionalized AuNPs may act as both molecular receptor and signal transducer in a single sensing process, which often simplifies the sensor design. Moreover, AuNPs exhibit many attributes that are superior to small molecules (e.g., their high absorptivity and dense mass). These features further facilitate the application of AuNPs in the construction of highly sensitive sensors. A great variety of analytes have been subjected to the sensing studies.

The sensitivity of AuNP-based sensors is correlated with a variety of factors, such as the analyte, the recognition partner, and the transduction mechanism. As

Table 8.2 Comparison of Detection Limits of Different AuNP-Based Chemical and Biological Sensors

Assay Method	*Analytes*	*Detection Limit*	*Reference*
Colorimetric	Metal ion (Pb2+)	2.5 nM	[70]
	Organic compound (adrenaline)	5 μM	[85]
	Oligonucleotide (ssDNA 30mer)	50 pM	[91]
	Protein (thermolysin)	~1 aM	[114]
Fluorescence	Metal ion (Hg2+)	10 nM	[122]
	Oligonucleotide (ssDNA 16mer)	0.2 μM	[126]
	Protein (avidin)	10 nM	[130]
Electrochemical	Volatile compound (toluene)	1 ppm	[140]
	Organic compound (glucose)	50 nM	[156]
	Oligonucleotide (ssDNA 27mer)	0.1 pM	[173]
	Protein (human IgG)	0.2 pM	[174]
SERS	Oligonucleotide (ssDNA 30 mer)	20 fM	[180]
	Protein (PSA)	30 fM	[183]
SPR	Organic compound (dopamine)	1 nM	[187]
	Oligonucleotide (ssDNA 39mer)	1.38 fM	[190]
	Protein (human IgG)	6.7 pM	[193]
QCM	Volatile compound (toluene)	10 ppm	[196]
	Oligonucleotide (ssDNA 27mer)	~1 fM	[206]
	Protein (streptavidin)	~20 pM	[209]
Bio-barcode	Oligonucleotide (ssDNA 27mer)	500 zM	[216]
	Protein (PSA)	30 aM	[210]

summarized in Table 8.2, the detection limit of AuNP sensors ranges from micromolar to zeptomolar, which is dependent not only on the target species, but also on the precise design of the sensors. Generally, the detection sensitivities are less than pico-/femto-molar, with DNA and protein as target molecules. It seems that a theoretical detection limit has been attained for the targets of this type, as it has been proposed that individual nanoscale sensors will be limited to picomolar-order sensitivity for practical time scales due to the analyte transport limitation [2], making directed transport of biomolecules essential for further enhancements in sensitivity.

To achieve highly efficient sensors, it is important to modulate the nanoparticle surface functionality for the selective capture of target analytes. Highly selective double-stranded DNA, antibody-antigen, and aptamer-analyte interactions have been utilized to engineer the recognition events. Despite their extraordinary specificity, these systems are not advantageous in the high-throughput screening of different analytes because a tremendous amount of pertinent recognition elements need to be fabricated for multianalyte detection. In this regard, the sensor array approach would play an important role, as selectivity rather than specificity is required. To this end, a limited number of individual sensors may provide nearly unlimited screening capability toward the target analytes.

Overall, the AuNP-based sensing studies described have mainly been focused on colorimetric and electrochemical protocols. Both methods afford pronounced detection sensitivity and extensive range of targets. By contrast, studies concerned with fluorescence-based sensing are relatively scarce, with current systems having high detection limits. AuNP-based fluorescence sensing systems are in principle superior to small organic molecular systems due to the intense absorptivity of AuNPs coupled with their superb quenching ability. This capability, however, has not been realized as of yet. Taken together, however, both the optoelectronic properties of AuNPs and their amplification ability hold great promise in producing chemical and biological sensors featuring high performance.

Acknowledgments

The authors acknowledge support from the NIH (GM GM077173).

References

[1] Diamond, D., *Principles of Chemical and Biological Sensors*, New York, NY: John Wiley & Sons, Inc., 1998. pp. 1–18.

[2] Sheehan, P. E. and Whitman, L. J., "Detection limits for nanoscale biosensors," *Nano Lett.*, Vol. 5, No. 4, 2005, pp. 803–807.

[3] Rosi, N. and Mirkin, C. A., "Nanostructures in Biodiagnostics," *Chem. Rev.*, Vol. 105, No. 4, 2005, pp. 1547–1562.

[4] Daniel, M.-C. and Astruc, D., "Gold Nanoparticles: Assembly, Supramolecular Chemistry, Quantum-Size-Related Properties, and Applications toward Biology, Catalysis, and Nanotechnology," *Chem. Rev.*, Vol. 104, No. 1, 2004, pp. 293–346.

[5] Thomas, K. G. and Kamat, P. V., "Chromophore-Functionalized Gold Nanoparticles," *Acc. Chem. Res.*, Vol. 36, No. 12, 2003, pp. 888–898.

[6] Katz, E. and Willner, I., "Integrated nanoparticle-biomolecule hybrid systems: synthesis, properties, and applications," *Angew. Chem. Int. Ed.*, Vol. 43, No. 45, 2004, pp. 6042–6108.

[7] You, C. C., et al., "Engineering the nanoparticle-biomacromolecule interface," *Soft Matter*, Vol. 2, No. 3, 2006, pp. 190–204.

[8] Faraday, M., "Experimental Relations of Gold (and other Metals) to Light," *Philos. Trans.*, Vol. 147, No., 1857, pp. 145–181.

[9] Schmid, G., et al., "$Au_{55}[P(C_6H_5)_3]_{12}Cl_6$-A Gold Cluster of An Exceptional Size," *Chem. Ber.*, Vol. 114, No. 11, 1981, pp. 3634–3642.

[10] Schmid, G., "Large Clusters and Colloids. Metals in the Embryonic State," *Chem. Rev.*, Vol. 92, No. 8, 1992, pp. 1709–1727.

[11] Weare, W. W., et al., "Improved Synthesis of Small (d_{CORE} = 1.5 nm) Phosphine-Stabilized Gold Nanoparticles," *J. Am. Chem. Soc.*, Vol. 122, No. 51, 2000, pp. 12890–12891.

[12] Brust, M., et al., "Synthesis of Thio-drivatised Gold Nanoparticles in a Two-phase Liquid-Liquid System," *J. Chem. Soc., Chem. Commun.*, Vol., No. 7, 1994, pp. 801–802.

[13] Leff, D. V., et al., "Thermodynamic Control of Gold Nanocrystal Size: Experiment and Theory," *J. Phys. Chem.*, Vol. 99, No. 18, 1995, pp. 7036–7041.

[14] Hostetler, M. J., et al., "Alkanethiolate Gold Cluster Molecules with Core Diameters from 1.5 to 5.2 nm: Core and Monolayer Properties as a Function of Core Size," *Langmuir*, Vol. 14, No. 1, 1998, pp. 17–30.

[15] Fink, J., et al., "Self-Organization of Nanosized Gold Particles," *Chem. Mater.*, Vol. 10, No. 3, 1998, pp. 922–926.

[16] Aslam, M., et al., "Novel One-Step Synthesis of Amine-Stabilized Aqueous Colloid Gold Nanoparticles," *J. Mater. Chem.*, Vol. 14, No., 2004, pp. 1795–1797.

[17] Hiramatsu, H. and Osterloh, F. E., "A Simple Large-Scale Synthesis of Nearly Monodisperse Gold and Silver Nanoparticles with Adjustable Sizes and with Exchangeable Surfactants," *Chem. Mater.*, Vol. 16, No. 13, 2004, pp. 2509–2511.

[18] Turkevich, J., et al., "A Study of the Nucleation and Growth Processes in the Synthesis of Colloidal Gold," *Discuss. Faraday Soc.*, Vol. 11, 1951, pp. 55–75.

[19] Frens, G., "Controlled Nucleation for Regulation of Particle-Size in Monodisperse Gold Suspensions," *Nature Phys. Sci.*, Vol. 241, No. 105, 1973, pp. 20–22.

[20] Grabar, K. C., et al., "Preparation and Characterization of Au Colloid Monolayers," *Anal. Chem.*, Vol. 67, No. 4, 1995, pp. 735–743.

[21] Schmid, G. and Simon, U., "Gold Nanoparticles: Assembly and Electrical Properties in 1-3 Dimensions," *Chem. Commun.*, No. 6, 2005, pp. 697–710.

[22] Petroski, J., et al., "Rapid Phosphine Exchange on 1.5-nm Gold Nanoparticles," *Inorg. Chem.*, Vol. 43, No. 5, 2004, pp. 1597–1599.

[23] Kanaras, A. G., et al., "Thioalkylated Tetraethylene Glycol: A New Ligand for Water Soluble Monolayer Protected Gold Clusters," *Chem. Commun.*, No. 20, 2002, pp. 2294–2295.

[24] Zheng, M., et al., "Ethylene Glycol Monolayer Protected Nanoparticles: Synthesis, Characterization, and Interactions with Biological Molecules," *Langmuir*, Vol. 20, No. 10, 2004, pp. 4226–4235.

[25] Bhargava, S. K., et al., "Gold Nanoparticle Formation during Bromoaurate Reduction by Amino Acids," *Langmuir*, Vol. 21, No. 13, 2005, pp. 5949–5956.

[26] Leff, D. V., et al., "Synthesis and Characterization of Hydrophobic, Organically-Soluble Gold Nanocrystals Functionalized with Primary Amines," *Langmuir*, Vol. 12, No. 20, 1996, pp. 4723–4730.

[27] Newman, J. D. S. and Blanchard, G. J., "Formation of Gold Nanoparticles Using Amine Reducing Agents," *Langmuir*, Vol. 22, No. 13, 2006, pp. 5882–5887.

[28] Duan, H. and Nie, S., "Etching Colloidal Gold Nanocrystals with Hyperbranched and Multivalent Polymers: A New Route to Fluorescent and Water-Soluble Atomic Clusters," *J. Am. Chem. Soc.*, Vol. 129, No. 9, 2007, pp. 2412–2413.

[29] Zhong, C. J., et al., "Size and Shape Evolution of Core-Shell Nanocrystals," *Chem. Commun.*, No. 13, 1999, pp. 1211–1212.

[30] Maye, M. M., et al., "Heating-Induced Evolution of Thiolate-Encapsulated Gold Nanoparticles: A Strategy for Size and Shape Manipulations," *Langmuir*, Vol. 16, No. 2, 2000, pp. 490–497.

[31] Tao, A. R., et al., "Shape control of colloidal metal nanocrystals," *Small*, Vol. 4, No. 3, 2008, pp. 310–325.

[32] Prasad, B. L. V., et al., "Digestive Ripening of Thiolated Gold Nanoparticles: The Effect of Alkyl Chain Length," *Langmuir*, Vol. 18, No. 20, 2002, pp. 7515–7520.

[33] Prasad, B. L. V., et al., "Digestive-Ripening Agents for Gold Nanoparticles: Alternatives to Thiols," *Chem. Mater.*, Vol. 15, No. 4, 2003, pp. 935–942.

[34] Sau, T. K., et al., "Size controlled Synthesis of Gold Nanoparticles Using Photochemically Prepared Seed Particles," *J. Nanoparticle Res.*, Vol. 3, No., 2001, pp. 257–261.

[35] Kurita, H., et al., "Size Reduction of Gold Particles in Aqueous Solution by Pulsed Laser Irradiation," *Appl. Phys. Lett.*, Vol. 72, No. 7, 1998, pp. 789–791.

[36] Templeton, A. C., et al., "Monolayer-Protected Cluster Molecules," *Acc. Chem. Res.*, Vol. 33, No. 1, 2000, pp. 27–36.

[37] Hong, R., et al., "In situ Observation of Place Exchange Reactions of Gold Nanoparticles. Correlation of Monolayer Structure and Stability," *Chem. Commun.*, No. 22, 2006, pp. 2347–2349.

[38] Boal, A. K. and Rotello, V. M., "Fabrication and Self-Optimization of Multivalent Receptors on Nanoparticle Scaffolds," *J. Am. Chem. Soc.*, Vol. 122, No. 4, 2000, pp. 734–735.

[39] Zachary, M. and Chechik, V., "Hopping of Thiolate Ligands between Au Nanoparticles Revealed by EPR Spectroscopy," *Angew. Chem. Int. Ed.*, Vol. 46, No. 18, 2007, pp. 3304–3307.

[40] Levy, R., et al., "Rational and Combinatorial Design of Peptide Capping Ligands for Gold Nanoparticles," *J. Am. Chem. Soc.*, Vol. 126, No. 32, 2004, pp. 10076–10084.

[41] Woehrle, G. H., et al., "Thiol-Functionalized, 1.5-nm Gold Nanoparticles through Ligand Exchange Reactions: Scope and Mechanism of Ligand Exchange," *J. Am. Chem. Soc.*, Vol. 127, No. 7, 2005, pp. 2172–2183.

[42] Rucareanu, S., et al., "4-(N,N-Dimethylamino)pyridine-Protected Au Nanoparticles: Versatile Precursors for Water- and Organic-Soluble Gold Nanoparticles," *Chem. Mater.*, Vol. 18, No., 2006, pp. 4674–4680.

[43] Tkachenko, A. G., et al., "Multifunctional Gold Nanoparticle-Peptide Complexes for Nuclear Targeting," *J. Am. Chem. Soc.*, Vol. 125, No. 16, 2003, pp. 4700–4701.

[44] El-Sayed, I. H., et al., "Selective Laser Photo-Thermal Therapy of Epithelial Carcinoma Using Anti-EGFR Antibody Conjugated Gold Nanoparticles," *Cancer Lett.*, Vol. 239, No. 1, 2006, pp. 129–135.

[45] Lin, S.-Y., et al., "Two-Step Functionalization of Neutral and Positively Charged Thiols onto Citrate-Stabilized Au Nanoparticles," *J. Phys. Chem. B*, Vol. 108, No. 7, 2004, pp. 2134–2139.

[46] Aslan, K. and Perez-Luna, V. H., "Surface Modification of Colloidal Gold by Chemisorption of Alkanethiols in the Presence of a Nonionic Surfactant," *Langmuir*, Vol. 18, No. 16, 2002, pp. 6059–6065.

[47] Jain, P. K., et al., "Calculated Absorption and Scattering Properties of Gold Nanoparticles of Different Size, Shape, and Composition: Applications in Biological Imaging and Biomedicine," *J. Phys. Chem. B*, Vol. 110, No. 14, 2006, pp. 7238–7248.

[48] Mie, G., "Beiträg zur Optik Trüber Medien, Speziell Kolloidaler Metallösungen," *Ann. Phys.*, Vol. 25, 1908, pp. 377–445.

[49] Kelly, K. L., et al., "The Optical Properties of Metal Nanoparticles: The Influence of Size, Shape, and Dielectric Environment," *J. Phys. Chem. B*, Vol. 107, No. 3, 2003, pp. 668–677.

[50] Eustis, S. and El-Sayed, M. A., "Why Gold Nanoparticles are More Precious than Pretty Gold: Noble Metal Surface Plasmon Resonance and Its Enhancement of the Radiative and Nonradiative Properties of Nanocrystals of Different Shapes," *Chem. Soc. Rev.*, Vol. 35, No. 3, 2006, pp. 209–217.

[51] Su, K.-H., et al., "Interparticle coupling effects on plasmon resonances of nanogold particles," *Nano Lett.*, Vol. 3, No. 8, 2003, pp. 1087–1090.

[52] Link, S., et al., "Alloy Formation of Gold-Silver Nanoparticles and the Dependence of the Plasomon Absorption on Their Composition," *J. Phys. Chem. B*, Vol. 103, No. 18, 1999, pp. 3529–3533.

[53] Liu, X., et al., "Extinction Coefficient of Gold Nanoparticles with Different Sizes and Different Capping Ligands," *Colloid Surf. B: Biointerfaces*, Vol. 58, No. 1, 2006, pp. 3–7.

[54] Jain, P. K., et al., "Au Nanoparticles Target Cancer," *Nano Today*, Vol. 2, No. 1, 2007, pp. 18–29.

[55] Zheng, J., et al., "Highly Fluorescent, Water-Soluble, Size-Tunable Gold Quantum Dots," *Phys. Rev. Lett.*, Vol. 93, No. 7, 2004, p. 077402.

[56] van Dijk, M. A., et al., "Far-Fiedl Optical Microscopy of Single Metal Nanoparticles," *Acc. Chem. Res.*, Vol. 38, No. 7, 2005, pp. 594–601.

[57] Lakowicz, J. R., "Radiative Decay Engineering 5: Metal-Enhanced Fluorescence and Plasmon Emission," *Anal. Biochem.*, Vol. 337, No. 2, 2005, pp. 171–194.

[58] Sapsford, K. E., et al., "Materials for Fluorescence Resonance Energy Transfer Analysis: Beyond Traditional Donor-Acceptor Combinations," *Angew. Chem. Int. Ed.*, Vol. 45, No. 28, 2006, pp. 4562–4589.

[59] Dulkeith, E., et al., "Fluorescence Quenching of Dye Molecules near Gold Nanoparticles: Radiative and Nonradiative Effects," *Phys. Rev. Lett.*, Vol. 89, No. 20, 2002, p. 203002.

[60] Kamat, P. V., et al., "Electrochemical Modulation of Fluorophore Emission on a Nanostructured Gold Film," *Angew. Chem. Int. Ed.*, Vol. 41, No. 15, 2002, pp. 2764–2767.

[61] Quinn, B. M., et al., "Electrochemical resolution of 15 oxidation states for monolayer protected gold nanoparticles," *J. Am. Chem. Soc.*, Vol. 125, No. 22, 2003, pp. 6644–6645.

[62] Antonello, S., et al., "Molecular electron-transfer properties of Au_{38} Clusters," *J. Am. Chem. Soc.*, Vol. 129, No. 32, 2007, pp. 9836–9837.

[63] Srivastava, S., et al., "Controlled plasmon resonance of gold nanoparticles self-assembled with PAMAM dendrimers," *Chem. Mater.*, Vol. 17, No. 3, 2005, pp. 487–490.

[64] Lin, S.-Y., et al., "Recognition of Potassium Ion in Water by 15-Crown-5 Functionalized Gold Nanoparticles," *Anal. Chem.*, Vol. 74, No. 2, 2002, pp. 330–335.

[65] Lin, S.-Y., et al., "A Cooperative Effect of Bifuctionalized Nnaoparticles on Recognition: Sensing Alkali Ions by Crown and Carboxylate Moieties in Aqueous Media," *Anal. Chem.*, Vol. 77, No. 15, 2005, pp. 4821–4828.

[66] Obare, S. O., et al., "Sensing Strategy for Lithium Ion Based on Gold Nanoparticles," *Langmuir*, Vol. 18, No. 26, 2002, pp. 10407–10410.

[67] Reynolds, A. J., et al., "Gold Glyconanoparticles for Mimics and Measurement of Metal Ion-Mediated Carbohydrate - Carbohydrate Interactions," *Langmuir*, Vol. 22, No. 3, 2006, pp. 1156–1163.

[68] Kim, Y. J., et al., "Gold nanoparticle-based sensing of "spectroscopically silent" heavy metal ions," *Nano Lett.*, Vol. 1, No. 4, 2001, pp. 165–167.

[69] Huang, C. C. and Chang, H. T., "Parameters for selective colorimetric sensing of mercury (II) in aqueous solutions using mercaptopropionic acid-modified gold nanoparticles," *Chem. Commun.*, No. 12, 2007, pp. 1215–1217.

[70] Lin, S.-Y., et al., "A simple strategy for prompt visual sensing by gold nanoparticles: general applications of interparticle hydrogen bonds," *Angew. Chem. Int. Ed.*, Vol. 45, No. 30, 2006, pp. 4948–4951.

[71] Yang, W. R., et al., "Fast colorimetric detection of copper ions using L-cysteine functionalized gold nanoparticles," *J. Nanosci. Nanotechnol.*, Vol. 7, No. 2, 2007, pp. 712–716.

[72] Si, S., et al., "One-dimensional assembly of peptide-functionalized gold nanoparticles: An approach toward mercury ion sensing," *J. Phys. Chem. C*, Vol. 111, No. 3, 2007, pp. 1248–1255.

[73] Lee, J.-S., et al., "Colorimetric detection of mercuric ion (Hg^{2+}) in aqueous media using DNA-functionalized gold nanoparticles," *Angew. Chem. Int. Ed.*, Vol. 46, No. 22, 2007, pp. 4093–4096.

[74] Liu, J. and Lu, Y., "A Colorimetric Lead Biosensor Using DNAzyme-Directed Assembly of Gold Nanoparticles," *J. Am. Chem. Soc.*, Vol. 125, No. 22, 2003, pp. 6642–6643.

[75] Liu, J. W. and Lu, Y., "Optimization of a Pb^{2+}-directed gold nanoparticle/DNAzyme assembly and its application as a colorimetric biosensor for Pb^{2+}," *Chem. Mater.*, Vol. 16, No. 17, 2004, pp. 3231–3238.

[76] Liu, J. W. and Lu, Y., "Accelerated color change of gold nanoparticles assembled by DNAzymes for simple and fast colorimetric Pb^{2+} detection," *J. Am. Chem. Soc.*, Vol. 126, No. 39, 2004, pp. 12298–12305.

[77] Mirkin, C. A., et al., "A DNA-Based Method for Rationally Assembling Nanoparticles into Macroscopic Materials," *Nature*, Vol. 382, No. 6592, 1996, pp. 607–609.

[78] Elghanian, R., et al., "Selective Colorimetric Detection of Polynucleotides Based on the Distance-Dependent Optical Properties of Gold Nanoparticles," *Science*, Vol. 277, No. 5329, 1997, pp. 1078–1081.

[79] Liu, J. and Lu, Y., "Stimuli-responsive disassembly of nanoparticle aggregates for light-up colorimetric sensing," *J. Am. Chem. Soc.*, Vol. 127, No. 36, 2005, pp. 12677–12683.

[80] Liu, J. W. and Lu, Y., "Adenosine-dependent assembly of aptazyme-functionalized gold nanoparticles and its application as a colorimetric biosensor," *Anal. Chem.*, Vol. 76, No. 6, 2004, pp. 1627–1632.

[81] Kubo, Y., "Isothiouronium-modified gold nanoparticles capable of colorimetric sensing of oxoanions in aqueous MeOH solution," *Tetrahedron Lett.*, Vol. 46, No. 25, 2005, pp. 4369–4372.

[82] Watanabe, S., et al., "Colorimetric Detection of Fluoride Ion in An Aqueous Solution Using a Thioglucose-Capped Gold Nanoparticle," *Tetrahedron Lett.*, Vol. 46, No. 51, 2005, pp. 8827–8829.

[83] Aslan, K., et al., "Nanogold-plasmon-resonance-based glucose sensing," *Anal. Biochem.*, Vol. 330, No. 1, 2004, pp. 145–155.

[84] Aslan, K., et al., "Nanogold plasmon resonance-based glucose sensing. 2. Wavelength-ratiometric resonance light scattering," *Anal. Chem.*, Vol. 77, No. 7, 2005, pp. 2007–2014.

[85] Matsui, J., et al., "Composite of Au nanoparticles and molecularly imprinted polymer as a sensing material," *Anal. Chem.*, Vol. 76, No. 5, 2004, pp. 1310–1315.

[86] Bunka, D. H. J. and Stockley, P. G., "Aptamers come of age - at last," *Nat. Rev. Microbiol.*, Vol. 4, No. 8, 2006, pp. 588–596.

[87] Liu, J. and Lu, Y., "Fast colorimetric sensing of adenosine and cocaine based on a general sensor design involving aptamers and nanoparticles," *Angew. Chem. Int. Ed.*, Vol. 45, No. 1, 2006, pp. 90–94.

[88] Liu, J. and Lu, Y., "Smart nanomaterials responsive to multiple chemical stimuli with controllable cooperativity," *Adv. Mater.*, Vol. 18, No. 13, 2006, pp. 1667–1671.

[89] Liu, J., et al., "A simple and sensitive 'dipstick' test in serum based on lateral flow separation of aptamer-linked nanostructures," *Angew. Chem. Int. Ed.*, Vol. 45, No. 47, 2006, pp. 7955–7959.

[90] Storhoff, J. J., et al., "One-pot colorimetric differentiation of polynucleotides with single base imperfections using gold nanoparticle probes," *J. Am. Chem. Soc.*, Vol. 120, No. 9, 1998, pp. 1959–1964.

[91] Reynolds, R. A., et al., "Homogeneous, Nanoparticle-Based Quantitative Colorimetric Detection of Oligonucleotides," *J. Am. Chem. Soc.*, Vol. 122, No. 15, 2000, pp. 3795–3796.

[92] Cao, Y. C., et al., "A two-color-change, nanoparticle-based method for DNA detection," *Talanta*, Vol. 67, No. 3, 2005, pp. 449–455.

[93] Thaxton, C. S., et al., "Gold nanoparticle probes for the detection of nucleic acid targets," *Clin. Chim. Acta*, Vol. 363, No. 1–2, 2006, pp. 120–126.

[94] Li, H. X. and Rothberg, L. J., "Label-free colorimetric detection of specific sequences in genomic DNA amplified by the polymerase chain reaction," *J. Am. Chem. Soc.*, Vol. 126, No. 35, 2004, pp. 10958–10961.

[95] Chakrabarti, R. and Klibanov, A. M., "Nanocrystals modified with peptide nucleic acids (PNAs) for selective self-assembly and DNA detection," *J. Am. Chem. Soc.*, Vol. 125, No. 41, 2003, pp. 12531–12540.

[96] Li, J., et al., "A Colorimetric Method for Point Mutation Detection Using High-Fidelity DNA Ligase," *Nucleic Acids Res.*, Vol. 33, No. 9, 2005, p. e168.

[97] Storhoff, J. J., et al., "Homogeneous detection of unamplified genomic DNA sequences based on colorimetric scatter of gold nanoparticle probes," *Nat. Biotechnol.*, Vol. 22, No. 7, 2004, pp. 883–887.

[98] Feldkamp, U. and Niemeyer, C. M., "Rational design of DNA nanoarchitectures," *Angew. Chem. Int. Ed.*, Vol. 45, No. 12, 2006, pp. 1856–1876.

[99] Li, H. and Rothberg, L., "Colorimetric detection of DNA sequences based on electrostatic interactions with unmodified gold nanoparticles," *Proc. Natl. Acad. Sci. USA*, Vol. 101, No. 39, 2004, pp. 14036–14039.

[100] Han, M. S., et al., "Colorimetric screening of DNA-binding molecules with gold nanoparticle probes," *Angew. Chem. Int. Ed.*, Vol. 45, No. 11, 2006, pp. 1807–1810.

[101] Han, M. S., et al., "A gold nanoparticle based approach for screening triplex DNA binders," *J. Am. Chem. Soc.*, Vol. 128, No. 15, 2006, pp. 4954–4955.

[102] Otsuka, H., et al., "Quantitative and Reversible Lectin-Induced Association of Gold Nanoparticles Modified with α-Lactosyl-ω-mercapto-poly(ethylene glycol)," *J. Am. Chem. Soc.*, Vol. 123, No. 34, 2001, pp. 8226–8230.

[103] Tsai, C. S., et al., "Gold nanoparticle-based competitive colorimetric assay for detection of protein-protein interactions," *Chem. Commun.*, No. 34, 2005, pp. 4273–4275.

[104] Schofield, C. L., et al., "Glyconanoparticles for the colorimetric detection of cholera toxin," *Anal. Chem.*, Vol. 79, No. 4, 2007, pp. 1356–1361.

[105] Nath, N. and Chilkoti, A., "A Colorimetric Gold Nanoparticle Sensor to Interrogate Biomolecular Interactions in Real Time on a Surface," *Anal. Chem.*, Vol. 74, No. 3, 2002, pp. 504–509.

[106] Nath, N. and Chilkoti, A., "Label-free biosensing by surface plasmon resonance of nanoparticles on glass: Optimization of nanoparticle size," *Anal. Chem.*, Vol. 76, No. 18, 2004, pp. 5370–5378.

[107] Huang, C.-C., et al., "Aptamer-Modified Gold Nanoparticles for Colorimetric Determination of Platelet-Derived Growth Factors and Their Receptors," *Anal. Chem.*, Vol. 77, No. 17, 2005, pp. 5735–5741.

[108] Wei, H., et al., "Simple and Sensitive Aptamer-Based Colorimetric Sensing of Protein Using Unmodified Gold Nanoparticle Probes," *Chem. Commun.*, No. 36, 2007, pp. 3735–3737.

[109] Pavlov, V., et al., "Aptamer-Functionalized Au Nanoparticles for the Amplified Optical Detection of Thrombin," *J. Am. Chem. Soc.*, Vol. 126, No. 38, 2004, pp. 11768–11769.

[110] Xiao, Y., et al., "Catalytic growth of Au nanoparticles by NAD(P)H cofactors: optical sensors for $NAD(P)^+$-dependent biocatalyzed transformations," *Angew. Chem. Int. Ed.*, Vol. 43, No. 34, 2004, pp. 4519–4522.

[111] Brust, M., et al., "Novel gold-dithiol nano-networks with nonmetallic electronic-properties," *Adv. Mater.*, Vol. 7, No. 9, 1995, pp. 795–799.

[112] You, C. C., et al., "Regulation of alpha-chymotrypsin activity on the surface of substrate-functionalized gold nanoparticles," *Chem. Commun.*, No. 27, 2006, pp. 2905–2907.

[113] Guarise, C., et al., "Gold Nanoparticle-Based Protease Assay," *Proc. Natl. Acad. Sci. USA*, Vol. 103, No. 11, 2006, pp. 3978–3982.

[114] Laromaine, A., et al., "Protease-Triggered Dispersion of Nanoparticle Assemblies," *J. Am. Chem. Soc.*, Vol. 129, No. 14, 2007, pp. 4156–4157.

[115] Xu, X.-Y., et al., "A Gold-Nanoparticle-Based Real-Time Colorimetric Screening Method for Endonuclease Activity and Inhibition," *Angew. Chem. Int. Ed.*, Vol. 46, No. 19, 2007, pp. 3468–3470.

[116] Wang, Z., et al., "Kinase-Catalyzed Modification of Gold Nanoparticles: A New Approach to Colometric Kinase Activity Screening," *J. Am. Chem. Soc.*, Vol. 128, No. 7, 2006, pp. 2214–2215.

[117] Choi, Y., et al., "Sensing Phosphatase Activity by Using Gold Nanoparticles," *Angew. Chem. Int. Ed.*, Vol. 46, No. 5, 2007, pp. 707–709.

[118] Zhao, W., et al., "Simple and Rapid Colorimetric Enzyme Sensing Assays Using Non-crosslinking Gold Nanoparticle Aggregation," *Chem. Commun.*, No. 36, 2007, pp. 3729–3731.

[119] Chah, S., et al., "Gold nanoparticles as a colorimetric sensor for protein conformational changes," *Chem. Biol.*, Vol. 12, No. 3, 2005, pp. 323–328.

[120] Pons, T., et al., "On the Quenching of Semiconductor Quantum Dot Photoluminescence by Proximal Gold Nanoparticles," *Nano Lett.*, Vol. 7, No. 10, 2007, pp. 3157–3164.

[121] Huang, T. and Murray, R. W., "Quenching of $[Ru(bpy)_3]^{2+}$ Fluorescence by Binding to Au Nanoparticles," *Langmuir*, Vol. 18, No. 18, 2002, pp. 7077–7081.

[122] Huang, C.-C. and Chang, H.-T., "Selective Gold-Nanoparticle-Based 'Turn-On' Fluorescent Sensors for Detection of Mercury(II) in Aqueous Solution," *Anal. Chem.*, Vol. 78, No. 24, 2006, pp. 8332–8338.

[123] Chen, S.-J. and Chang, H.-T., "Nile red-adsorbed gold nanoparticles for selective determination of thiols based on energy transfer and aggregation," *Anal. Chem.*, Vol. 76, No. 13, 2004, pp. 3727–3734.

[124] He, X. R., et al., "Gold nanoparticle-based fluorometric and colorimetric sensing of copper(II) ions," *Adv. Mater.*, Vol. 17, No. 23, 2005, pp. 2811–2815.

[125] Ipe, B. I., et al., "Functionalized Gold Nanoparticles as Phosphorescent Nanomaterials and Sensors," *J. Am. Chem. Soc.*, Vol. 128, No. 6, 2006, pp. 1907–1913.

[126] Dubertret, B., et al., "Single-mismatch detection using gold-quenched fluorescent oligonucleotides," *Nat. Biotechnol.*, Vol. 19, No. 4, 2001, pp. 365–370.

[127] Maxwell, D. J., et al., "Self-assembled nanoparticle probes for recognition and detection of biomolecules," *J. Am. Chem. Soc.*, Vol. 124, No. 32, 2002, pp. 9606–9612.

[128] Ray, P. C., et al., "Gold nanoparticle based FRET asssay for the detection of DNA cleavage," *J. Phys. Chem. B*, Vol. 110, No. 42, 2006, pp. 20745–20748.

[129] Dyadyusha, L., et al., "Quenching of CdSe Quantum Dot Emission, a New Approach for Biosensing," *Chem. Commun.*, No. 25, 2005, pp. 3201–3203.

[130] Oh, E., et al., "Inhibition Assay of Biomolecules Based on Fluorescence Resonance Energy Transfer (FRET) Between Quantum Dots and Gold Nanoparticles," *J. Am. Chem. Soc.*, Vol. 127, No. 10, 2005, pp. 3270–3271.

[131] Oh, E., et al., "Nanoparticle-based energy transfer for rapid and simple detection of protein glycosylation," *Angew. Chem. Int. Ed.*, Vol. 45, No. 47, 2006, pp. 7959–7963.

[132] You, C. C., et al., "Detection and identification of proteins using nanoparticle-fluorescent polymer 'chemical nose' sensors," *Nat. Nanotechnol.*, Vol. 2, No. 5, 2007, pp. 318–323.

[133] You, C. C., et al., "Tunable inhibition and denaturation of alpha-chymotrypsin with amino acid-functionalized gold nanoparticles," *J. Am. Chem. Soc.*, Vol. 127, No. 37, 2005, pp. 12873–12881.

[134] De, M., et al., "Biomimetic interactions of proteins with functionalized nanoparticles: a thermodynamic study," *J. Am. Chem. Soc.*, Vol. 129, No. 35, 2007, pp. 10747–10753.

[135] Katz, E., et al., "Electroanalytical and bioelectroanalytical systems based on metal and semiconductor nanoparticles," *Electroanalysis*, Vol. 16, No. 1–2, 2004, pp. 19–44.

[136] Yu, A. M., et al., "Nanostructured electrochemical sensor based on dense gold nanoparticle films," *Nano Lett.*, Vol. 3, No. 9, 2003, pp. 1203–1207.

[137] Raj, C. R., et al., "Gold Nanoparticle Arrays for the Voltammetric Sensing of Dopamine," *J. Electroanal. Chem.*, Vol. 543, No. 1, 2003, pp. 127–133.

[138] Roy, P. R., et al., "Simultaneous electrochemical detection of uric acid and ascorbic acid at a poly(N,N-dimethylaniline) film-coated GC electrode," *J. Electroanal. Chem.*, Vol. 561, No., 2004, pp. 75–82.

[139] Zamborini, F. P., et al., "Electron hopping conductivity and vapor sensing properties of flexible network polymer films of metal nanoparticles," *J. Am. Chem. Soc.*, Vol. 124, No. 30, 2002, pp. 8958–8964.

[140] Wohltjen, H. and Snow, A. W., "Colloidal metal-insulator-metal ensemble chemiresistor sensor," *Anal. Chem.*, Vol. 70, No. 14, 1998, pp. 2856–2859.

[141] Evans, S. D., et al., "Vapour Sensing Using Hybrid Organic-Inorganic Nanostructured Materials," *J. Mater. Chem.*, Vol. 10, No. 1, 2000, pp. 183–188.

[142] Joseph, Y., et al., "Self-assembled gold nanoparticle/alkanedithiol films: preparation, electron microscopy, XPS-analysis, charge transport, and vapor-sensing properties," *J. Phys. Chem. B*, Vol. 107, No. 30, 2003, pp. 7406–7413.

[143] Wang, L. Y., et al., "Sensing arrays constructed from nanoparticle thin films and interdigitated microelectrodes," *Sensors*, Vol. 6, No. 6, 2006, pp. 667–679.

[144] Wang, L. Y., et al., "Array of molecularly mediated thin film assemblies of nanoparticles: Correlation of vapor sensing with interparticle spatial properties," *J. Am. Chem. Soc.*, Vol. 129, No. 7, 2007, pp. 2161–2170.

[145] Krasteva, N., et al., "Self-Assembled Gold Nanoparticle/Dendrimer Composite Films for Vapor Sensing Applications," *Nano Lett.*, Vol. 2, No. 5, 2002, pp. 551–555.

[146] Singh, A., et al., "Spider silk as an active scaffold in the assembly of gold nanoparticles and application of the gold-silk bioconjugate in vapor sensing," *Small*, Vol. 3, No. 3, 2007, pp. 466–473.

[147] Shipway, A. N., et al., "Bis-bipyridinium cyclophane receptor-Au nanoparticle superstures for electrochemical sensing applications," *Chem. Mater.*, Vol. 11, No. 1, 1999, pp. 13–15.

[148] Lahav, M., et al., "Au-nanoparticle-bis-bipyridinium cyclophane superstructures: assembly, characterization and sensoric applications," *J. Chem. Soc., Perkin Trans. 2*, No. 9, 1999, pp. 1925–1931.

[149] Lahav, M., et al., "An enlarged bis-bipyridinium cyclophane-Au nanoparticle superstructure for selective electrochemical sensing applications," *J. Electroanal. Chem.*, Vol. 482, No. 2, 2000, pp. 217–221.

[150] Lahav, M., et al., "Au-colloid-'molecular square' superstructures: novel electrochemical sensing interfaces," *Chem. Commun.*, No. 19, 1999, pp. 1937–1938.

[151] Blonder, R., et al., "Three-dimensional redox-active layered composites of Au-Au, Ag-Ag and Au-Ag colloids," *Chem. Commun.*, No. 13, 1998, pp. 1393–1394.

[152] Kharitonov, A. B., et al., "An Au nanoparticle/bispyridinium cyclophane-functionalized ion-sensitive filed-effect transistor for the sensing of a drenaline," *Anal. Chem.*, Vol. 71, No. 23, 1999, pp. 5441–5443.

[153] Geng, J. F., et al., "Suppressed electron hopping in a Au nanoparticle/H_2S system: development towards a H_2S nanosensor," *Chem. Commun.*, No. 14, 2005, pp. 1895–1897.

[154] Thompson, D. T., "Using gold nanoparticles for catalysis," *Nanotoday*, Vol. 2, No. 4, 2007, pp. 40–43.

[155] Raj, C. R. and Jena, B. K., "Efficient electrocatalytic oxidation of NADH at gold nanoparticles self-assembled on three-dimensional sol-gel network," *Chem. Commun.*, No. 15, 2005, pp. 2005–2007.

[156] Jena, B. K. and Raj, C. R., "Enzyme-free amperometric sensing of glucose by using gold nanoparticles," *Chem. Eur. J.*, Vol. 12, No. 10, 2006, pp. 2702–2708.

[157] Jena, B. K. and Raj, C. R., "Synthesis of flower-like gold nanoparticles and their electrocatalytic activity towards the oxidation of methanol and the reduction of oxygen," *Langmuir*, Vol. 23, No. 7, 2007, pp. 4064–4070.

[158] Crumbliss, A. L., et al., "Colloidal gold as a biocompatible immobilization matrix suitable for the fabrication of enzyme electrodes by electrodeposition," *Biotech. Bioeng.*, Vol. 40, No. 4, 1992, pp. 483–490.

[159] Xu, X. X., et al., "Disposable nitrite sensor based on hemoglobin-colloidal gold nanoparticle modified screen-printed electrode," *Anal. Lett.*, Vol. 36, No. 11, 2003, pp. 2427–2442.

[160] Shulga, O. and Kirchhoff, J. R., "An acetylcholinesterase enzyme electrode stabilized by an electrodeposited gold nanoparticle layer," *Electrochem. Commun.*, Vol. 9, No. 5, 2007, pp. 935–940.

[161] Bharathi, S. and Nogami, M., "A Glucose Biosensor Based on Electrodeposited Biocomposites of Gold Nanoparticles and Glucose Oxidase Enzyme," *Analyst*, Vol. 126, No. 11, 2001, pp. 1919–1922.

[162] You, C. C., et al., "Modulation of the catalytic behavior of alpha-chymotrypsin at monolayer-protected nanoparticle surfaces," *J. Am. Chem. Soc.*, Vol. 128, No. 45, 2006, pp. 14612–14618.

[163] Pandey, P., et al., "Application of thiolated gold nanoparticles for the enhancement of glucose oxidase activity," *Langmuir*, Vol. 23, No. 6, 2007, pp. 3333–3337.

[164] Xiao, Y., et al., "'Plugging into enzymes': nanowiring of redox enzymes by a gold nanoparticle," *Science*, Vol. 299, No. 5614, 2003, pp. 1877–1881.

[165] Castaneda, M. T., et al., "Electrochemical sensing of DNA using gold nanoparticles," *Electroanalysis*, Vol. 19, No. 7–8, 2007, pp. 743–753.

[166] Park, S. J., et al., "Array-based electrical detection of DNA with nanoparticle probes," *Science*, Vol. 295, No. 5559, 2002, pp. 1503–1506.

[167] Ozsoz, M., et al., "Electrochemical genosensor based on colloidal gold nanoparticles for the detection of factor V leiden mutation using disposable pencil graphite electrodes," *Anal. Chem.*, Vol. 75, No. 9, 2003, pp. 2181–2187.

[168] Cai, H., et al., "Electrochemical detection of DNA hybridization based on silver enhanced gold nanoparticle label," *Anal. Chim. Acta*, Vol. 469, No. 2, 2002, pp. 165–172.

[169] Wang, J., et al., "Amplified voltammetric detection of DNA hybridization via oxidation of ferrocene caps on gold nanoparticle/streptavidin conjugates," *Anal. Chem.*, Vol. 75, No. 15, 2003, pp. 3941–3945.

[170] Baca, A. J., et al., "Attachment of ferrocene-capped gold nanoparticle-streptavidin conjugates onto electrode surfaces covered with biotinylated biomolecules for enhanced voltammetric analysis," *Electroanalysis*, Vol. 16, No. 1–2, 2004, pp. 73–80.

[171] Wang, J., et al., "Capture of p53 by Electrodes Modified with Consensus DNA Duplexes and Amplified Voltammetric Detection Using Ferrocene-Capped Gold Nanoparticle/Streptavidin Conjugates," *Anal. Chem.*, Vol. 80, No. 3, 2008, pp. 769–774.

[172] Zhang, J., et al., "Sequence-specific detection of femtomolar DNA via a chronocoulometric DNA sensor (CDS): Effects of nanoparticle-mediated amplification and nanoscale control of DNA assembly at electrodes," *J. Am. Chem. Soc.*, Vol. 128, No. 26, 2006, pp. 8575–8580.

[173] Li, D., et al., "Amplified electrochemical detection of DNA through the aggregation of Au nanoparticles on electrodes and the incorporation of methylene blue into the DNA-croslinked structure," *Chem. Commun.*, No. 34, 2007, pp. 3544–3546.

[174] Velev, O. D. and Kaler, E. W., "In situ assembly of colloidal particles into miniaturized biosensors," *Langmuir*, Vol. 15, No. 11, 1999, pp. 3693–3698.

[175] Dequaire, M., et al., "An electrochemical metalloimmunoassay based on a colloidal gold label," *Anal. Chem.*, Vol. 72, No. 22, 2000, pp. 5521–5528.

[176] Mao, X., et al., "Cyclic accumulation of nanoparticles: A new strategy for electrochemical immunoassay based on the reversible reaction between dethiobiotin and avidin," *Anal. Chim. Acta*, Vol. 557, No. 1, 2006, pp. 159–163.

[177] Nie, S. M. and Emory, S. R., "Probing single molecules and single nanoparticles by surface-enhanced Raman scattering," *Science*, Vol. 275, No. 5303, 1997, pp. 1102–1106.

[178] Aroca, R. F., et al., "Surface-enhanced Raman scattering on colloidal nanostructures," *Adv. Colloid Interf.*, Vol. 116, No. 1, 2005, pp. 45–61.

[179] Toderas, F., et al., "Controlling gold nanoparticle assemblies for efficient surface-enhanced Raman scattering and localized surface plasmon resonance sensors," *Nanotechnology*, Vol. 18, No. 25, 2007, p. 255702.

[180] Cao, Y. C., et al., "Nanoparticles with Raman Spectroscopic Fingerprints for DNA and RNA Detection," *Science*, Vol. 297, No. 5586, 2002, pp. 1536–1540.

[181] Sun, L., et al., "Surface-enhanced Raman scattering based nonfluorescent probe for multiplex DNA detection," *Anal. Chem.*, Vol. 79, No. 11, 2007, pp. 3981–3988.

[182] Cao, Y. C., et al., "Raman dye-labeled nanoparticle probes for proteins," *J. Am. Chem. Soc.*, Vol. 125, No. 48, 2003, pp. 14676–14677.

[183] Grubisha, D. S., et al., "Femtomolar detection of prostate-specific antigen: An immunoassay based on surface-enhanced Raman scattering and immunogold labels," *Anal. Chem.*, Vol. 75, No. 21, 2003, pp. 5936–5943.

[184] Qian, X., et al., "In vivo tumor targeting and spectroscopic detection with surface-enhanced Raman nanoparticle tags," *Nat. Biotechnol.*, Vol. 26, No. 1, 2008, pp. 83–90.

[185] Homola, J., et al., "Surface plasmon resonance sensors: review," *Sens. Actuator B-Chem.*, Vol. 54, No. 1–2, 1999, pp. 3–15.

[186] Wang, J., "Nanomaterial-based amplified transduction of biomolecular interactions," *Small*, Vol. 1, No. 11, 2005, pp. 1036–1043.

[187] Matsui, J., et al., "SPR sensor chip for detection of small molecules using molecularly imprinted polymer with embeded gold nanoparticles," *Anal. Chem.*, Vol. 77, No. 13, 2005, pp. 4282–4285.

[188] He, L., et al., "Colloidal Au-enhanced surface plasmon resonance for ultrasensitive detection of DNA hybridization," *J. Am. Chem. Soc.*, Vol. 122, No. 38, 2000, pp. 9071–9077.

[189] Fang, S. P., et al., "Attomole microarray detection of MicroRNAs by nanoparticle-amplified SPR imaging measurements of surface polyadenylation reactions," *J. Am. Chem. Soc.*, Vol. 128, No. 43, 2006, pp. 14044–14046.

[190] Yao, X., et al., "Sub-attomole oligonucleotide and p53 cDNA determinations via a high-resolution surface plasmon resonance combined with oligonucleotide-capped gold nanoparticle signal amplification," *Anal. Biochem.*, Vol. 354, No. 2, 2006, pp. 220–228.

[191] Bailey, R. C., et al., "Real-time multicolor DNA detection with chemoresponsive diffraction gratings and nanoparticle probes," *J. Am. Chem. Soc.*, Vol. 125, No. 44, 2003, pp. 13541–13547.

[192] Hirsch, L. R., et al., "A whole blood immunoassay using gold nanoshells," *Anal. Chem.*, Vol. 75, No. 10, 2003, pp. 2377–2381.

[193] Lyon, L. A., et al., "Colloidal Au-Enhanced Surface Plasmon Resonance Immunosensing," *Anal. Chem.*, Vol. 70, No. 24, 1998, pp. 5177–5183.

[194] Pieper-Furst, U., et al., "Gold nanoparticle-enhanced surface plasmon resonance measurement with a highly sensitive quantification for human tissue inhibitor of metalloproteinases-2," *Anal. Chim. Acta*, Vol. 550, No. 1–2, 2005, pp. 69–76.

[195] Marx, K. A., "Quartz crystal microbalance: A useful tool for studying thin polymer films and complex biomolecular systems at the solution-surface interface," *Biomacromolecules*, Vol. 4, No. 5, 2003, pp. 1099–1120.

[196] Han, L., et al., "Core-Shell Nanostructured Nanoparticle Films as Chemically Sensitive Interfaces," *Anal. Chem.*, Vol. 73, No. 18, 2001, pp. 4441–4449.

[197] Grate, J. W., et al., "Sorptive behavior of monolayer-protected gold nanoparticle films: Implications for chemical vapor sensing," *Anal. Chem.*, Vol. 75, No. 8, 2003, pp. 1868–1879.

[198] Krasteva, N., et al., "Vapor sorption and electrical response of Au-nanoparticle-dendrimer composites," *Adv. Func. Mater.*, Vol. 17, No. 6, 2007, pp. 881–888.

[199] Mao, X. L., et al., "A nanoparticle amplification based quartz crystal microbalance DNA sensor for detection of Escherichia coli O157 : H7," *Biosens. Bioelectron.*, Vol. 21, No. 7, 2006, pp. 1178–1185.

[200] Lin, L., et al., "Study on colloidal Au-enhanced DNA sensing by quartz crystal microbalance," *Biochem. Biophy. Res. Commun.*, Vol. 274, No. 3, 2000, pp. 817–820.

[201] Zhou, X.-C., et al., "Amplified Microgravimetric Gene Sensor Using Au Nanoparticle Modified Oligonucleotides," *Chem. Commun.*, No. 11, 2000, pp. 953–954.

[202] Patolsky, F., et al., "Dendritic amplification of DNA analysis by oliogonucleotide-functionalized Au-nanoparticles," *Chem. Commun.*, No. 12, 2000, pp. 1025–1026.

[203] Willner, I., et al., "Amplified detection of single-base mismatches in DNA using microgravimetric quartz-crystal-microbalance transduction," *Talanta*, Vol. 56, No. 5, 2002, pp. 847–856.

[204] Nie, L. B., et al., "Enhanced DNA detection based on the amplification of gold nanoparticles using quartz crystal microbalance," *Nanotechnology*, Vol. 18, No. 30, 2007, p. 305501.

[205] Liu, T., et al., "A novel microgravimetric DNA sensor with high sensitivity," *Biochem. Biophy. Res. Commun.*, Vol. 304, No. 1, 2003, pp. 98–100.

[206] Weizmann, Y., et al., "Amplified detection of DNA and analysis of single-base mismatches by the catalyzed deposition of gold on Au-nanoparticles," *Analyst*, Vol. 126, No. 9, 2001, pp. 1502–1504.

[207] Liu, T., et al., "Sensitivity enhancement of DNA sensors by nanogold surface modification," *Biochem. Biophy. Res. Commun.*, Vol. 295, No. 1, 2002, pp. 14–16.

[208] Su, M., et al., "Microcantilever resonance-based DNA detection with nanoparticle probes," *Appl. Phys. Lett.*, Vol. 82, No. 20, 2003, pp. 3562–3564.

[209] Kim, N. H., et al., "Highly sensitive biomolecule detection on a quartz crystal microbalance using gold nanoparticles as signal amplification probes," *Anal. Sci.*, Vol. 23, No. 2, 2007, pp. 177–181.

[210] Nam, J. M., et al., "Nanoparticle-based bio-bar codes for the ultrasensitive detection of proteins," *Science*, Vol. 301, No. 5641, 2003, pp. 1884–1886.

[211] Georganopoulou, D. G., et al., "Nanoparticle-based detection in cerebral spinal fluid of a soluble pathogenic biomarker for Alzheimer's disease," *Proc. Natl. Acad. Sci. U.S.A.*, Vol. 102, No. 7, 2005, pp. 2273–2276.

[212] Stoeva, S. I., et al., "Multiplexed Detection of Protein Cancer Markers with Biobarcoded Nanoparticle Probes," *J. Am. Chem. Soc.*, Vol. 128, No. 26, 2006, pp. 8378–8379.

[213] Oh, B. K., et al., "A fluorophore-based bio-barcode amplification assay for proteins," *Small*, Vol. 2, No. 1, 2006, pp. 103–108.

[214] Nam, J. M., et al., "Colorimetric bio-barcode amplification assay for cytokines," *Anal. Chem.*, Vol. 77, No. 21, 2005, pp. 6985–6988.

[215] Nam, J. M., et al., "Detection of Proteins Using a Colorimetric Bio-Barcode Assay," *Nat. Protocols*, Vol. 2, No. 6, 2007, pp. 1438–1444.

[216] Nam, J. M., et al., "Bio-bar-code-based DNA detection with PCR-like sensitivity," *J. Am. Chem. Soc.*, Vol. 126, No. 19, 2004, pp. 5932–5933.

[217] Stoeva, S. I., et al., "Multiplexed DNA detection with biobarcoded nanoparticle probes," *Angew. Chem. Int. Ed.*, Vol. 45, No. 20, 2006, pp. 3303–3306.

CHAPTER 9

Plasmon-Resonant Gold Nanorods: Photophysical Properties Applied Toward Biological Imaging and Therapy

Qingshan Wei and Alexander Wei

9.1 Introduction

Anisotropic gold nanoparticles are ideally suited as contrast agents for the optical imaging of biological tissues. Unlike many other inorganic nanomaterials, colloidal gold is essentially inert and has a long history of clinical use, not only as immunocytochemical probes for ex vivo applications [1–4] but also as colloidal adjuvants for in vivo radiotherapies [5–8], and more recently in animal studies for rheumatoid arthritis [9–11]. Moreover, recent developments in nanomaterials synthesis have enabled gold nanoparticles to be engineered into structures with tunable surface plasmon modes and with optical resonances ranging from visible to near-infrared (NIR) wavelengths [12]. Several types of gold nanostructures are currently being investigated as contrast agents for various optical imaging modalities, but those with plasmon resonances in the NIR region between 750 and 1300 nm are particularly favorable for biomedical imaging, as shorter wavelengths are extinguished by hemoglobin or other endogenous pigments and longer wavelengths are strongly attenuated by water [13]. Gold nanorods (GNRs) are especially attractive due to the tunability of their plasmon resonances, and also their straightforward and highly reproducible synthesis. GNRs support a higher absorption cross section at NIR frequencies per unit volume than most other nanostructures and have narrower linewidths at comparable resonance frequencies due to reduced radiative damping effects [14]. With respect to synthesis, GNRs are efficiently prepared in micellar surfactant solutions using seeded growth conditions, with various modifications developed for fine control over aspect ratio, scalability and uniformity, optical and colloidal stability, and absorption and scattering properties. The latter define the types of optical imaging modalities that can be empowered by the use of GNRs as contrast agents.

In this chapter, we review the current level of knowledge on the chemistry and photophysical properties of GNRs, followed by their applications toward biological imaging. Numerous examples of biological applications will be discussed to illustrate the breadth of possibilities that have been inspired by the versatility of these useful nanomaterials.

9.2 Synthesis

In recent years, numerous methods have been developed toward the preparation of GNRs with controlled diameters and length-to-width (aspect) ratios. Mesoscopic (micron to submicron) GNRs have been fabricated using "top-down" lithographic methods such as electron-beam lithography [15], focused-ion beam milling [16], and microtomy (nanoskiving) [17], or by templated electrodeposition into nanoporous aluminum oxide [18–24] or polycarbonate [25] membranes. However, these methods are less useful for preparing smaller GNRs with lengths below 100 nm, a more compatible size range for biomedical and in vivo applications. Instead, GNRs can be synthesized in a scalable fashion by the reduction of gold chloride ($HAuCl_4$) in aqueous solutions containing micellar cationic surfactants, such as cetyltrimethylammonium bromide (CTAB). These methods are extremely popular for the tunability of reaction parameters that determine the aspect ratio and subsequent optical properties of GNRs. The CTAB-mediated synthesis of GNRs has gone through several stages of development. Seminal contributions by Wang and coworkers demonstrated the synthesis of GNRs in CTAB solutions by electrochemical reduction of gold ions or by the electrolysis of gold electrodes, with controlled aspect ratios from 2.5 to 6.0 and optical extinctions extending well into the NIR range [26–29]. Photochemical reduction of $HAuCl_4$ has also proven to be quite useful for GNR synthesis [30–37], as well as more recently developed methods based on microwave [38–40] and proton beam irradiation [41].

At present, the most popular method for synthesizing GNRs with NIR absorption involves the chemical reduction of $HAuCl_4$ using a mild, organic reductant such as ascorbic acid, nucleated by small gold nanoparticle "seeds" [42, 43]. The seeded growth concept for GNR synthesis was first established in 2001 by Murphy and coworkers, and has rapidly gone through numerous stages of development [44–46]. Initial studies involved the addition of citrate-stabilized nanoparticles to growth solutions containing $HAuCl_4$ and CTAB, with ascorbic acid as a reducing agent and silver nitrate ($AgNO_3$) as an additive (Figure 9.1) [42, 47]. Variations in the reaction conditions and seeding strategies yielded GNRs with diameters of 15–20 nm and controlled aspect ratios as high as 20, but these dispersions often contained a significant fraction of spherical nanoparticles. Replacing citrate-stabilized seeds with CTAB-stabilized seeds increases the GNR yields to over 90 percent [48].

The aspect ratio and NIR-absorbing properties of GNRs can be tuned either by controlling the relative concentration of seeds or by the amount of $AgNO_3$ [42, 47, 48, 50], which was later established to have a passivating role through the underpotential deposition of a silver monolayer, primarily onto the {110} facets along the length of the GNRs [51]. The kinetics of GNR growth are rapid and nearly complete within minutes of seed addition, and typically produce dumbbell-shaped GNRs with slightly flared ends with lengths well below 100 nm and absorptions in the range of 750–900 nm, due to their longitudinal plasmon resonances (see next section). However, the reduction of $HAuCl_4$ by ascorbic acid is often incomplete and

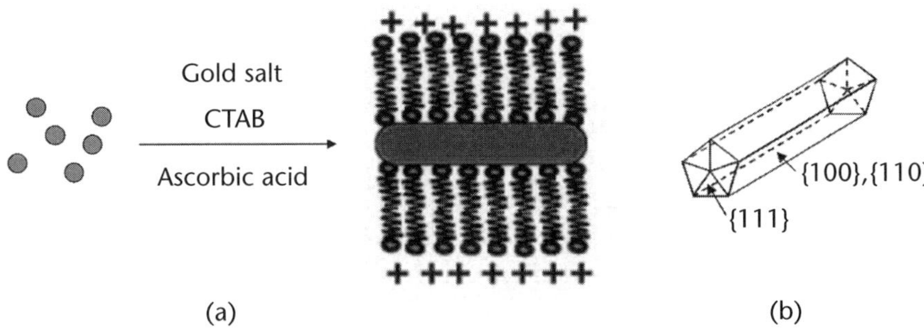

Figure 9.1 (a) Scheme for seed-mediated growth of GNRs; (b) crystalline facets on a typical GNR [49]. Reprinted with permission from the Materials Research Society and American Chemical Society.

can lead to a slower, secondary growth stage, in which the GNRs are "fattened" by the galvanic displacement of silver from the GNR sides. This can gradually shift the plasmon resonance from NIR to visible wavelengths, resulting in an "optical drift" by as much as 100 nm. This secondary growth process can be suppressed by ensuring the consumption of residual $HAuCl_4$, either by adding sodium sulfide (Na_2S) after the nanorod synthesis to quench further growth [52] or by adjusting the amount of ascorbic acid to ensure complete reduction.[1]

GNRs with higher aspect ratios and submicron lengths can be prepared by a consecutive seeded growth process [53–56] or by serial addition of growth solution [57, 58]. These growth conditions do not require the addition of $AgNO_3$ and can be further promoted by introducing small amounts of nitric acid [59, 60], although the exact role of the latter additive is presently unknown. Alternative surfactants to CTAB with larger cationic headgroups [48, 61–63] or polymeric ligands [64] can also be used to increase GNR aspect ratio.

With regard to the GNR growth mechanism, a full understanding is lacking, although several hypotheses have been suggested. One of these concerns the role of CTAB and its possible preference for certain crystalline facets on the surfaces of the gold nanoparticle seeds [65]. Preferential adsorption to the {100} facets will lead to faster growth along the {110} common axis shared by {111} facets, resulting in the production of {110} facets along the sides of the GNRs at the expense of {111} surface area. An electric field-directed growth mechanism has also been proposed, in which Au^I-CTAB complexes are transported to the nanorod tips by convective forces driven by electric field gradients [66]. The role of the $AgNO_3$ is also of great interest: the competitive deposition of Ag ions slows down the overall growth rate and can account for the high uniformity and yield of GNRs. Furthermore, the electroless (underpotential) deposition of Ag occurs preferentially on high-energy {110} facets, promoting anisotropic growth [51]. The GNR growth kinetics are also influenced by the relative concentrations of the nucleating particle, $HAuCl_4$, CTAB, $AgNO_3$, and ascorbic acid, as well as the pH and reaction temperature, all of which can lead to significant changes in particle shapes, sizes, and yields [50, 67–71].

1. Zubarev, E. R., personal communication.

9.3 Optical Properties

9.3.1 Absorption

The tremendous interest in GNRs in the past decade stems in large part from their intense and wavelength-tunable optical properties. These are intimately associated with an electrodynamic phenomenon known as surface plasmons, which embody the collective oscillations of conduction electrons when excited by light. In the case of gold nanoparticles (which are much smaller than the wavelength of visible light), the plasmons are bounded and will resonate at specific electromagnetic frequencies, and are thus characterized by very large optical cross sections. These localized surface plasmon resonances (LSPRs) are highly sensitive to particle size, shape, material composition, and the local dielectric environment. A number of recent monographs and reviews provide a detailed discussion on the many factors that significantly impact the LSPR of metal nanoparticles [72–86].

For small isotropic nanoparticles, the LSPR can be simply described as a single dipole mode according to Mie theory [87].[2] However, the reduced symmetry of anisotropic particles such as GNRs results in at least two resonance modes, a longitudinal resonance (LR) along the GNR axis and a transverse resonance (TR) normal to that axis. The LR and TR modes were first defined for ellipsoidal particles by Gans in the early twentieth century as an extension of Mie theory [88]. The extinction cross section (C_{ext}) of an ellipsoid can be mathematically expressed as

$$C_{ext} = \frac{2\pi V}{3\lambda}\varepsilon_m^{3/2}\sum_j \frac{\left(1/P_j^2\right)\varepsilon_2}{\left(\varepsilon_1 + \frac{1-P_j}{P_j}\varepsilon_m\right)^2 + \varepsilon_2^2} \tag{9.1}$$

where V is the particle volume, ε_m is the dielectric constant of the surrounding medium, $\varepsilon = \varepsilon_1 + i\varepsilon_2$ is the complex dielectric function of the metal, and P_j are depolarization factors associated with dimensions A, B, and C (A = length; B, C = width). These factors are defined for GNRs as

$$P_A = \frac{1-e^2}{e^2}\left[\frac{1}{2e}\ln\left(\frac{1+e}{1-e}\right) - 1\right] \tag{9.2}$$

$$P_B = P_C = \frac{1-P_A}{2} \tag{9.3}$$

where $e = \sqrt{1 - \frac{1}{R^2}}$ represents the ellipticity and R is the aspect ratio, or A/B.

El-Sayed and coworkers adapted the Mie-Gans equation to derive a simple, semiempirical relationship between the GNR longitudinal resonance wavelength (λ_{LR}) and aspect ratio R [89–91]:

2. Mie theory is more accurately defined as a complete analytical solution of Maxwell's equations for the electromagnetic scattering by polarizable bodies.

$$\lambda_{LR} = (53.71R - 42.29)\varepsilon_m + 495.14 \tag{9.4}$$

This relationship indicates that λ_{LR} shifts from the visible to NIR and mid-IR wavelengths with increasing R, and is valid within the first degree of approximation. However, significant disparities exist between (9.4) and experimental absorption values. This is not surprising given the assumption of GNRs as ideally prolate ellipsoids, and also because of polydispersity in particle aspect ratio as well as unaccounted modulations in the dielectric function at the GNR surface. A better fit of experimental measurements to (9.4) can be achieved by adjusting one or more physical parameters, such as a higher effective dielectric medium to offset the presence of charge near the GNR surface [92].

The plasmon resonance modes of GNRs can also be calculated numerically, such as by the discrete dipole approximation (DDA) [93–96] or finite-difference time-domain (FDTD) [15, 97] methods, which take into account the true shape of GNRs. Again, linear relationships between λ_{LR} and R can be established within a limited range [93], but the calculations also reveal that λ_{LR} is highly dependent on particle shape [98], diameter [89, 99], and the dielectric medium [100–104]. In contrast, the transverse resonance wavelength (λ_{TR}) is only mildly affected by changes in GNR shape and aspect ratio, usually staying within the range of 515–525 nm.

The tunable LR is most easily appreciated by the variations in color of GNRs as a function of aspect ratio R. Shorter GNRs appear blue, while longer GNRs appear red, indicating the minima in extinction at those wavelengths (Figure 9.2(a)); more precisely, the colors are the consequence of strong absorption at orange and green wavelengths. These are on the opposite side of the color wheel of blue and red (Figure 9.2(b)), and correspond, respectively, to λ_{LR} for short GNRs and λ_{TR} for long GNRs [105].

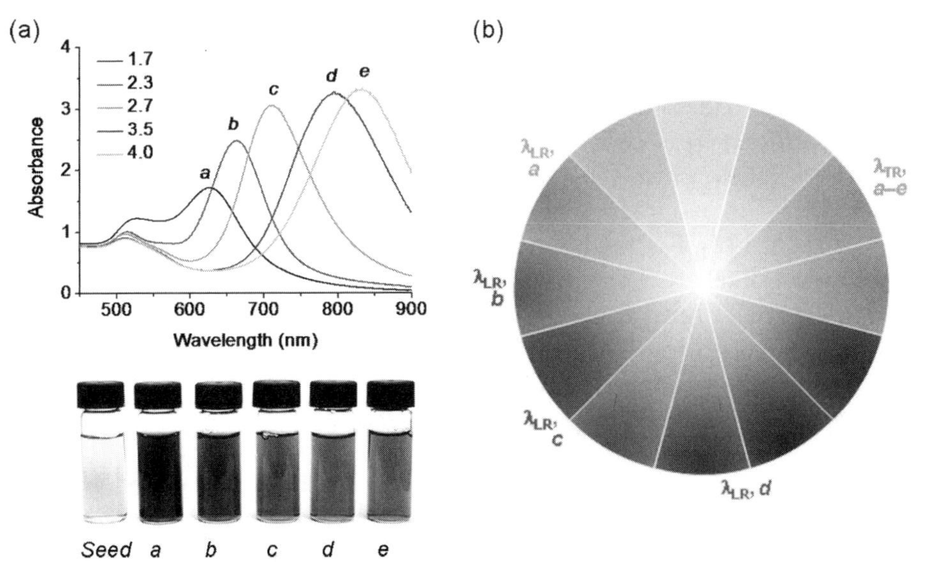

Figure 9.2 (a) Optical absorption spectra of GNRs with different aspect ratios; (b) color wheel with reference to λ_{LR} (and λ_{TR}) for GNR samples *a–e*. (See Color Plate 17.)

The LR mode is highly sensitive to environmental factors. The anisotropy of GNRs intrinsically renders them polarization-dependent, which gives rise to a $\cos^2$ relationship between the GNR long axis and polarized incident light [106, 107]. This angular dependency on light absorption has been observed experimentally using GNRs aligned in polymer films [106, 108]: the LR mode is at its strongest when the polarized light is aligned parallel to the GNRs, whereas the TR mode becomes dominant if the polarization is perpendicular to the GNR axis. The LR wavelength is also strongly influenced by changes in the surface dielectric by chemical adsorption or surface modifications [52, 109–111]. Metal nanoparticles are well known to experience LSPR shifts due to surface adsorption, and nanorods are the most sensitive among these [112]. This has led to the development of GNR-based multiplex biosensors, using shifts in LR for optical detection (Section 9.5.3) [110, 113]. Other factors known to influence the LR wavelength include surface roughness [114], electron charging [115, 116], and interparticle coupling (aggregation) effects [117–119]. Multipole plasmon resonances are also reported in relatively long rods [120–122].

9.3.2 Plasmon-Resonant Scattering

Resonant light scattering detection is one of the most straightforward and versatile methods for visualizing and tracking nanoparticles. Plasmon-resonant scattering from GNRs has been investigated by confocal and darkfield microscopy [17, 123–125] and is also modeled using numerical approaches [126–130]. Time-resolved light scattering from individual GNRs adsorbed loosely onto glass substrates has been monitored at a high frame rate, revealing orientational diffusion on the millisecond timescale but local residency (stiction) times on the order of seconds [131]. The low particle volumes of GNRs prepared by seeded growth make their scattering cross-sections relatively small compared with their absorbances [128]. On the other hand, the small size of GNRs supports a narrow plasmon resonance linewidth, whereas those produced by NIR-absorbing spherical nanoparticles are much broader due to size-dependent damping effects [5]. The scattering signals from GNRs increase with particle diameter, commensurate with an increase in volume [97]. In contrast, the resonant scattering does not increase linearly with length but achieves a maximum when the aspect ratio is close to 2, then gradually decreases [127, 128, 130]. Far-field optical microscopy techniques based on elastic light scattering will likely remain a useful tool for decades to come, but other methods have also been developed for the direct observation of LSPRs in GNRs. These include scanning near-field optical microscopy (SNOM) [132–136], two-dimensional transient absorption mapping [137], high-resolution cathodoluminescence spectroscopy [138], and photoemission electron microscopy [139].

9.3.3 Linear Photoluminescence

The absorption and scattering properties of gold nanoparticles are well established, but their photoemission properties are much less so. Indeed, photoluminescence (PL) is considered a rather unusual property for metals, which are better known for their ability to quench fluorescent molecules or particles by back-electron transfer.

Nevertheless, weak yet detectable PL can be generated from bulk Au [140] and from Au nanoparticles and GNRs using laser excitation [141–143]. PL can also be efficiently generated by UV excitation of very small (<2 nm) gold nanoclusters [144, 145], whose discretized energy states are absent in larger colloidal nanoparticles.

El-Sayed and coworkers excited GNRs at 480 nm (above plasmon resonance) to produce linear photoemission spectra with λ_{em} ranging from 548–588 nm. The emission wavelength was observed to increase linearly with aspect ratio, whereas the quantum efficiency (ϕ_{em}) had a quadratic dependency on GNR length [141]. Plasmons were determined to be important in PL amplification, with the ϕ_{em} of GNRs estimated to be more than 10^6 times compared with bulk Au, due to resonant coupling with local electromagnetic fields. Subsequent studies attributed the increase in PL to ultrafast, plasmon-enhanced emissions [142, 143]. The effect of higher aspect ratios ($R > 3.5$) on PL is somewhat less clear and in partial conflict with the earlier study [141]. In a report by the same group, the PL intensity (λ_{ex} = 480 nm; λ_{em} ca. 600 nm) decreased with R, which was attributed to the reduced overlap between LR and the interband transition [146]. This was also accompanied by the appearance of a second emission peak at 740 nm, close to the band edge of Au. A second, independent report indicated that the intensity of this emission band increased when using even longer GNRs (R = 13) at lower energy excitation (λ_{ex} up to 690 nm) [147].

9.3.4 Nonlinear Optical Properties

GNRs exhibit several nonlinear optical (NLO) properties, generated upon plasmon-resonant excitation with ultrashort (femtosecond) laser pulses. Two-photon luminescence (TPL), hyper-Rayleigh scattering (HRS), and second harmonic generation (SHG) have all attracted a great deal of attention for their capacity to produce optical contrast at visible wavelengths using NIR excitation and with very low autofluorescence. TPL involves the simultaneous absorption of two photons (typically in the NIR range), followed by a three-step process: (1) excitation of electrons from the *d*- to the *sp*-band to generate electron-hole pairs, (2) scattering of electrons and holes on the picosecond timescale with partial energy transfer to the phonon lattice, and (3) electron-hole recombination resulting in photoemission [140]. As with single-photon PL, the intrinsic TPL efficiency of bulk gold is poor, but TPL signals from GNRs can be greatly amplified by resonant coupling of the incident excitation with the LR mode (Figure 9.3(a)) [148, 149]. The two-photon absorption cross section of GNRs produced by seeded growth methods is on the order of 2×10^3 GM, intermediate between that of typical dye molecules (~10^2 GM) [150, 151] and semiconductor quantum dots (~10^4 GM) [152]. Other Au nanostructures such as nanospheres [153], nanoplates [154], nanoshells [155], and nanoparticle dimers [156, 157] have also been found to exhibit TPL activity, but GNRs produced by seeded growth methods have the highest TPL intensity per unit volume, as well as the added feature of polarization-dependent excitation [148, 158].

The TPL intensity of GNRs is quadratically dependent on excitation power as expected, but has little correlation with excitation frequency (Figure 9.3(b, c)) [148]. The emission spectra are broad and contain several peaks associated with

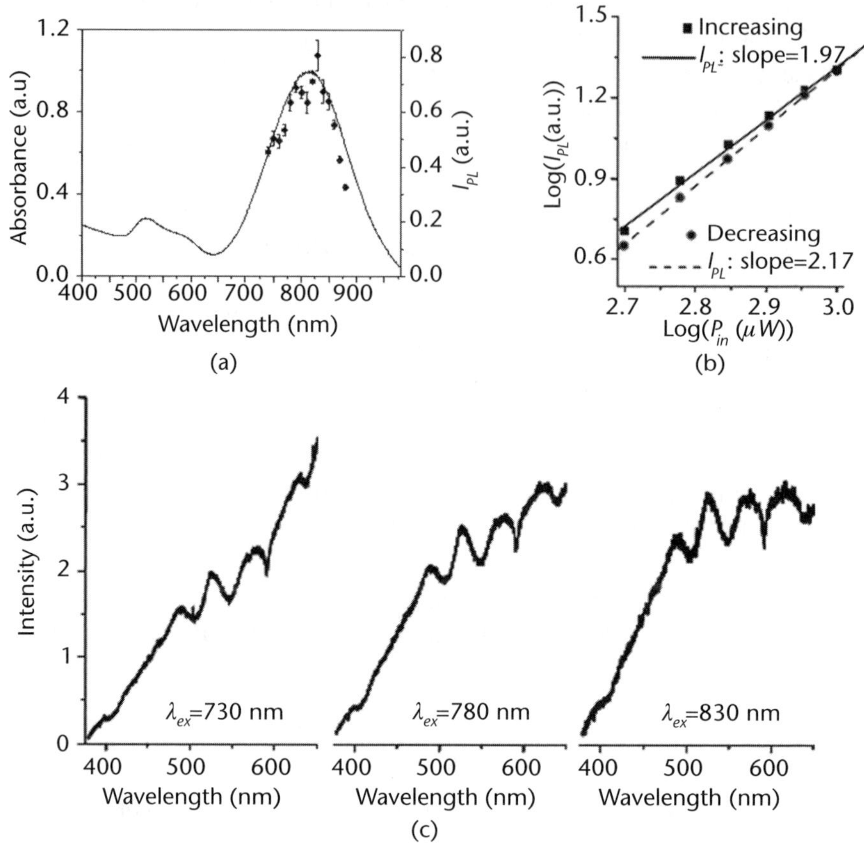

Figure 9.3 TPL generated from GNRs, using a femtosecond-pulsed Ti:sapphire laser: (a) Excitation intensities superimposed onto GNR absorption spectrum; (b) quadratic dependence of PL intensity with excitation power; (c) TPL emission spectra from GNRs in aqueous solution, excited at 730, 780, and 830 nm, respectively [148].

interband transitions. The TPL of individual GNRs have also been examined by SNOM and shown to depend strongly on the local density of states, with maximum PL enhancement at the tips where the electromagnetic field is strongest [159, 160]. Furthermore, the TPL intensity of single GNRs has a $\cos^4$ dependency on the polarization of incident light, another characteristic of a nonlinear absorption process [148]. Higher-order, multiphoton emissions have been reported in Au nanostripes fabricated by focused-ion beam milling [16] and Au nanowire arrays [161], as well as third-order absorption coefficients of GNRs embedded in a silica matrix [162]. These studies contribute toward our fundamental understanding of the nonlinear absorption properties of GNRs.

The second-order polarizability of GNRs has been measured by hyper-Rayleigh scattering (HRS) [163]. Unlike TPL, the HRS signal is frequency-doubled and the incident polarization is retained. The HRS response is plasmon-enhanced and has been modeled as a discrete, linear aggregate of spherical nanoparticles, whose strong interparticle couplings increase the HRS signal by an order of magnitude compared with the sum of individual nanospheres. Second harmonic generation (SHG) is another closely related, plasmon-enhanced NLO response, and has been investigated in oriented GNR arrays as a function of excitation polarization and wavelength [164, 165]. The emergence and characterization of these NLO properties provide fertile ground for biological imaging applications, as will be discussed in the next section.

9.3.5 Other Optical Properties

The tunable plasmonic responses of GNRs endow them with exciting potential for various bioanalytical applications, such as surface-enhanced Raman scattering (SERS) and surface-enhanced fluorescence (SEF). SERS is based on the Raman vibrational modes of chemical species adsorbed onto the surfaces of plasmon-resonant nanoparticles. The normally weak Raman intensities can be amplified by many orders of magnitude using local, plasmon-enhanced electromagnetic fields; consequently, the signal strength is highly dependent on the plasmon resonance of the supporting nanostructure. GNRs have been shown to support SERS using a NIR excitation source with estimated enhancement factors ranging from 10^7 to 10^9, up to 10^5 times larger than from Au nanoparticles irradiated under identical (nonresonant) conditions [166, 167]. Not surprisingly, the SERS response of GNRs is also very sensitive to aspect ratio, with differences of up to 100-fold in signal enhancement between resonant and nonresonant conditions [168]. The interparticle spacing between GNRs can also be important, as it determines the strength of coupled plasmon modes and can generate "hot spots" with extremely high local enhancements [169]. GNR aggregates have been prepared simply by salt-induced flocculation [170], whereas substrates with adjustable packing densities have been prepared using layer-by-layer (LbL) assembly [171, 172], by two-dimensional self-assembly at solvent interfaces [173], and by one-dimensional (end-to-end) assembly with a pronounced shift in λ_{LR} [174]. In addition to local field enhancement, the electronic interaction between the Au substrate and absorbed molecules can also contribute to SERS, commonly referred to as a chemical enhancement effect [175, 176].

SEF has been carefully investigated for fluorophores on colloidal nanoparticle surfaces [177–180], but less attention has been paid toward GNRs [181, 182]. SEF is very sensitive to the distance between fluorophores and nanoparticles, as a result of the competition between local field enhancement and quenching effects due to back-electron or resonant energy transfer. The latter effects are at their maximum when the fluorophores are within a few nanometers (<5 nm) of the metal surface, but a slight increase in separation can result in an emission enhancement of up to 100-fold [183]. Both SEF and fluorescence energy transfer are strongly dependent on the overlap between the LSPR and the molecule's absorption and emission spectra. For example, rhodamine B ($\lambda_{ex}/\lambda_{em}$ = 520/570 nm) adsorbed onto GNRs with λ_{LR} = 700 nm experienced less than 10 percent quenching by resonant energy transfer, but almost 100 percent quenching on Au nanospheres [181]. Interestingly, the electronic coupling between the dye and GNR can split λ_{LR} into two peaks, with a large plasmon shift up to 120 nm [182]. This splitting was highly dependent on the dye concentration as well as the dye–nanorod distance.

9.4 Surface Chemistry and Biocompatibility

Surface engineering plays a critical role in the development of GNRs for biomedical applications. Nanoparticle-based agents need to meet at least several criteria in order to be considered useful for in vivo applications: (1) dispersion stability in blood and other physiological fluids; (2) functionalization methods for site-selective targeting and/or cell uptake; (3) resistance against nonspecific cell uptake and protein adsorption; (4) sufficiently long circulation lifetimes to allow efficient delivery to the region of interest; (5) low cytotoxicity and inflammatory response. In addition, the engineered nanomaterial must be robust against chemical degradation while under biological exposure to avoid compromising its ability to meet these criteria. Together, these present a formidable obstacle course through which very few materials have successfully navigated. Consequently, the surface chemistry of GNRs (and of nanoparticles in general) requires as much attention and development as the nanomaterials themselves, if they are to meet their full biomedical potential. In this section, we survey the various surface chemistries developed for GNRs and their intended use in biological systems.

9.4.1 Bioconjugation Methods

It is not difficult to appreciate the utility of GNRs functionalized with biomolecular recognition elements. Decades of research have already been devoted to the bioconjugation of colloidal gold nanoparticles, many of which have been targeted toward cell-surface biomarkers for ex vivo immunolabeling studies by optical or electron microscopy [1]. However, many of those protocols cannot be adapted in a straightforward manner toward the bioconjugation of GNRs, particularly those synthesized or stabilized in micellar CTAB solutions [184]. As will become clear later, the presence of this cationic and toxic surfactant introduces some significant challenges in the preparation of functionalized GNRs, which can fulfill the criteria described earlier.

The physical or electrostatic absorption of anionic polyelectrolytes (PE) such as polystyrenesulfonate is the most direct and practical method of coating CTAB-stabilized GNRs (Figure 9.4(a)). PE-coated GNRs have been shown to form stable dispersions at various pH or ionic strength, and are also stable against dilution effects [185]. The latter is important because soluble CTAB can be removed from aqueous suspensions of GNRs by multiple centrifugation-redispersion cycles or by extraction with chloroform, but when CTAB falls below the critical micelle concentration (ca. 1 mM) [186], the GNRs become destabilized and quickly flocculate. In most cases, the polyanionic coating prevents GNRs from agglomerating and also reverses their zeta potential from positive to negative, which substantially improves their compatibility with biological media. The PE coating can also serve as a "primer" layer for antibodies [187] or small proteins such as myoglobin [188, 189], transferrin [185], or streptavidin [190, 191] via physisorption at a relatively low pH. Recent examples of GNRs functionalized by this approach have been targeted against epidermal growth factor receptor (EGFR) [192, 193], prostate specific antigen (PSA) [194], and the δ-opioid receptor [195]. It is worth mentioning that multilayer PE coatings have also been used to load various molecular cargos onto GNRs, including dye

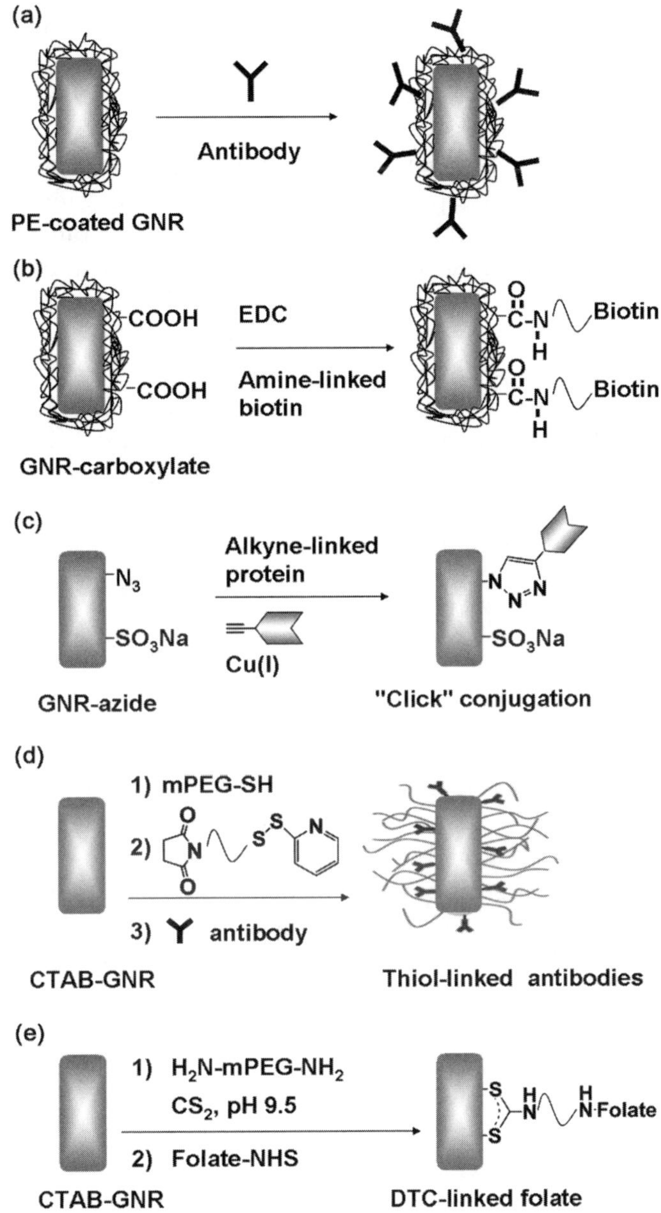

Figure 9.4 Surface functionalization and bioconjugation methods developed for GNRs: (a) electrostatic physisorption onto PE-coated GNRs [187]; (b) covalent attachment via carbodiimide coupling [197]; (c) "click" bioconjugation [198]; (d) chemisorption using thiols [200]; (e) chemisorption using dithiocarbamates (DTCs) [224]. Reprinted with permission from the American Chemical Society.

molecules [182] and hydrophobic proteins such as bovine serum albumin (BSA) [196].

Covalent crosslinking further increases the stability of bioconjugated GNRs, although the long-term stability of the physisorbed polyelectrolyte remains an open question for the time being. Amine- and acetylene-terminated biomolecules have been incorporated onto GNRs via carbodiimide coupling [197] and "click" bioconjugation [198], using intermediate PE coatings bearing activated *N*-hydroxysuccinimide (NHS) carboxylate esters or azides, respectively (Figure 9.4(b,c)).

Chemisorption offers an alternative route for the surface bioconjugation of GNRs and other Au nanoparticles. Thiols (–SH) are presently the most widely used functional group [199], and have been conjugated to proteins [200], oligonucleotides [201, 202], DNA aptamers [203], and oligopeptides [204] for their immobilization on GNR surfaces (Figure 9.4(d)). Low molecular-weight species such as alkanedithiols [205], biotin [206, 207], mercaptoacetic acid [208–210], cysteine [117, 209, 211–213], and glutathione [117, 211, 212] can also be introduced for subsequent biofunctionalization. A very interesting consequence of the chemisorptive approach is that many of these ligands adsorb preferentially onto the tips of GNRs, either on the {111} facets or their edges. This anisotropic functionalization has enabled GNRs to be assembled in end-to-end fashion, with a strong effect on their plasmon resonances (Section 9.3.5) [117, 202, 205–210, 212, 213]. End-to-end assembly can be coupled with biomolecular recognition events, and has been used as an optical switch for biosensing applications (Section 9.5.3.1) [117, 174, 202, 205, 210].

Despite their popularity for the functionalization of Au surfaces, chemisorbed thiols may have limited stability when exposed to physiological conditions [214, 215]. A number of reports have demonstrated that chemisorbed alkanethiols are readily displaced by surface exchange by other molecules [216–218] (including biogenic thiols such as glutathione) [219] and desorb at an appreciable rate under oxidative conditions [220] or in the presence of electrolytes [221]. These pathways compromise the integrity of alkanethiol-based self-assembled monolayers [215, 217], with less than positive consequences for in vivo applications.

Robust alternatives to thiol chemisorption are currently under investigation. One promising development involves ligands based on the dithiocarbamate (DTC) group ($-NCS_2^-$), which can be formed in situ by the condensation of alkylamines with CS_2 under moderately basic conditions (Figure 9.4(e)) [222]. This is a useful addition to existing bioconjugation methods, as it provides the option of attaching amine-terminated ligands directly onto Au surfaces. DTC chemisorption has been demonstrated on GNRs using amine-terminated polyethyeleneglycol (PEG) [223] and diamine oligoethyleneglycols conjugated to folic acid [224, 279]. Other recent examples involving DTC chemisorption include the conjugation of amine-terminated DNA oligonucleotides [225] and proline-terminated oligopeptides [226].

Finally, it is worth noting that CTAB-stabilized GNRs have also been coated with a silica layer using the well-known Stöber method [184, 227–231]. Mesoporous silica coatings have also been prepared by adjusting the amount of CTAB around the nucleating GNR [232]. The surface modification of silica is well known and may represent yet another direction for bioconjugation, given sufficient chemical stability and control over dispersion stability.

9.4.2 Cytotoxicity and Nonspecific Cell Uptake

The cytotoxicity of nanomaterials has been a broadly discussed issue and has attracted a great deal of attention worldwide [233]. With respect to GNRs, cytotoxicity studies have been few but are increasing in number, paving the way toward their potential biomedical applications. The membrane-compromising effects of the cationic surfactant CTAB is a primary concern due to its high acute cytotoxicity ($IC_{50} < 10\,\mu M$) and ability to inhibit mitochondrial activity [234, 235], so considerable attention has been paid to reduce its presence [236–238]. CTAB-stabilized GNRs coated with anionic PE [239, 197], serum proteins [238], or exchanged with phosphatidylcholine [230] or synthetic cationic lipids [240] all have reduced cytotoxicity profiles, due in part to the shielding effect of those physisorbed materials. On the other hand, in vitro studies have shown that the CTAB-stabilized GNRs themselves are not necessarily cytotoxic, if the excess CTAB is removed from the solution. For example, CTAB-coated GNRs were observed to be internalized by K562 or KB cells (from human leukemia or nasopharyngeal carcinoma cell lines, respectively) but did not produce an appreciable cytotoxic response over several days of incubation [223, 236]. Nevertheless, the nonspecific uptake of GNRs mediated by CTAB is undesirable, and efforts are currently underway to ensure its complete removal.

Chemisorptive approaches have also been used to improve the biocompability of GNRs. Treatment of CTAB-stabilized GNRs with thiol-terminated poly(ethylene glycol) (PEG-SH) [200, 237, 241] or with amine-terminated PEGs in the presence of CS_2 (in situ PEG-DTC formation) [223] have been shown to be inert to cell uptake and amenable to in vivo biodistribution studies, with a circulation half life on the order of several hours [159]. PEG-coated GNRs form stable dispersions in buffered solutions, can be extensively dialyzed for the rigorous removal of CTAB [223, 162], and have low cytotoxicity even at high concentrations, with 90 percent cell viability reported for a GNR concentration of 0.5 mM [237].

9.5 Biological Applications of Gold Nanorods

Like many other inorganic nanomaterials discussed throughout this volume, plasmon-resonant GNRs have several key advantages over conventional NIR dyes and chromophores for in vitro and in vivo applications. Their linear and nonlinear optical cross sections are many times larger than organic molecules, and their photophysical responses are essentially invulnerable to photobleaching effects. Moreover, GNRs are capable of producing intense photothermal effects, a property not typically associated with conventional imaging agents or fluorophores. The concept of using NIR-absorbing nanoparticles as highly localized heat sources has inspired a tidal wave of possibilities for combining diagnostic imaging with photoactivated therapies, nowadays referred to by the portmanteau "theragnostics." Here we survey a wide range of studies that apply the optical and photothermal properties of GNRs in a biological context.

9.5.1 Contrast Agents for Imaging

9.5.1.1 Dark-Field Microscopy

The ever-increasing sensitivity and resolving power of optical and optoelectronic systems has renewed an interest in imaging modalities based on resonant light scattering, both in the visible and the NIR range. Plasmon-resonant scatterers are well matched with dark-field microscopy, a popular tool for imaging biological samples. GNRs have a certain appeal as scattering contrast agents because they support dual plasmon modes in the visible and NIR range. The latter can be expected to produce a polarization-dependent response (Section 9.3.1), although this feature has yet to be exploited for biological imaging. GNRs have been used in dark-field microscopy for targeted cancer cell imaging: for example, antibody-labeled GNRs were observed to label malignant carcinoma cell lines by recognition of their cell-surface EFGRs, whereas their affinity for normal human keratinocytes was low [192]. In this case, the TR mode of GNRs produced an easily detectable orange-red scattering with white light excitation. The same strategy has been used to monitor the targeted nuclear delivery of GNRs conjugated with transferrin [185] or cell-penetrating peptides [204]. Dark-field microscopy with white-light illumination can also support multiplex labeling strategies, as demonstrated by the simultaneous detection of GNRs with different aspect ratios, targeted toward separate cell-surface biomarkers on human breast epithelial cells [113]. Dark-field GNR imaging can even be used to measure tissue properties: longer GNRs (R~15) were embedded in a cardiac fibroblast network to track local deformations induced by mechanical stress (Figure 9.5) [242]. Strain distributions were measured by monitoring the positions of GNRs in real time [242, 243].

9.5.1.2 Two-Photon Luminescence Microscopy

Interest in nanomaterials for NLO imaging has grown very rapidly in the past five years, in sync with the greater availability of multiphoton confocal microscopy. Semiconductor quantum-dot nanocrystals [152, 244] and quantum rods [245–247], nanosized carbon dots [248], and gold nanoshells [249] have all proven to have useful NLO properties and can serve as contrast agents for biological imaging in multiphoton microscopy. GNRs exhibit appreciable luminescence under both linear and nonlinear excitation conditions (Sections 9.3.3 and 9.3.4) [141, 146], but the latter is better suited for biological imaging for the following reasons: (1) as men-

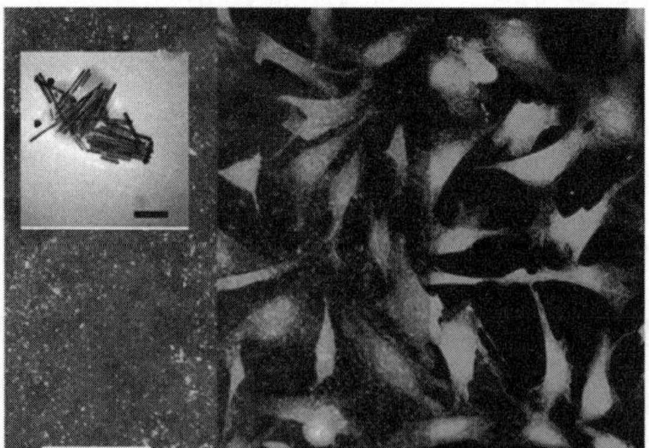

Figure 9.5 Partially overlapping dark-field and fluorescence images of GNRs incubated with cardiac fibroblasts [242]. TEM image of GNRs shown in upper-left inset. Reprinted with permission from the American Chemical Society. (See Color Plate 18.)

tioned previously, NIR illumination has greater transmittivity through biological structures and can therefore achieve greater penetration depth than visible light; (2) multiphoton excitation produces a much lower autofluorescence background, with a commensurate increase in signal-to-noise ratio; (3) NLO signal intensities are highly power dependent, which increases the 3D spatial resolution and minimizes collateral photodamage.

The utility of GNRs as TPL contrast agents has been demonstrated both in vitro and in vivo [148]. In a seminal in vivo TPL imaging study by Cheng and coworkers, a dilute solution of CTAB-stabilized GNRs were delivered into an anesthetized mouse by tail vein injection, then detected some minutes later passing through ear blood vessels after dilution in the blood pool (Figure 9.6) [148]. Continuous TPL monitoring revealed that the GNRs were cleared from the bloodstream within 30 minutes presumably due to opsonization, but subsequent in vivo TPL studies with PEG-conjugated GNRs indicate a much longer blood residency time, with a circulation half life of several hours.[3] A three-dimensional TPL imaging modality has also been developed for tissues using GNRs as contrast agents [193], with penetration depths up to 75 μm in a tissue phantom [193].

In vitro TPL imaging can be performed in real time or over the course of many hours, and has been used to track the trajectory and eventual fate of individual GNRs incubated with KB cells [223, 224]. CTAB-stabilized GNRs were internalized by KB cells within a few hours and observed to migrate toward the nucleus with a bidirectional motion, suggestive of co-transport with endosomes along microtubules [223]. In contrast, GNRs coated with PEG chains by in situ DTC formation were not taken up by KB cells, as characterized by the near-absence of TPL signals. Folic acid-conjugated GNRs have been targeted to the high-affinity folate receptor expressed on the surfaces of KB cells and observed by TPL imaging to accumulate on the outer cell membrane for many hours prior to their receptor-mediated endocytosis and delivery to the perinuclear region [224]. This image-guided deliv-

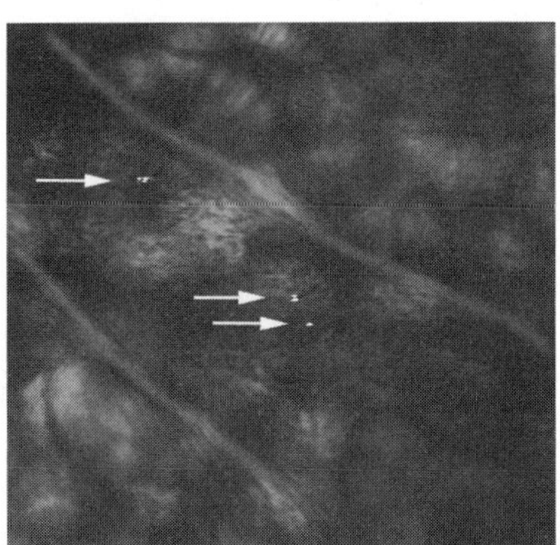

Figure 9.6 Still-frame TPL image of several GNRs (indicated by arrows) passing through a mouse ear blood vessel, several minutes after a tail vein injection [148]. Blood vessel walls in transmission overlay enhanced for clarity.

3. Tong, L., and Cheng, J.-X., personal communication.

ery provides an opportunity not just to identify and target cancer cells for photothermally induced cell death (discussed later), but also to time the delivery of NIR dosage for maximum efficacy.

9.5.1.3 Optical Coherence Tomography

Optical coherence tomography (OCT) is a recently established biomedical imaging technology capable of 2–3-mm depth penetration, with axial resolution on the order of 10 μm and lateral resolution in the low micron range [250–252]. OCT is noninvasive and analogous in several respects to ultrasound imaging, except that reflections of NIR light are detected rather than sound. OCT is primarily used in clinical opthalmology, but recent technological advances have made it possible to image nontransparent tissues, extending its application toward a broader range of medical specialties. But unlike other noninvasive imaging modalities such as ultrasound, magnetic resonance imaging (MRI), or x-ray computed tomography (CT), OCT can image cellular and even subcellular structures, with 10–25 times greater spatial resolution than that produced by ultrasound imaging, and up to 100 times better than MRI or CT [253].

OCT typically generates images based on morphology-dependent scattering, but can also produce images by differential absorption contrast (spectroscopic mode) or by differences in absorption/scattering profiles. These OCT variations can profit enormously from NIR-active contrast agents. Plasmon-resonant nanoparticles such as gold nanoshells [254–257], nanocages [258, 259], and GNRs [260–263] are among the most promising contrast agents, based on their NIR extinction properties. However, GNRs differ from the others in that their optical response is dominated by their absorption cross section. GNRs have been employed in conventional backscattering OCT, but a very high concentration is needed to produce detectable contrast [262].

GNRs are much better suited to support OCT modalities based on differential absorption or backscattering albedo (the ratio of backscattering to total extinction), which have the advantage of producing contrast in tissues with intrinsically high scattering cross-sections. An OCT modality based on low backscattering albedo has been demonstrated with GNRs in highly backscattering tissue phantoms, with an estimated detection limit as low as 30 ppm [260]. The narrow absorption linewidths of GNRs can also be used to enhance spectroscopic-domain OCT, and were recently investigated as contrast agents in an excised sample of human breast invasive ductal carcinoma [261]. The GNR distribution was parameterized by evaluating the evolution of the backscattered light spectrum over a range of tissue depths. The polarization-dependent extinction of GNRs has not yet been exploited for OCT imaging, but is anticipated to provide further enhancements to absorption-based modalities, and offers untapped potential for polarization-sensitive OCT.

9.5.1.4 Photoacoustic Imaging

The optoacoustic properties of plasmon-resonant gold nanoparticles originate from photoinduced cavitation effects. This process can be summarized as follows: (1) thermalization of conduction electrons on the subpicosecond timescale [74]; (2)

electron-phonon relaxation on the picosecond timescale and thermalization of the phonon lattice, with a subsequent rise in temperature by hundreds to thousands of degrees; (3) transient microbubble expansion upon reaching the kinetic spinodal of the superheated medium, initiated on the nanosecond timescale [264, 265]; (4) microbubble collapse, resulting in shockwaves and other forms of acoustic emission. The expansion and collapse of a cavitation bubble takes place on a microsecond timescale and are easily detected by ultrasonic transducers.

Photoacoustic tomography (PAT) is an emerging noninvasive imaging technique based on NIR-induced photoacoustic effects [266]. Images are obtained by the reconstruction of the optical energy absorption distributed across an array of acoustic transducers. The advantage of PAT over pure optical or ultrasonic imaging technique relies on the combined merits of optical irradiation and acoustic detection. Laser pulse irradiation provides a site-directed illumination with micron-level spatial resolution, as compared with the millimeter resolution of ultrasound waves. On the other hand, the low diffusion of propagating acoustic waves is advantageous over reflected optical signals, which suffer from scattering by biological tissue [267]. The depth resolution of PAT can be several centimeters in biological tissue [268], whereas pure optical imaging is limited to millimeter penetration depths [269].

NIR-absorbing gold nanoparticles have only recently been employed as exogenous in vivo contrast agents for PAT, which normally relies on the intrinsic differences in optical absorption by different tissue for producing contrast. In one recent example, PAT images of nude mice were significantly enhanced by the injection of GNRs, which could provide variations in signal intensity with concentration differences as low as 1.25 pM (Figure 9.7) [270]. This limit of sensitivity is 75 times greater than the detection of superparamagnetic iron oxide nanoparticles by MRI. Other examples involving GNRs in PAT include quantitative flow analysis in biological tissues [271] and the distribution kinetics of drug delivery systems [272]. Gold nanoshells (>100 nm) and nanocages of more compact size (<50 nm) have also been used as PAT contrast agents and detected in rat brains after intravenous injection, with observable vascular contrast within minutes [273, 274].

9.5.2 Photothermal Therapy

Metal nanoparticles are highly efficient converters of light energy into heat, making them promising agents for the targeted photothermolysis of cells. Numerous in vitro examples have been reported using Au nanoparticles conjugated to

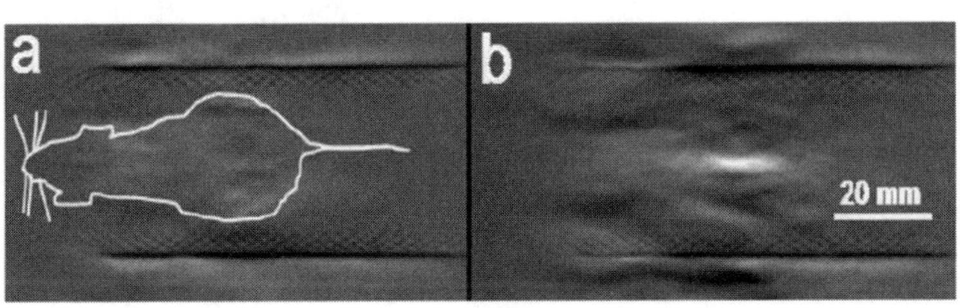

Figure 9.7 Photoacoustic tomography of a nude mouse (a) before and (b) after injection of GNRs [270]. Reprinted with permission from the American Chemical Society.

biomolecular recognition elements. The threshold laser fluence required for photoinduced damage can be remarkably low: an early report by Lin and coworkers demonstrated that antibody-labeled Au nanoparticles targeted toward CD8+ lymphocytes could deliver a death blow with just a single 20-ns laser pulse of 0.35 J/cm^2 [275]. For photothermolysis in vivo, NIR irradiation is preferred due to their greater penetration depth into biological tissue [13]. A seminal report by Halas and West illustrated the use of NIR-active gold nanoshells for in vivo photothermal imaging and therapy in a tumor mouse model [276]. PEG-coated nanoshells administered in the vicinity of tumors could induce photothermal ablation following exposure to NIR laser irradiation, which raised the local temperature by nearly 40K [276]. A subsequent study indicated that mice subjected to nanoshell-mediated photothermal therapy had a 100 percent survival rate with complete tumor reduction (N=7), whereas control mice all died within 10–20 days [277].

GNRs are also highly efficient converters of NIR light energy into heat and have been explored for the targeted photothermolysis of tumor cells [192, 224, 278, 279], parasitic protozoans [280], macrophage [281], and pathogenic bacteria [282]. While the issue of cell-selective delivery is of primary importance for future theragnostic applications, attention must also be paid toward the mechanisms of photoinduced cell injury. In particular, necrosis is often assumed to be the result of hyperthermia, for which a few degrees is sufficient to cause cell and tissue malfunction. However, this is not necessarily the case at the single-cell level. A recent study by Wei and Cheng has shown that GNRs bound to tumor cell membranes can serve as "optoporation" agents and induce cell necrosis by promoting an intracellular influx of Ca ions (Figure 9.8) [279]. This is explained most straightfowardly by the injury of the cell membrane due to local cavitation dynamics [264, 265], although a number of biomolecular mechanisms can also contribute toward the disruption of intracellular homeostasis.

The photothermal properties of GNRs suggest another attractive therapeutic application: molecular release triggered by NIR light. Photoinduced release of DNA previously adsorbed onto GNRs has been reported by several groups [283–285]. The release mechanism has been attributed to the reshaping of GNRs [283, 285] as well as the photoinduced dissociation of thiolated DNA from the GNR surface [284]. Importantly, the released DNA remains biologically active as proven in subsequent transfection experiments, resulting in GFP expression [284]. Poly-

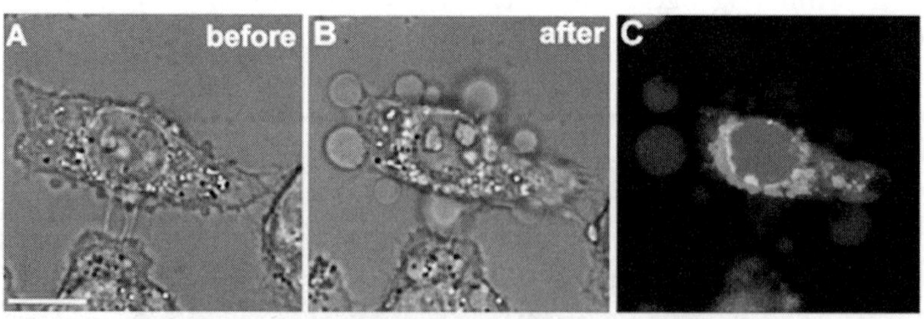

Figure 9.8 (a, b) Folate-conjugated GNRs (red) targeted to the membranes of KB cells, before and after a 1-min exposure to a scanning NIR laser (12 J/cm^2). (c) Evidence for "optoporation" was obtained by using ethidium bromide (red) and a fluorescent dye indicating high levels of intracellular Ca^{2+} (green) [279]. Reprinted with permission from Wiley-VCH Publishing. (See Color Plate 19.)

mer-coated GNRs are also appealing from the perspective of drug delivery and controlled release. Thermoresponsive polymers such as poly(*N*-isopropylacrylamide), or PNIPAAm, can be actuated in response to light when adsorbed onto GNRs or by loading GNRs into PNIPAAm hydrogels [286]. GNRs adsorbed onto PNIPAAm microspheres have also been prepared by electrostatic absorption, with reversible volume transitions and LSPR shifts observed upon photothermal stimulation [287–290]. Photoresponsive GNR–PNIPAAm hydrogels loaded with bioactive substances may have potential for controlled drug release but are presently limited by the uneven distribution of GNRs within the hydrogel matrix, resulting in a nonuniform photothermal response. As an alternative, PNIPAAm chains can be grafted directly onto GNRs via surface-initiated atom transfer radical polymerization (SI-ATRP) [291]. These polymer-conjugated GNRs have a well-defined core-shell morphology and a unit particle size below 100 nm, and may be more appropriate intermediates for the preparation of hydrogels with uniform photoresponsive behavior.

9.5.3 Ex Vivo Bioanalytical Applications

The longitudinal SPR of GNRs is highly sensitive to surface adsorption and environmental changes, making them excellent substrates for optically based bioanalytical applications. A few of these have already been discussed in the context of in vitro biosensing [113]; however, some of the most powerful and widely used diagnostic methods are performed offline. Here we focus on ex vivo bioanalytical applications whose scope can be further augmented by the incorporation of GNRs.

9.5.3.1 LSPR-Based Biosensors

Bioanalytical methods based on the LSPR of plasmon-resonant nanoparticles typically fall into two categories: colorimetric response to analytes triggered by nanoparticle aggregation and LSPR shifts caused by changes in local refractive index. GNRs have been successfully used in both types of sensing modalities. Low-aspect ratio GNRs are particularly well suited for detecting analytes that can trigger their end-to-end aggregation. Their longitudinal resonances produce much stronger redshifts than that observed for isotropic nanoparticles of comparable size (and can thus support lower limits of detection) but are still readily measured using conventional optical detection systems [208]. Aggregation-induced LSPR shifts can also be adapted for multiplexing strategies; for example, sequence-selective oligonucleotide detection based on GNR-GNR versus GNR-nanosphere assembly has been demonstrated [202]. Interestingly, the GNR-nanosphere coupling produced a greater redshift than GNR-GNR assemblies under similar sampling conditions. This counterintuitive observation may be attributed to the kinetics of nanoparticle aggregation and the preferential chemisorption of the thiolated antisense oligonucleotide on the GNR tips: the frequency of collision with isotropic gold nanospheres is higher than the rate of self-aggregation.

Thiolated amino acids such as cysteine and glutathione have also been reported to induce GNR aggregation selectively (see Figure 9.9) [117]. The combination of the primary thiol and the α-amino acid functionality is required to induce a strong

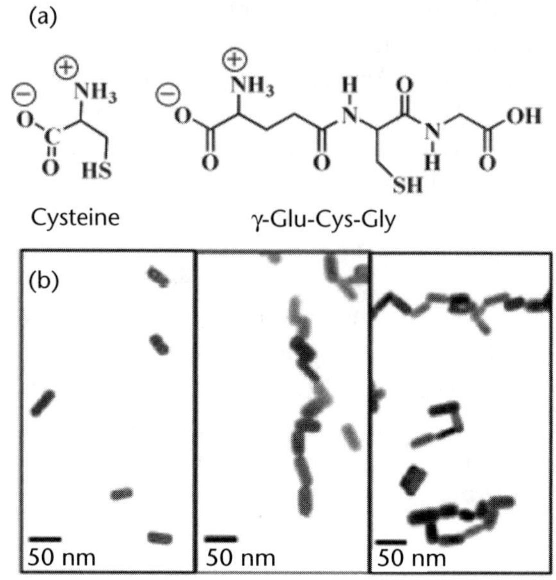

Figure 9.9 Selective detection of cysteine and glutathione by end-to-end aggregation of GNRs [117]: (a) Structures of cysteine and glutathione; (b) TEM images of GNRs in the absence (left) and presence (middle and right) of cysteine. Reprinted with permission from the American Chemical Society.

colorimetric response. Antibody-antigen recognition can also be used to trigger the self-assembly of GNRs at low antigen concentrations, with detection limits as low as 60 ng/mL during a 2-min sampling cycle [187]. Inorganic ions such as Fe^{2+} can cause the aggregation of PSS-coated GNRs [292], and even alkali ions such as Na^{+} and K^{+} ions can be used to selectively induce GNR aggregation by appending thiolated crown ether derivatives onto the GNR surfaces [293]. But not all metal ions are detected by a redshift in LSPR: Hg^{2+} ions have been shown to be a selective etchant of GNRs due to the amalgamation of mercury and gold, and can reduce their aspect ratio to produce a chemoselective blueshift [294]. This detection modality is sufficiently sensitive to detect trace Hg^{2+} in tap water by simple addition to a GNR dispersion.

Chemical and biomolecular analytes can also produce sizable LSPR shifts in GNRs via receptor-mediated surface adsorption, which produces a change in local refractive index. GNRs are typically immobilized on glass substrates and separated by at least one particle length to minimize plasmon coupling effects [295]. These systems have been applied to streptavidin-biotin binding in serum [101, 296] and for antibody-antigen recognition on freely suspended GNRs [110] or on core–shell GNR–silica films [297]. The kinetics of biomolecular adsorption have also been studied by using time-resolved LSPR shifts of GNRs immobilized along the walls of a flow cell channel [298]. The sensitivity of adsorption-induced LSPR shifts can be further enhanced by the interrogation of single GNRs rather than ensemble measurements. Single-GNR scattering spectra recorded by dark-field microscopy have been monitored for LSPR shifts induced by analyte adsorption to biomolecular receptors [299].

9.5.3.2 SERS-Based Sensors

While the SERS activities of GNRs have been extensively investigated (Section 9.3.5) [166–174], at present there are only a few demonstrations for bioanalytical applications. One recent in vitro study investigated the potential of CTAB-stabilized GNRs as SERS tags for cancer diagnostics, using anti-EFGR for targeting oral carcinoma cells distributed in a population of healthy cells (Figure 9.10) [300]. CTAB provided a convenient Raman vibrational signature for identifying cancer cells. Another SERS-related effort is under development for detecting nuclear translocation events using GNRs functionalized with rationally designed peptide ligands [204]. The in vivo use of dye-functionalized gold nanoparticles as immunolabels for SERS-based imaging has recently been demonstrated [301] and will likely inspire further developments in this area using NIR-active GNRs.

9.6 Outlook

Current developments of plasmon-resonant GNRs as biological sensors and theragnostic agents place them on a fast track toward technologies with exciting potential for biomedical diagnostics and image-guided therapies. With respect to imaging, optical microscopies based on linear and multiphoton processes such as TPL can be used to investigate GNR-based theragnostics in cells and tissues with micron spatial resolution, whereas emerging in vivo imaging modalities such as OCT and PAT stand to make tremendous gains by employing GNRs as NIR-active contrast agents. Preclinical evaluation of functionalized GNRs remains an outstanding issue: While colloidal Au nanoparticles have been employed as adjuvants

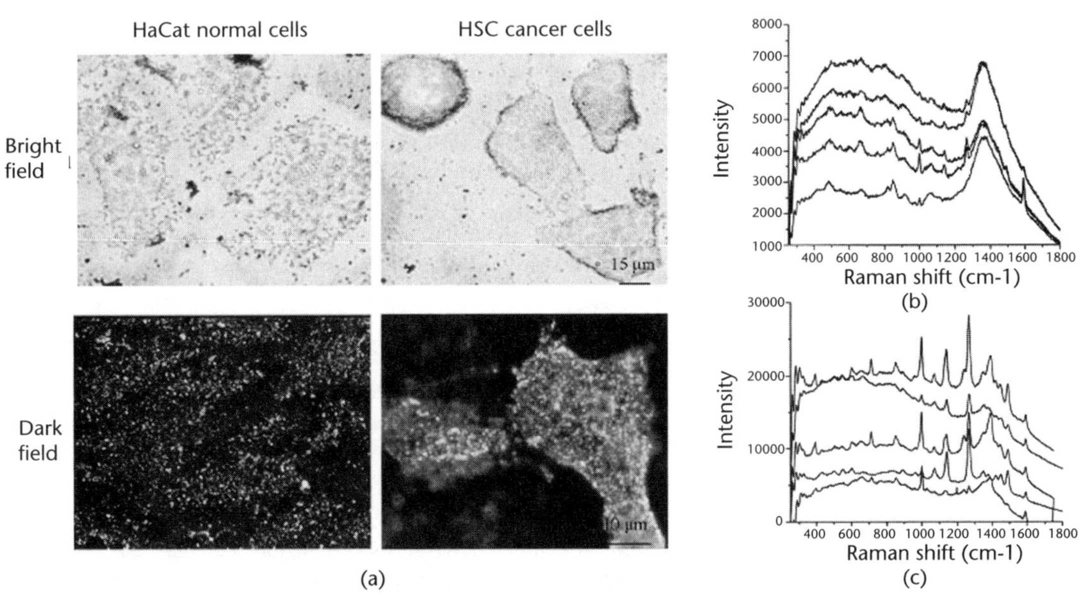

Figure 9.10 Antibody-functionalized GNRs for SERS imaging [300]: (a) Bright- and dark-field images of anti-EGFR-conjugated GNRs on normal human keratinocytes (HaCat) and malignant squamous carcinoma (HSC) cells. (b, c) SERS spectra of GNRs incubated with HaCat and HSC cells, respectively. Reprinted with permission from the American Chemical Society.

in clinical radiotherapies for many years [5–8], functionalized GNRs will be regarded as novel combination products and will require the same pharmacokinetic testing as any other chemical entity. Indeed, the photothermal activity of GNRs underscores the importance of optimizing their biodistribution, adsorption, and excretion to minimize unintended photodamage to healthy tissues and organs. Surface chemistry has a vital role in the development of safe and clinically useful nanomaterials and may prove to be the critical determinant for meeting regulatory standards. Successful advances in nanomedicine will require active collaborations between research scientists and engineers for further optimization of GNR-based technologies, clinicians and veterinarians for translational research on patient outcomes as well as medium- to long-term health effects, and government agencies for providing the necessary support and infrastructure to catalyze the transition from promising nanotechnologies to biomedical practice.

References

[1] Hayat, M. A., *Colloidal Gold: Principles, Methods, and Applications*, San Diego: Academic Press, 1989.

[2] Swanson, J. N., "Repeated Colloidal Gold Tests in Rheumatoid Arthritis," *Annals of the Rheumatic Disorders*, Vol. 8, No. 3, 1949, pp. 232–237.

[3] Glomm, W. R., "Functionalized Gold Nanoparticles for Applications in Bionanotechnology," *Journal of Dispersion Science and Technology*, Vol. 26, No. 3, 2005, pp. 389–414.

[4] Thaxton, C. S., Georganopoulou, D. G., and Mirkin, C. A., "Gold Nanoparticle Probes for the Detection of Nucleic Acid Targets," *Clinica Chimica Acta*, Vol. 363, No. 1–2, 2006, pp. 120–126.

[5] Root, S. W., et al., "The Distribution and Radiation Effects of Intravenously Administered Colloidal Au^{198} in Man," *Cancer*, Vol. 7, No. 5, 1954, pp. 856–866.

[6] Moses, C., Kent, E., and Boatman, J. B., "Experimental and Clinical Studies with Radioactive Colloidal Gold in the Therapy of Serous Effusions Arising from Cancer," *Cancer*, Vol. 8, No. 2, 1955, pp. 417–423.

[7] Seal, S. H., et al., "The Treatment of Malignant Effusions with Radioactive Colloidal Gold (Au-198) - Review of 66 Cases," *American Journal of Obstetrics and Gynecology*, Vol. 75, No. 5, 1958, pp. 1027–1033.

[8] Rubin, P., and Levitt, S. H., "The Response of Disseminated Reticulum Cell Sarcoma to the Intravenous Injection of Colloidal Radioactive Gold," *Journal of Nuclear Medicine*, Vol. 5, No. 8, 1964, pp. 581–594.

[9] Durkes, T. E., "Gold Bead Implants," *Problems in Veterinary Medicine*, Vol. 4, No. 1, 1992, pp. 207–211.

[10] Jæger, G. T., et al., "Two Years Follow-up Study of the Pain-Relieving Effect of Gold Bead Implantation in Dogs with Hip-Joint Arthritis," *Acta Veterinaria Scandinavica*, Vol. 49, No. 1, 2007, pp. 9–14.

[11] Tsai, C. Y., et al., "Amelioration of Collagen-Induced Arthritis in Rats by Nanogold," *Arthritis and Rheumatism*, Vol. 56, No. 2, 2007, pp. 544–554.

[12] Xia, Y., and Halas, N. J., "Shape-Controlled Synthesis and Surface Plasmonic Properties of Metallic Nanostructures," *MRS Bulletin*, Vol. 30, 2005, pp. 338–343.

[13] Weissleder, R., "A Clearer Vision for in Vivo Imaging," *Nature Biotechnology*, Vol. 19, No. 4, 2001, pp. 316–317.

[14] Sönnichsen, C., et al., "Drastic Reduction of Plasmon Damping in Gold Nanorods," *Physical Review Letters*, Vol. 88, No. 7, 2002, 077402.

[15] Ueno, K., et al., "Spectrally-Resolved Atomic-Scale Length Variations of Gold Nanorods," *Journal of the American Chemical Society*, Vol. 128, No. 44, 2006, pp. 14226–14227.

[16] Muhlschlegel, P., et al., "Resonant Optical Antennas," *Science*, Vol. 308, No. 5728, 2005, pp. 1607–1609.

[17] Xu, Q., et al., "Surface Plasmon Resonances of Free-Standing Gold Nanowires Fabricated by Nanoskiving," *Angewandte Chemie International Edition*, Vol. 45, No. 22, 2006, pp. 3631–3635.

[18] Foss, C. A., et al., "Template-Synthesized Nanoscopic Gold Particles: Optical Spectra and the Effects of Particle Size and Shape," *Journal of Physical Chemistry*, Vol. 98, No. 11, 1994, pp. 2963–2971.

[19] van der Zande, B. M. I., et al., "Aqueous Gold Sols of Rod-Shaped Particles," *Journal of Physical Chemistry B*, Vol. 101, No. 6, 1997, pp. 852–854.

[20] van der Zande, B. M. I., et al., "Colloidal Dispersions of Gold Rods: Synthesis and Optical Properties," *Langmuir*, Vol. 16, No. 2, 2000, pp. 451–458.

[21] Sander, M. S., and Tan, L. S., "Nanoparticle Arrays on Surfaces Fabricated Using Anodic Alumina Films as Templates," *Advanced Functional Materials*, Vol. 13, No. 5, 2003, pp. 393–397.

[22] Losic, D., et al., "Fabrication of Gold Nanorod Arrays by Templating from Porous Alumina," *Nanotechnology*, Vol. 16, No. 10, 2005, pp. 2275–2281.

[23] Moon, J. M., and Wei, A., "Uniform Gold Nanorod Arrays from Polyethylenimine-Coated Alumina Templates," *Journal of Physical Chemistry B*, Vol. 109, No. 49, 2005, pp. 23336–23341.

[24] Wolfrum, B. M., Yulia, et al., "Fabrication of Large-Scale Patterned Gold-Nanopillar Arrays on a Silicon Substrate Using Imprinted Porous Alumina Templates," *Small*, Vol. 2, No. 11, 2006, pp. 1256–1260.

[25] Cepak, V. M., and Martin, C. R., "Preparation and Stability of Template-Synthesized Metal Nanorod Sols in Organic Solvents," *Journal of Physical Chemistry B*, Vol. 102, No., 1998, pp. 9985–9990.

[26] Yu, Y. Y., et al., "Gold Nanorods: Electrochemical Synthesis and Optical Properties," *Journal of Physical Chemistry B*, Vol. 101, No. 34, 1997, pp. 6661–6664.

[27] Chang, S. S., et al., "The Shape Transition of Gold Nanorods," *Langmuir*, Vol. 15, No. 3, 1999, pp. 701–709.

[28] Yao, H., et al., "High Aspect Ratio Gold Nanorods Grown Normal to High-Energy Surfaces," *Chemistry Letters*, Vol. 31, No. 4, 2002, pp. 458–459.

[29] Huang, C.-J., et al., "Synthesis of the Gold Nanodumbbells by Electrochemical Method," *Journal of Colloid and Interface Science*, Vol. 303, No., 2006, pp. 430–436.

[30] Esumi, K., Matsuhisa, K., and Torigoe, K., "Preparation of Rodlike Gold Particles by UV Irradiation Using Cationic Micelles as a Template," *Langmuir*, Vol. 11, No., 1995, pp. 3285–3287.

[31] Kameo, A., et al., "Fiber-Like Gold Particles Prepared in Cationic Micelles by UV Irradiation: Effect of Alkyl Chain Length of Cationic Surfactant on Particle Size," *Journal of Colloid and Interface Science*, Vol. 241, No., 2001, pp. 289–292.

[32] Kim, F., Song, J. H., and Yang, P., "Photochemical Synthesis of Gold Nanorods," *Journal of the American Chemical Society*, Vol. 124, No. 48, 2002, pp. 14316–14317.

[33] Niidome, Y., et al., "Rapid Synthesis of Gold Nanorods by the Combination of Chemical Reduction and Photoirradiation Processes; Morphological Changes Depending on the Growing Processes," *Chemical Communications*, No. 18, 2003, pp. 2376–2377.

[34] Miranda, O. R., and Ahmadi, T. S., "Effects of Intensity and Energy of CW UV Light on the Growth of Gold Nanorods," *Journal of Physical Chemistry B*, Vol. 109, No. 33, 2005, pp. 15724–15734.

[35] Niidome, Y., et al., "Effects of Ammonium Salts and Anionic Amphiphiles on the Photochemical Formation of Gold Nanorods," *Colloids and Surface A*, Vol. 257–258, 2005, pp. 161–164.

[36] Miranda, O. R., Dollahon, N. R., and Ahmadi, T. S., "Critical Concentrations and Role of Ascorbic Acid (Vitamin C) in the Crystallization of Gold Nanorods within Hexadecyltrimethyl Ammonium Bromide (CTAB)/Tetraoctyl Ammonium Bromide (TOAB) Micelles," *Crystal Growth and Design*, Vol. 6, No. 12, 2006, pp. 2747–2753.

[37] Nishioka, K., Niidome, Y., and Yamada, S., "Photochemical Reactions of Ketones to Synthesize Gold Nanorods," *Langmuir*, Vol. 23, No. 20, 2007, pp. 10353–10356.

[38] Zhu, Y.-J., and Hu, X.-L., "Microwave-Polyol Preparation of Single-Crystalline Gold Nanorods and Nanowires," *Chemistry Letters*, Vol. 32, No. 12, 2003, pp. 1140–1141.

[39] Liu, F.-K., et al., "Microwave Rapid Heating for the Synthesis of Gold Nanorods," *Materials Letters*, Vol. 58, No. 3–4, 2004, pp. 373–377.

[40] Tsuji, M., et al., "Synthesis of Gold Nanorods and Nanowires by a Microwave-Polyol Method," *Materials Letters*, Vol. 58, No. 17–18, 2004, pp. 2326–2330.

[41] Kim, Y.-J., Cho, G., and Song, J. H., "Ag^+ Concentration Effect on the Shape of Au Nanomaterials under Proton Beam Irradiation," *Nuclear Instruments and Methods in Physics Research Section B*, Vol. 254, No. 1, 2007, pp. 73–77.

[42] Jana, N. R., Gearheart, L., and Murphy, C. J., "Seed-Mediated Growth Approach for Shape-Controlled Synthesis of Spheroidal and Rod-Like Gold Nanoparticles Using a Surfactant Template," *Advanced Materials*, Vol. 13, No. 18, 2001, pp. 1389–1393.

[43] Jana, N. R., Gearheart, L., and Murphy, C. J., "Wet Chemical Synthesis of High Aspect Ratio Cylindrical Gold Nanorods," *Journal of Physical Chemistry B*, Vol. 105, No. 19, 2001, pp. 4065–4067.

[44] Murphy, C. J., et al., "Surfactant-Directed Synthesis and Optical Properties of One-Dimensional Plasmonic Metallic Nanostructures," *MRS Bulletin*, Vol. 30, No. 5, 2005, pp. 349–355.

[45] Murphy, C. J., et al., "Anisotropic Metal Nanoparticles: Synthesis, Assembly, and Optical Applications," *Journal of Physical Chemistry B*, Vol. 109, No. 29, 2005, pp. 13857–13870.

[46] Murphy, C. J., et al., "One-Dimensional Colloidal Gold and Silver Nanostructures," *Inorg. Chem.*, Vol. 45, No. 19, 2006, pp. 7544–7554.

[47] Murphy, C. J., and Jana, N. R., "Controlling the Aspect Ratio of Inorganic Nanorods and Nanowires," *Advanced Materials*, Vol. 14, No. 1, 2002, pp. 80–82.

[48] Nikoobakht, B., and El-Sayed, M. A., "Preparation and Growth Mechanism of Gold Nanorods (NRs) Using Seed-Mediated Growth Method," *Chemistry of Materials*, Vol. 15, No. 10, 2003, pp. 1957–1962.

[49] Orendorff, C. J., and Murphy, C. J., "Quantitation of Metal Content in the Silver-Assisted Growth of Gold Nanorods," *Journal of Physical Chemistry B*, Vol. 110, No. 9, 2006, pp. 3990–3994.

[50] Sau, T. K., and Murphy, C. J., "Seeded High Yield Synthesis of Short Au Nanorods in Aqueous Solution," *Langmuir*, Vol. 20, No. 15, 2004, pp. 6414–6420.

[51] Liu, M., and Guyot-Sionnest, P., "Mechanism of Silver(I)-Assisted Growth of Gold Nanorods and Bipyramids," *Journal of Physical Chemistry B*, Vol. 109, No. 47, 2005, pp. 22192–22200.

[52] Zweifel, D. A., and Wei, A., "Sulfide-Arrested Growth of Gold Nanorods," *Chemistry of Materials*, Vol. 17, No. 16, 2005, pp. 4256–4261.

[53] Jana, N. R., Gearheart, L., and Murphy, C. J., "Wet Chemical Synthesis of Silver Nanorods and Nanowires of Controllable Aspect Ratio," *Chemical Communications*, No. 7, 2001, pp. 617–618.

[54] Busbee, B. D., Obare, S. O., and Murphy, C. J., "An Improved Synthesis of High-Aspect-Ratio Gold Nanorods," *Advanced Materials*, Vol. 15, No. 5, 2003, pp. 414–416.

[55] Gao, J., Bender, C. M., and Murphy, C. J., "Dependence of the Gold Nanorod Aspect Ratio on the Nature of the Directing Surfactant in Aqueous Solution," *Langmuir*, Vol. 19, No. 21, 2003, pp. 9065–9070.

[56] Gole, A., and Murphy, C. J., "Seed-Mediated Synthesis of Gold Nanorods: Role of the Size and Nature of the Seed," *Chemistry of Materials*, Vol. 16, No. 19, 2004, pp. 3633–3640.

[57] Chen, H. M., et al., "Controlling the Length and Shape of Gold Nanorods," *Journal of Physical Chemistry B*, Vol. 109, No. 42, 2005, pp. 19553–19555.

[58] Chen, H. M., et al., "Controlling Length of Gold Nanowires with Large-Scale: X-Ray Absorption Spectroscopy Approaches to the Growth Process," *Journal of Physical Chemistry C*, Vol. 111, No. 50, 2007, pp. 18550–18557.

[59] Wu, H. Y., et al., "Seed-Mediated Synthesis of High Aspect Ratio Gold Nanorods with Nitric Acid," *Chemistry of Materials*, Vol. 17, No. 25, 2005, pp. 6447–6451.

[60] Wu, H. Y., Huang, W. L., and Huang, M. H., "Direct High-Yield Synthesis of High Aspect Ratio Gold Nanorods," *Crystal Growth and Design*, Vol. 7, No. 4, 2007, pp. 831–835.

[61] Kou, X., et al., "Growth of Gold Nanorods and Bipyramids Using Ctcab Surfactant," *Journal of Physical Chemistry B*, Vol. 110, No. 33, 2006, pp. 16377–16383.

[62] Kou, X., et al., "Growth of Gold Bipyramids with Improved Yield and Their Curvature-Directed Oxidation," *Small*, Vol. 3, No. 12, 2007, pp. 2103–2113.

[63] Kou, X., et al., "One-Step Synthesis of Large-Aspect-Ratio Single-Crystalline Gold Nanorods by Using CTPAB and CTBAB Surfactants," *Chemistry - A European Journal*, Vol. 13, No. 10, 2007, pp. 2929–2936.

[64] Lqbal, M., Chung, Y.-I., and Tae, G., "An Enhanced Synthesis of Gold Nanorods by the Addition of Pluronic (F-127) Via a Seed Mediated Growth Process," *Journal of Materials Chemistry*, Vol. 17, No. 4, 2007, pp. 335–342.

[65] Johnson, C. J., et al., "Growth and Form of Gold Nanorods Prepared by Seed-Mediated, Surfactant-Directed Synthesis," *Journal of Materials Chemistry*, Vol. 12, No. 6, 2002, pp. 1765–1770.

[66] Pérez-Juste, J., et al., "Electric-Field-Directed Growth of Gold Nanorods in Aqueous Surfactant Solutions," *Advanced Functional Materials*, Vol. 14, No. 6, 2004, pp. 571–579.

[67] Sau, T. K., and Murphy, C. J., "Room Temperature, High-Yield Synthesis of Multiple Shapes of Gold Nanoparticles in Aqueous Solution," *Journal of the American Chemical Society*, Vol. 126, No. 28, 2004, pp. 8648–8649.

[68] Gou, L., and Murphy, C. J., "Fine-Tuning the Shape of Gold Nanorods," *Chemistry of Materials*, Vol. 17, No. 14, 2005, pp. 3668–3672.

[69] Jana, N. R., "Gram-Scale Synthesis of Soluble, near-Monodisperse Gold Nanorods and Other Anisotropic Nanoparticles," *Small*, Vol. 1, No. 8–9, 2005, pp. 875–882.

[70] Zijlstra, P., et al., "High-Temperature Seedless Synthesis of Gold Nanorods," *Journal of Physical Chemistry B*, Vol. 110, No. 39, 2006, pp. 19315–19318.

[71] Millstone, J. E., et al., "Observation of a Quadrupole Plasmon Mode for a Colloidal Solution of Gold Nanoprisms," *Journal of the American Chemical Society*, Vol. 127, No. 15, 2005, pp. 5312–5313.

[72] Kreibig, U., and Vollmer, M., *Optical Properties of Metal Clusters*, New York: Springer, 1995.

[73] Link, S., and El-Sayed, M. A., "Spectral Properties and Relaxation Dynamics of Surface Plasmon Electronic Oscillations in Gold and Silver Nanodots and Nanorods," *Journal of Physical Chemistry B*, Vol. 103, No. 40, 1999, pp. 8410–8426.

[74] Link, S., and El-Sayed, M. A., "Shape and Size Dependence of Radiative, Non-Radiative and Photothermal Properties of Gold Nanocrystals," *International Reviews in Physical Chemistry*, Vol. 19, No. 3, 2000, pp. 409–453.

[75] Kelly, K. L., et al., "The Optical Properties of Metal Nanoparticles: The Influence of Size, Shape, and Dielectric Environment," *Journal of Physical Chemistry B*, Vol. 107, No. 3, 2003, pp. 668–677.

[76] Link, S., and El-Sayed, M. A., "Optical Properties and Ultrafast Dynamics of Metallic Nanocrystals," *Annual Review of Physical Chemistry*, Vol. 54, No. 1, 2003, pp. 331–366.

[77] Liz-Marzán, L. M., and Mulvaney, P., "The Assembly of Coated Nanocrystals," *Journal of Physical Chemistry B*, Vol. 107, No. 30, 2003, pp. 7312–7326.

[78] Sosa, I. O., Noguez, C., and Barrera, R. G., "Optical Properties of Metal Nanoparticles with Arbitrary Shapes," *Journal of Physical Chemistry B*, Vol. 107, No. 26, 2003, pp. 6269–6275.

[79] Daniel, M. C., and Astruc, D., "Gold Nanoparticles: Assembly, Supramolecular Chemistry, Quantum-Size-Related Properties, and Applications toward Biology, Catalysis, and Nanotechnology," *Chemical Reviews*, Vol. 104, No. 1, 2004, pp. 293–346.

[80] Wei, A., In *Nanoparticles: Scaffolds and Building Blocks*, pp. 173–200, V. M. Rotello (ed.), New York: Kluwer Academic, 2004.

[81] Eustis, S., and El-Sayed, M. A., "Why Gold Nanoparticles Are More Precious Than Pretty Gold: Noble Metal Surface Plasmon Resonance and Its Enhancement of the Radiative and Nonradiative Properties of Nanocrystals of Different Shapes," *Chemical Society Reviews*, Vol. 35, No. 3, 2006, pp. 209–217.

[82] Liz-Marzán, L. M., "Tailoring Surface Plasmons through the Morphology and Assembly of Metal Nanoparticles," *Langmuir*, Vol. 22, No. 1, 2006, pp. 32–41.

[83] Moores, A., and Goettmann, F., "The Plasmon Band in Noble Metal Nanoparticles: An Introduction to Theory and Applications," *New Journal of Chemistry*, Vol. 30, No. 8, 2006, pp. 1121–1132.

[84] Murray, W. A., and Barnes, W. L., "Plasmonic Materials," *Advanced Materials*, Vol. 19, No. 22, 2007, pp. 3771–3782.

[85] Noguez, C., "Surface Plasmons on Metal Nanoparticles: The Influence of Shape and Physical Environment," *Journal of Physical Chemistry C*, Vol. 111, No. 10, 2007, pp. 3806–3819.

[86] Nehl, C. L., and Hafner, J. H., "Shape-Dependent Plasmon Resonances of Gold Nanoparticles," *Journal of Materials Chemistry*, Vol. 18, No. 21, 2008, pp. 2415–2419.

[87] Mie, G., "Beiträge Zur Optik Trüber Medien, Speziell Kolloidaler Metallösungen," *Annals of Physics*, Vol. 25, No. 3, 1908, pp. 377–445.

[88] Gans, R., " ber Die Form Ultramikroskopischer Goldteilchen," *Annals of Physics*, Vol. 37, No. 5, 1912, pp. 881–900.

[89] Link, S., Mohamed, M. B., and El-Sayed, M. A., "Simulation of the Optical Absorption Spectra of Gold Nanorods as a Function of Their Aspect Ratio and the Effect of the Medium Dielectric Constant," *Journal of Physical Chemistry B*, Vol. 103, No. 16, 1999, pp. 3073–3077.

[90] Yan, B., Yang, Y., and Wang, Y., "Comment On "Simulation of the Optical Absorption Spectra of Gold Nanorods as a Function of Their Aspect Ratio and the Effect of the Medium Dielectric Constant"," *Journal of Physical Chemistry B*, Vol. 107, No. 34, 2003, pp. 9159–9159.

[91] Link, S., and El-Sayed, M. A., "Simulation of the Optical Absorption Spectra of Gold Nanorods as a Function of Their Aspect Ratio and the Effect of the Medium Dielectric Constant," *Journal of Physical Chemistry B*, Vol. 109, No. 20, 2005, pp. 10531–10532.

[92] Sprunken, D. P., et al., "Influence of the Local Environment on Determining Aspect-Ratio Distributions of Gold Nanorods in Solution Using Gans Theory," *Journal of Physical Chemistry C*, Vol. 111, No. 39, 2007, pp. 14299–14306.

[93] Brioude, A., Jiang, X. C., and Pileni, M. P., "Optical Properties of Gold Nanorods: DDA Simulations Supported by Experiments," *Journal of Physical Chemistry B*, Vol. 109, No. 27, 2005, pp. 13138–13142.

[94] Kooij, E. S., and Poelsema, B., "Shape and Size Effects in the Optical Properties of Metallic Nanorods," *Physical Chemistry Chemical Physics*, Vol. 8, No. 28, 2006, pp. 3349–3357.

[95] Prescott, S. W., and Mulvaney, P., "Gold Nanorod Extinction Spectra," *Journal of Applied Physics*, Vol. 99, No. 12, 2006, 123504.

[96] Melikyan, A., and Minassian, H., "Calculation of Longitudinal Surface Plasmon Frequencies in Noble Metal Nanorods," *Chemical Physics Letters*, Vol. 452, No. 1–3, 2008, pp. 139–143.

[97] Ni, W., et al., "Tailoring Longitudinal Surface Plasmon Wavelengths, Scattering and Absorption Cross Sections of Gold Nanorods," *ACS Nano*, Vol. 2, No. 4, 2008, pp. 677–686.

[98] Xu, X., and Cortie, M. B., "Shape Change and Color Gamut in Gold Nanorods, Dumbbells, and Dog Bones," *Advanced Functional Materials*, Vol. 16, No. 16, 2006, pp. 2170–2176.

[99] Bryant, G. W., Garcia de Abajo, F. J., and Aizpurua, J., "Mapping the Plasmon Resonances of Metallic Nanoantennas," *Nano Letters*, Vol. 8, No. 2, 2008, pp. 631–636.

[100] Yang, J., et al., "Organic Solvent Dependence of Plasma Resonance of Gold Nanorods: A Simple Relationship," *Chemical Physics Letters*, Vol. 416, No. 4–6, 2005, pp. 215–219.

[101] Chen, C.-D., et al., "Sensing Capability of the Localized Surface Plasmon Resonance of Gold Nanorods," *Biosensors and Bioelectronics*, Vol. 22, No. 6, 2007, pp. 926–932.

[102] Ueno, K., et al., "Spectral Sensitivity of Uniform Arrays of Gold Nanorods to Dielectric Environment," *Journal of Physical Chemistry C*, Vol. 111, No. 11, 2007, pp. 4180–4184.

[103] Chen, H., et al., "Shape- and Size-Dependent Refractive Index Sensitivity of Gold Nanoparticles," *Langmuir*, Vol. 24, No. 10, 2008, pp. 5233–5237.

[104] Huang, H., et al., "Preparation and Optical Properties of Worm-Like Gold Nanorods," *Journal of Colloid and Interface Science*, Vol. 322, No. 1, 2008, pp. 136–142.

[105] Orendorff, C. J., Sau, T. K., and Murphy, C. J., "Shape-Dependent Plasmon-Resonant Gold Nanoparticles," *Small*, Vol. 2, No. 5, 2006, pp. 636–639.

[106] Pérez-Juste, J., et al., "Optical Control and Patterning of Gold-Nanorod-Poly(Vinyl Alcohol) Nanocomposite Films," *Advanced Functional Materials*, Vol. 15, No. 7, 2005, pp. 1065–1071.

[107] Hu, M., et al., "Gold Nanostructures: Engineering Their Plasmonic Properties for Biomedical Applications," *Chemical Society Reviews*, Vol. 35, No. 11, 2006, pp. 1084–1094.

[108] Murphy, C. J., and Orendorff, C. J., "Alignment of Gold Nanorods in Polymer Composites and on Polymer Surfaces," *Advanced Materials*, Vol. 17, No. 18, 2005, pp. 2173–2177.

[109] Liu, M., and Guyot-Sionnest, P., "Preparation and Optical Properties of Silver Chalcogenide Coated Gold Nanorods," *Journal of Materials Chemistry*, Vol. 16, No. 40, 2006, pp. 3942–3945.

[110] Yu, C., and Irudayaraj, J., "Multiplex Biosensor Using Gold Nanorods," *Analytical Chemistry*, Vol. 79, No. 2, 2007, pp. 572–579.

[111] Hansen, M. N., Chang, L.-S., and Wei, A., "Resorcinarene-Encapsulated Gold Nanorods: Solvatochromatism and Magnetic Nanoshell Formation," *Supramolecular Chemistry*, Vol. 20, No. 1, 2008, pp. 35–40.

[112] McFarland, A. D., and Van Duyne, R. P., "Single Silver Nanoparticles as Real-Time Optical Sensors with Zeptomole Sensitivity," *Nano Letters*, Vol. 3, No. 8, 2003, pp. 1057–1062.

[113] Yu, C., Nakshatri, H., and Irudayaraj, J., "Identity Profiling of Cell Surface Markers by Multiplex Gold Nanorod Probes," *Nano Letters*, Vol. 7, No. 8, 2007, pp. 2300–2306.

[114] Pecharromán, C., et al., "Redshift of Surface Plasmon Modes of Small Gold Rods Due to Their Atomic Roughness and End-Cap Geometry," *Physical Review B*, Vol. 77, No. 3, 2008, 035418.

[115] Mulvaney, P., et al., "Drastic Surface Plasmon Mode Shifts in Gold Nanorods Due to Electron Charging," *Plasmonics*, Vol. 1, No. 1, 2006, pp. 61–66.

[116] Juluri, B. K., et al., "Effects of Geometry and Composition on Charge-Induced Plasmonic Shifts in Gold Nanoparticles," *Journal of Physical Chemistry C*, Vol. 112, No. 19, 2008, pp. 7309–7317.

[117] Sudeep, P. K., Joseph, S. T. S., and Thomas, K. G., "Selective Detection of Cysteine and Glutathione Using Gold Nanorods," *Journal of the American Chemical Society*, Vol. 127, No. 18, 2005, pp. 6516–6517.

[118] Jain, P. K., Eustis, S., and El-Sayed, M. A., "Plasmon Coupling in Nanorod Assemblies: Optical Absorption, Discrete Dipole Approximation Simulation, and Exciton-Coupling Model," *Journal of Physical Chemistry B*, Vol. 110, No. 37, 2006, pp. 18243–18253.

[119] Vial, S., et al., "Plasmon Coupling in Layer-by-Layer Assembled Gold Nanorod Films," *Langmuir*, Vol. 23, No. 8, 2007, pp. 4606–4611.

[120] Payne, E. K., et al., "Multipole Plasmon Resonances in Gold Nanorods," *Journal of Physical Chemistry B*, Vol. 110, No. 5, 2006, pp. 2150–2154.

[121] Encina, E. R., and Coronado, E. A., "Resonance Conditions for Multipole Plasmon Excitations in Noble Metal Nanorods," *Journal of Physical Chemistry C*, Vol. 111, No. 45, 2007, pp. 16796–16801.

[122] Khlebtsov, B. N., and Khlebtsov, N. G., "Multipole Plasmons in Metal Nanorods: Scaling Properties and Dependence on Particle Size, Shape, Orientation, and Dielectric Environment," *Journal of Physical Chemistry C*, Vol. 111, No. 31, 2007, pp. 11516–11527.

[123] Sönnichsen, C., et al., "Drastic Reduction of Plasmon Damping in Gold Nanorods," *Physical Review Letters*, Vol. 88, No. 7, 2002, pp. 077402.

[124] Le, Q., et al., "Single Gold Nanorod Detection Using Confocal Light Absorption and Scattering Spectroscopy," *IEEE Journal of Selected Topics in Quantum Electronics*, Vol. 13, No. 6, 2007, pp. 1730–1738.

[125] Chner, T., et al., "A Novel Approach to Detect and Characterize the Scattering Patterns of Single Au Nanoparticles Using Confocal Microscopy," *Journal of Microscopy*, Vol. 229, 2008, pp. 337–343.

[126] Kuwata, H., et al., "Resonant Light Scattering from Metal Nanoparticles: Practical Analysis Beyond Rayleigh Approximation," *Applied Physics Letters*, Vol. 83, No. 22, 2003, pp. 4625–4627.

[127] Lee, K. S., and El-Sayed, M. A., "Dependence of the Enhanced Optical Scattering Efficiency Relative to That of Absorption for Gold Metal Nanorods on Aspect Ratio, Size, End-Cap Shape, and Medium Refractive Index," *Journal of Physical Chemistry B*, Vol. 109, No. 43, 2005, pp. 20331–20338.

[128] Jain, P. K., et al., "Calculated Absorption and Scattering Properties of Gold Nanoparticles of Different Size, Shape, and Composition: Applications in Biological Imaging and Biomedicine," *Journal of Physical Chemistry B*, Vol. 110, No. 14, 2006, pp. 7238–7248.

[129] Zhu, J., et al., "Shape Dependent Resonance Light Scattering Properties of Gold Nanorods," *Materials Science and Engineering B*, Vol. 121, No. 3, 2005, pp. 199–203.

[130] Eremina, E., Eremin, Y., and Wriedt, T., "Analysis of the Light Scattering Properties of a Gold Nanorod on a Plane Surface Via Discrete Sources Method," *Optics Communications*, Vol. 273, No. 1, 2007, pp. 278–285.

[131] Sönnichsen, C., and Alivisatos, A. P., "Gold Nanorods as Novel Nonbleaching Plasmon-Based Orientation Sensors for Polarized Single-Particle Microscopy," *Nano Letters*, Vol. 5, No. 2, 2005, pp. 301–304.

[132] Imura, K., Nagahara, T., and Okamoto, H., "Imaging of Surface Plasmon and Ultrafast Dynamics in Gold Nanorods by Near-Field Microscopy," *Journal of Physical Chemistry B*, Vol. 108, No. 42, 2004, pp. 16344–16347.

[133] Imura, K., Nagahara, T., and Okamoto, H., "Near-Field Optical Imaging of Plasmon Modes in Gold Nanorods," *The Journal of Chemical Physics*, Vol. 122, No. 15, 2005, 154701.

[134] Imura, K., and Okamoto, H., "Reciprocity in Scanning Near-Field Optical Microscopy: Illumination and Collection Modes of Transmission Measurements," *Optics Letters*, Vol. 31, No. 10, 2006, pp. 1474–1476.

[135] Okamoto, H., and Imura, K., "Near-Field Imaging of Optical Field and Plasmon Wavefunctions in Metal Nanoparticles," *Journal of Materials Chemistry*, Vol. 16, No. 40, 2006, pp. 3920–3928.

[136] Imura, K., and Okamoto, H., "Ultrafast Photoinduced Changes of Eigenfunctions of Localized Plasmon Modes in Gold Nanorods," *Physical Review B*, Vol. 77, No. 4, 2008, 041401(R).

[137] Seferyan, H. Y., et al., "Diagnostics of Spectrally Resolved Transient Absorption: Surface Plasmon Resonance of Metal Nanoparticles," *Journal of Physical Chemistry C*, Vol. 111, No. 50, 2007, pp. 18525–18532.

[138] Vesseur, E. J. R., et al., "Direct Observation of Plasmonic Modes in Au Nanowires Using High-Resolution Cathodoluminescence Spectroscopy," *Nano Letters*, Vol. 7, No. 9, 2007, pp. 2843–2846.

[139] Douillard, L., et al., "Short Range Plasmon Resonators Probed by Photoemission Electron Microscopy," *Nano Letters*, Vol. 8, No. 3, 2008, pp. 935–940.

[140] Mooradian, A., "Photoluminescence of Metals," *Physical Review Letters*, Vol. 22, No. 5, 1969, pp. 185–187.

[141] Mohamed, M. B., et al., "The 'Lightning' Gold Nanorods: Fluorescence Enhancement of over a Million Compared to the Gold Metal," *Chemical Physics Letters*, Vol. 317, No. 6, 2000, pp. 517–523.

[142] Varnavski, O. P., et al., "Relative Enhancement of Ultrafast Emission in Gold Nanorods," *Journal of Physical Chemistry B*, Vol. 107, No. 14, 2003, pp. 3101–3104.

[143] Dulkeith, E., et al., "Plasmon Emission in Photoexcited Gold Nanoparticles," *Physical Review B*, Vol. 70, No. 20, 2004, 205424.

[144] Zheng, J., Petty, J. T., and Dickson, R. M., "High Quantum Yield Blue Emission from Water-Soluble Au-8 Nanodots," *Journal of the American Chemical Society*, Vol. 125, No. 26, 2003, pp. 7780–7781.

[145] Zheng, J., Zhang, C., and Dickson, R. M., "Highly Fluorescent, Water-Soluble, Size-Tunable Gold Quantum Dots," *Physical Review Letters*, Vol. 93, No. 7, 2004, 077402.

[146] Eustis, S., and El-Sayed, M., "Aspect Ratio Dependence of the Enhanced Fluorescence Intensity of Gold Nanorods: Experimental and Simulation Study," *Journal of Physical Chemistry B*, Vol. 109, No. 34, 2005, pp. 16350–16356.

[147] Li, C.-Z., et al., "Fluorescence Properties of Gold Nanorods and Their Application for DNA Biosensing," *Chemical Communications*, No. 31, 2005, pp. 3924–3926.

[148] Wang, H., et al., "In Vitro and in Vivo Two-Photon Luminescence Imaging of Single Gold Nanorods," *Proceedings of the National Academy of Sciences*, Vol. 102, No. 44, 2005, pp. 15752–15756.

[149] Boyd, G. T., Yu, Z. H., and Shen, Y. R., "Photoinduced Luminescence from the Noble Metals and Its Enhancement on Roughened Surfaces," *Physical Review B*, Vol. 33, No. 12, 1986, pp. 7923–7936.

[150] Zipfel, W. R., Williams, R. M., and Webb, W. W., "Nonlinear Magic: Multiphoton Microscopy in the Biosciences," *Nature Biotechnology*, Vol. 21, No. 11, 2003, pp. 1369–1377.

[151] Albota, M. A., Xu, C., and Webb, W. W., "Two-Photon Fluorescence Excitation Cross Sections of Biomolecular Probes from 690 to 960 nm," *Applied Optics*, Vol. 37, No. 31, 1998, pp. 7352–7356.

[152] Larson, D. R., et al., "Water-Soluble Quantum Dots for Multiphoton Fluorescence Imaging in Vivo," *Science*, Vol. 300, No. 5624, 2003, pp. 1434–1436.

[153] Ramakrishna, G., et al., "Quantum-Sized Gold Clusters as Efficient Two-Photon Absorbers," *Journal of the American Chemical Society*, Vol. 130, No. 15, 2008, pp. 5032–5033.

[154] Imura, K., Nagahara, T., and Okamoto, H., "Photoluminescence from Gold Nanoplates Induced by Near-Field Two-Photon Absorption," *Applied Physics Letters*, Vol. 88, No. 2, 2006, 023104.

[155] Park, J., et al., "Two-Photon-Induced Photoluminescence Imaging of Tumors Using Near-Infrared Excited Gold Nanoshells," *Optics Express*, Vol. 16, No. 3, 2008, pp. 1590–1599.

[156] Schuck, P. J., et al., "Improving the Mismatch between Light and Nanoscale Objects with Gold Bowtie Nanoantennas," *Physical Review Letters*, Vol. 94, No. 1, 2005, pp. 017402–017404.

[157] Ueno, K., et al., "Clusters of Closely Spaced Gold Nanoparticles as a Source of Two-Photon Photoluminescence at Visible Wavelengths," *Advanced Materials*, Vol. 20, No. 1, 2008, pp. 26–30.

[158] Bouhelier, A., et al., "Surface Plasmon Characteristics of Tunable Photoluminescence in Single Gold Nanorods," *Physical Review Letters*, Vol. 95, No. 26, 2005, 267405.

[159] Imura, K., Nagahara, T., and Okamoto, H., "Plasmon Mode Imaging of Single Gold Nanorods," *Journal of the American Chemical Society*, Vol. 126, No. 40, 2004, pp. 12730–12731.

[160] Imura, K., Nagahara, T., and Okamoto, H., "Near-Field Two-Photon-Induced Photoluminescence from Single Gold Nanorods and Imaging of Plasmon Modes," *Journal of Physical Chemistry B*, Vol. 109, No. 27, 2005, pp. 13214–13220.

[161] Wang, Q. Q., et al., "Highly Efficient Avalanche Multiphoton Luminescence from Coupled Au Nanowires in the Visible Region," *Nano Letters*, Vol. 7, No. 3, 2007, pp. 723–728.

[162] Lamarre, J.-M., et al., "Anisotropic Nonlinear Optical Absorption of Gold Nanorods in a Silica Matrix," *Optics Communications*, Vol. 281, No. 2, 2008, pp. 331–340.

[163] Nappa, J., et al., "Hyper-Rayleigh Scattering of Gold Nanorods and Their Relationship with Linear Assemblies of Gold Nanospheres," *Faraday Discussions*, Vol. 125, 2004, pp. 145–156.

[164] Hubert, C., et al., "Role of Surface Plasmon in Second Harmonic Generation from Gold Nanorods," *Applied Physics Letters*, Vol. 90, No. 18, 2007, 181105.

[165] Celebrano, M., et al., "Mapping Local Field Enhancements at Nanostructured Metal Surfaces by Second-Harmonic Generation Induced in the Near Field," *Journal of Microscopy*, Vol. 229, 2008, pp. 233–239.

[166] Orendorff, C. J., et al., "Surface-Enhanced Raman Spectroscopy of Self-Assembled Monolayers: Sandwich Architecture and Nanoparticle Shape Dependence," *Analytical Chemistry*, Vol. 77, No. 10, 2005, pp. 3261–3266.

[167] Nikoobakht, B., Wang, J., and El-Sayed, M. A., "Surface-Enhanced Raman Scattering of Molecules Adsorbed on Gold Nanorods: Off-Surface Plasmon Resonance Condition," *Chemical Physics Letters*, Vol. 366, No. 1–2, 2002, pp. 17–23.

[168] Orendorff, C. J., et al., "Aspect Ratio Dependence on Surface Enhanced Raman Scattering Using Silver and Gold Nanorod Substrates," *Physical Chemistry Chemical Physics*, Vol. 8, No. 1, 2006, pp. 165–170.

[169] Nikoobakht, B., and El-Sayed, M. A., "Surface-Enhanced Raman Scattering Studies on Aggregated Gold Nanorods," *Journal of Physical Chemistry A*, Vol. 107, No. 18, 2003, pp. 3372–3378.

[170] Jana, N. R., and Pal, T., "Anisotropic Metal Nanoparticles for Use as Surface-Enhanced Raman Substrates," *Advanced Materials*, Vol. 19, No. 13, 2007, pp. 1761–1765.

[171] Hu, X., et al., "Fabrication, Characterization, and Application in SERS of Self-Assembled Polyelectrolyte-Gold Nanorod Multilayered Films," *Journal of Physical Chemistry B*, Vol. 109, No. 41, 2005, pp. 19385–19389.

[172] Yun, S., et al., "Linker-Molecule-Free Gold Nanorod Layer-by-Layer Films for Surface-Enhanced Raman Scattering," *Analytical Chemistry*, Vol. 79, No. 22, 2007, pp. 8584–8589.

[173] Wang, Y., et al., "Facile Fabrication of Large Area of Aggregated Gold Nanorods Film for Efficient Surface-Enhanced Raman Scattering," *Journal of Colloid and Interface Science*, Vol. 318, No. 1, 2008, pp. 82–87.

[174] Kawamura, G., Yang, Y., and Nogami, M., "Facile Assembling of Gold Nanorods with Large Aspect Ratio and Their Surface-Enhanced Raman Scattering Properties," *Applied Physics Letters*, Vol. 90, No. 26, 2007, 261908.

[175] Animesh, K. O., Gautam, C., and Anushree, R., "A Study on Adsorption of Acetonitrile on Gold Nanorods by Non-Resonant Raman Measurements and Density Functional Theory Calculations," *Nanotechnology*, Vol. 19, No. 9, 2008, 095706.

[176] Félidj, N., et al., "Far-Field Raman Imaging of Short-Wavelength Particle Plasmons on Gold Nanorods," *Plasmonics*, Vol. 1, No. 1, 2006, pp. 35–39.

[177] Pompa, P. P., et al., "Metal-Enhanced Fluorescence of Colloidal Nanocrystals with Nanoscale Control," *Nature Nanotechnology*, Vol. 1, No. 2, 2006, pp. 126–130.

[178] Chen, Y., Munechika, K., and Ginger, D. S., "Dependence of Fluorescence Intensity on the Spectral Overlap between Fluorophores and Plasmon Resonant Single Silver Nanoparticles," *Nano Letters*, Vol. 7, No. 3, 2007, pp. 690–696.

[179] Zhang, J., et al., "Metal-Enhanced Single-Molecule Fluorescence on Silver Particle Monomer and Dimer: Coupling Effect between Metal Particles," *Nano Letters*, Vol. 7, No. 7, 2007, pp. 2101–2107.

[180] Xie, F., Baker, M. S., and Goldys, E. M., "Enhanced Fluorescence Detection on Homogeneous Gold Colloid Self-Assembled Monolayer Substrates," *Chemistry of Materials*, Vol. 20, No. 5, 2008, pp. 1788–1797.

[181] Darbha, G. K., Ray, A., and Ray, P. C., "Gold Nanoparticle-Based Miniaturized Nanomaterial Surface Energy Transfer Probe for Rapid and Ultrasensitive Detection of Mercury in Soil, Water, and Fish," *ACS Nano*, Vol. 1, No. 3, 2007, pp. 208–214.

[182] Ni, W., et al., "Coupling between Molecular and Plasmonic Resonances in Freestanding Dye-Gold Nanorod Hybrid Nanostructures," *Journal of the American Chemical Society*, Vol. 130, No. 21, 2008, pp. 6692–6693.

[183] Lakowicz, J., et al., "Advances in Surface-Enhanced Fluorescence," *Journal of Fluorescence*, Vol. 14, No. 4, 2004, pp. 425–441.

[184] Nikoobakht, B., and El-Sayed, M. A., "Evidence for Bilayer Assembly of Cationic Surfactants on the Surface of Gold Nanorods," *Langmuir*, Vol. 17, No. 20, 2001, pp. 6368–6374.

[185] Ding, H., et al., "Gold Nanorods Coated with Multilayer Polyelectrolyte as Contrast Agents for Multimodal Imaging," *Journal of Physical Chemistry C*, Vol. 111, No. 34, 2007, pp. 12552–12557.

[186] Berr, S. S., "Solvent Isotope Effects on Alkytrimethylammonium Bromide Micelles as a Function of Alkyl Chain Length," *The Journal of Physical Chemistry*, Vol. 91, No. 18, 1987, pp. 4760–4765.

[187] Wang, C., et al., "Biorecognition-Driven Self-Assembly of Gold Nanorods: A Rapid and Sensitive Approach toward Antibody Sensing," *Chemistry of Materials*, Vol. 19, No. 24, 2007, pp. 5809–5811.

[188] Tom, R. T., et al., "Hemoprotein Bioconjugates of Gold and Silver Nanoparticles and Gold Nanorods: Structure-Function Correlations," *Langmuir*, Vol. 23, No. 3, 2007, pp. 1320–1325.

[189] Kitagawa, R., et al., "Formation of Gold Nanorod-Myoglobin Aggregates by Electrostatic Interactions and Their Photochemical Properties," *Japanese Journal of Applied Physics*, Vol. 47, No. 2, 2008, pp. 1374–1376.

[190] Spetzler, D., et al., "Microsecond Time Scale Rotation Measurements of Single F_1-ATPase Molecules," *Biochemistry*, Vol. 45, No. 10, 2006, pp. 3117–3124.

[191] Copland, J. A., et al., "Bioconjugated Gold Nanoparticles as a Molecular Based Contrast Agent: Implications for Imaging of Deep Tumors Using Optoacoustic Tomography," *Molecular Imaging and Biology*, Vol. 6, No. 5, 2004, pp. 341–349.

[192] Huang, X., et al., "Cancer Cell Imaging and Photothermal Therapy in the Near-Infrared Region by Using Gold Nanorods," *Journal of the American Chemical Society*, Vol. 128, No. 6, 2006, pp. 2115–2120.

[193] Durr, N. J., et al., "Two-Photon Luminescence Imaging of Cancer Cells Using Molecularly Targeted Gold Nanorods," *Nano Letters*, Vol. 7, No. 4, 2007, pp. 941–945.

[194] Liu, X., et al., "A One-Step Homogeneous Immunoassay for Cancer Biomarker Detection Using Gold Nanoparticle Probes Coupled with Dynamic Light Scattering," *Journal of the American Chemical Society*, Vol. 130, No. 9, 2008, pp. 2780–2782.

[195] Black, K. C., et al., "Gold Nanorods Targeted to Delta Opioid Receptor: Plasmon-Resonant Contrast and Photothermal Agents," *Molecular Imaging*, Vol. 7, No. 1, 2008, pp. 50–57.

[196] Takahashi, H., et al., "Surface Modification of Gold Nanorods Using Layer-by-Layer Technique for Cellular Uptake," *Journal of Nanoparticle Research*, Vol. 10, No. 1, 2008, pp. 221–228.

[197] Gole, A., and Murphy, C. J., "Biotin-Streptavidin-Induced Aggregation of Gold Nanorods: Tuning Rod-Rod Orientation," *Langmuir*, Vol. 21, No. 23, 2005, pp. 10756–10762.

[198] Gole, A., and Murphy, C. J., "Azide-Derivatized Gold Nanorods: Functional Materials For "Click" Chemistry," *Langmuir*, Vol. 24, No. 1, 2008, pp. 266–272.

[199] Love, J. C., et al., "Self-Assembled Monolayers of Thiolates on Metals as a Form of Nanotechnology," *Chemical Reviews*, Vol. 105, No. 4, 2005, pp. 1103–1170.

[200] Liao, H., and Hafner, J. H., "Gold Nanorod Bioconjugates," *Chemistry of Materials*, Vol. 17, No. 18, 2005, pp. 4636–4641.

[201] Dujardin, E., et al., "DNA-Driven Self-Assembly of Gold Nanorods," *Chemical Communications*, No. 14, 2001, pp. 1264–1265.

[202] Pan, B., et al., "End-to-End Self-Assembly and Colorimetric Characterization of Gold Nanorods and Nanospheres Via Oligonucleotide Hybridization," *Nanotechnology*, Vol. 16, No. 9, 2005, pp. 1776–1780.

[203] Huang, Y. F., Chang, H. T., and Tan, W., "Cancer Cell Targeting Using Multiple Aptamers Conjugated on Nanorods," *Analytical Chemistry*, Vol. 80, No. 3, 2008, pp. 567–572.

[204] Oyelere, A. K., et al., "Peptide-Conjugated Gold Nanorods for Nuclear Targeting," *Bioconjugate Chemistry*, Vol. 18, No. 5, 2007, pp. 1490–1497.

[205] Shibu Joseph, S. T., et al., "Gold Nanorods to Nanochains: Mechanistic Investigations on Their Longitudinal Assembly Using α,ω-Alkanedithiols and Interplasmon Coupling," *Journal of Physical Chemistry B*, Vol. 110, No. 1, 2006, pp. 150–157.

[206] Caswell, K. K., et al., "Preferential End-to-End Assembly of Gold Nanorods by Biotin-Streptavidin Connectors," *Journal of the American Chemical Society*, Vol. 125, No. 46, 2003, pp. 13914–13915.

[207] Zareie, M. H., Xu, X., and Cortie, M. B., "In Situ Organization of Gold Nanorods on Mixed Self-Assembled-Monolayer Substrates," *Small*, Vol. 3, No. 1, 2007, pp. 139–145.

[208] Thomas, K. G., et al., "Uniaxial Plasmon Coupling through Longitudinal Self-Assembly of Gold Nanorods," *Journal of Physical Chemistry B*, Vol. 108, No. 35, 2004, pp. 13066–13068.

[209] Varghese, N., et al., "A Calorimetric Investigation of the Assembly of Gold Nanorods to Form Necklaces," *Chemical Physics Letters*, Vol. 450, No. 4–6, 2008, pp. 340–344.

[210] Chang, J.-Y., et al., "Oriented Assembly of Au Nanorods Using Biorecognition System," *Chemical Communications*, Vol., No. 8, 2005, pp. 1092–1094.

[211] Kou, X., et al., "Glutathione- and Cysteine-Induced Transverse Overgrowth on Gold Nanorods," *Journal of the American Chemical Society*, Vol. 129, No. 20, 2007, pp. 6402–6404.

[212] Zhang, S., et al., "Nanonecklaces Assembled from Gold Rods, Spheres, and Bipyramids," *Chemical Communications*, Vol., No. 18, 2007, pp. 1816–1818.

[213] Hu, X., et al., "Well-Ordered End-to-End Linkage of Gold Nanorods," *Nanotechnology*, Vol. 16, No. 10, 2005, pp. 2164–2169.

[214] Mrksich, M., et al., "Using Microcontact Printing to Pattern the Attachment of Mammalian Cells to Self-Assembled Monolayers of Alkanethiolates on Transparent Films of Gold and Silver," *Experimental Cell Research*, Vol. 235, No. 2, 1997, pp. 305–313.

[215] Flynn, N. T., et al., "Long-Term Stability of Self-Assembled Monolayers in Biological Media," *Langmuir*, Vol. 19, No. 26, 2003, pp. 10909–10915.

[216] Schlenoff, J. B., Li, M., and Ly, H., "Stability and Self-Exchange in Alkanethiol Monolayers," *Journal of the American Chemical Society*, Vol. 117, No. 50, 1995, pp. 12528–12536.

[217] Demers, L. M., et al., "A Fluorescence-Based Method for Determining the Surface Coverage and Hybridization Efficiency of Thiol-Capped Oligonucleotides Bound to Gold Thin Films and Nanoparticles," *Analytical Chemistry*, Vol. 72, No. 22, 2000, pp. 5535–5541.

[218] Castelino, K., Kannan, B., and Majumdar, A., "Characterization of Grafting Density and Binding Efficiency of DNA and Proteins on Gold Surfaces," *Langmuir*, Vol. 21, No. 5, 2005, pp. 1956–1961.

[219] Hong, R., et al., "Glutathione-Mediated Delivery and Release Using Monolayer Protected Nanoparticle Carriers," *Journal of the American Chemical Society*, Vol. 128, No. 4, 2006, pp. 1078–1079.

[220] Schoenfisch, M. H., and Pemberton, J. E., "Air Stability of Alkanethiol Self-Assembled Monolayers on Silver and Gold Surfaces," *Journal of the American Chemical Society*, Vol. 120, No. 18, 1998, pp. 4502–4513.

[221] Dasog, M., and Scott, R. W. J., "Understanding the Oxidative Stability of Gold Monolayer-Protected Clusters in the Presence of Halide Ions under Ambient Conditions," *Langmuir*, Vol. 23, No. 6, 2007, pp. 3381–3387.

[222] Zhao, Y., et al., "Dithiocarbamate Assembly on Gold," *Journal of the American Chemical Society*, Vol. 127, No. 20, 2005, pp. 7328–7329.

[223] Huff, T. B., et al., "Controlling the Cellular Uptake of Gold Nanorods," *Langmuir*, Vol. 23, No. 4, 2007, pp. 1596–1599.

[224] Huff, T. B., et al., "Hyperthermic Effects of Gold Nanorods on Tumor Cells," *Nanomedicine*, Vol. 2, No. 1, 2007, pp. 125–132.

[225] Sharma, J., et al., "A Facile in Situ Generation of Dithiocarbamate Ligands for Stable Gold Nanoparticle-Oligonucleotide Conjugates," *Chemical Communications*, Vol., No. 18, 2008, pp. 2140–2142.

[226] Zhu, H., et al., "Assembly of Dithiocarbamate-Anchored Monolayers on Gold Surfaces in Aqueous Solutions," *Langmuir*, Vol. 24, 2008.

[227] Boev, V. I., et al., "Flexible Ureasil Hybrids with Tailored Optical Properties through Doping with Metal Nanoparticles," *Langmuir*, Vol. 20, No. 23, 2004, pp. 10268–10272.

[228] Pérez-Juste, J., Correa-Duarte, M. A., and Liz-Marzán, L. M., "Silica Gels with Tailored, Gold Nanorod-Driven Optical Functionalities," *Applied Surface Science*, Vol. 226, No. 1–3, 2004, pp. 137–143.

[229] Pastoriza-Santos, I., Perez-Juste, J., and Liz-Marzán, L. M., "Silica-Coating and Hydrophobation of CTAB-Stabilized Gold Nanorods," *Chemistry of Materials*, Vol. 18, No. 10, 2006, pp. 2465–2467.

[230] Takahashi, H., et al., "Modification of Gold Nanorods Using Phosphatidylcholine to Reduce Cytotoxicity," *Langmuir*, Vol. 22, No. 1, 2006, pp. 2–5.

[231] Wang, C., Ma, Z., and Su, Z., "Synthesis and Self-Assembly of Silica-Coated Anisotropic Gold Nanoparticle Films," *Nanotechnology*, Vol. 17, No. 8, 2006, pp. 1819–1824.

[232] Gorelikov, I., and Matsuura, N., "Single-Step Coating of Mesoporous Silica on Cetyltrimethyl Ammonium Bromide-Capped Nanoparticles," *Nano Letters*, Vol. 8, No. 1, 2008, pp. 369–373.

[233] Lewinski, N., Colvin, V., and Drezek, R., "Cytotoxicity of Nanoparticles," *Small*, Vol. 4, No. 1, 2008, pp. 26–49.

[234] Cortesi, R., et al., "Effect of Cationic Liposome Composition on *in Vitro* Cytotoxicity and Protective Effect on Carried DNA," *International Journal of Pharmaceutics*, Vol. 139, No. 1–2, 1996, pp. 69–78.

[235] Bragadin, M., and Dell'Antone, P., "Mitochondrial Bioenergetics as Affected by Cationic Detergents," *Archives of Environmental Contamination and Toxicology*, Vol. 30, No. 2, 1996, pp. 280–284.

[236] Connor, E. E., et al., "Gold Nanoparticles Are Taken up by Human Cells but Do Not Cause Acute Cytotoxicity," *Small*, Vol. 1, No. 3, 2005, pp. 325–327.

[237] Niidome, T., et al., "PEG-Modified Gold Nanorods with a Stealth Character for in Vivo Applications," *Journal of Controlled Release*, Vol. 114, No. 3, 2006, pp. 343–347.

[238] Hauck, T. S., Ghazani, A. A., and Chan, W. C. W., "Assessing the Effect of Surface Chemistry on Gold Nanorod Uptake, Toxicity, and Gene Expression in Mammalian Cells," *Small*, Vol. 4, No. 1, 2008, pp. 153–159.

[239] Gole, A., and Murphy, C. J., "Polyelectrolyte-Coated Gold Nanorods: Synthesis, Characterization and Immobilization," *Chemistry of Materials*, Vol. 17, No. 6, 2005, pp. 1325–1330.

[240] Niidome, Y., et al., "Surface Modification of Gold Nanorods with Synthetic Cationic Lipids," *Chemical Communications*, No. 36, 2007, pp. 3777–3779.

[241] Pierrat, S., et al., "Self-Assembly of Small Gold Colloids with Functionalized Gold Nanorods," *Nano Letters*, Vol. 7, No. 2, 2007, pp. 259–263.

[242] Stone, J. W., et al., "Using Gold Nanorods to Probe Cell-Induced Collagen Deformation," *Nano Letters*, Vol. 7, No. 1, 2007, pp. 116–119.

[243] Orendorff, C. J., et al., "Light Scattering from Gold Nanorods: Tracking Material Deformation," *Nanotechnology*, Vol. 16, No. 11, 2005, pp. 2601–2605.

[244] Bharali, D. J., et al., "Folate-Receptor-Mediated Delivery of InP Quantum Dots for Bioimaging Using Confocal and Two-Photon Microscopy," *Journal of the American Chemical Society*, Vol. 127, No. 32, 2005, pp. 11364–11371.

[245] Fu, A., et al., "Semiconductor Quantum Rods as Single Molecule Fluorescent Biological Labels," *Nano Letters*, Vol. 7, No. 1, 2007, pp. 179–182.

[246] Yong, K. T., et al., "Quantum Rod Bioconjugates as Targeted Probes for Confocal and Two-Photon Fluorescence Imaging of Cancer Cells," *Nano Letters*, Vol. 7, No. 3, 2007, pp. 761–765.

[247] Yong, K.-T., et al., "Multiplex Imaging of Pancreatic Cancer Cells by Using Functionalized Quantum Rods," *Advanced Materials*, Vol. 20, No. 8, 2008, pp. 1412–1417.

[248] Cao, L., et al., "Carbon Dots for Multiphoton Bioimaging," *Journal of the American Chemical Society*, Vol. 129, No. 37, 2007, pp. 11318–11319.

[249] Park, J., et al., "Two-Photon-Induced Photoluminescence Imaging of Tumors Using Near-Infrared Excited Gold Nanoshells," *Optics Express*, Vol. 16, No. 3, 2008, pp. 1590–1599.

[250] Fujimoto, J. G., et al., "Optical Biopsy and Imaging Using Optical Coherence Tomography," *Nature Medicine*, Vol. 1, No. 9, 1995, pp. 970–972.

[251] Low, A. F., et al., "Technology Insight: Optical Coherence Tomography-Current Status and Future Development," *Nature Clinical Practice Cardiovascular Medicine*, Vol. 3, No. 3, 2006, pp. 154–162.

[252] Zysk, A. M., et al., "Optical Coherence Tomography: A Review of Clinical Development from Bench to Bedside," *Journal of Biomedical Optics*, Vol. 12, No. 5, 2007, 051403.

[253] Fujimoto, J. G., "Optical Coherence Tomography for Ultrahigh Resolution in Vivo Imaging," *Nature Biotechnology*, Vol. 21, No. 11, 2003, pp. 1361–1367.

[254] Barton, J. K., et al., "Nanoshells as an Optical Coherence Tomography Contrast Agent," *Proceedings of the SPIE*, Vol. 5316, 2004, pp. 99–106.

[255] Loo, C., et al., "Nanoshell-Enabled Photonics-Based Imaging and Therapy of Cancer," *Technology in Cancer Research and Treatment*, Vol. 3, No. 1, 2004, pp. 33–40.

[256] Agrawal, A., et al., "Quantitative Evaluation of Optical Coherence Tomography Signal Enhancement with Gold Nanoshells," *Journal of Biomedical Optics*, Vol. 11, No. 4, 2006, pp. 041121–041128.

[257] Gobin, A. M., et al., "Near-Infrared Resonant Nanoshells for Combined Optical Imaging and Photothermal Cancer Therapy," *Nano Letters*, Vol. 7, No. 7, 2007, pp. 1929–1934.

[258] Cang, H., et al., "Gold Nanocages as Contrast Agents for Spectroscopic Optical Coherence Tomography," *Optics Letters*, Vol. 30, No. 22, 2005, pp. 3048–3050.

[259] Chen, J., et al., "Gold Nanocages: Bioconjugation and Their Potential Use as Optical Imaging Contrast Agents," *Nano Letters*, Vol. 5, No. 3, 2005, pp. 473–477.

[260] Oldenburg, A. L., et al., "Plasmon-Resonant Gold Nanorods as Low Backscattering Albedo Contrast Agents for Optical Coherence Tomography," *Optics Express*, Vol. 14, No. 15, 2006, pp. 6724–6738.

[261] Oldenburg, A. L., et al., "Plasmon-Resonant Gold Nanorods Provide Spectroscopic OCT Contrast in Excised Human Breast Tumors," *Proceedings of the SPIE*, Vol. 6867, 2008, 68670E.

[262] Troutman, T. S., Barton, J. K., and Romanowski, M., "Optical Coherence Tomography with Plasmon Resonant Nanorods of Gold," *Optics Letters*, Vol. 32, No. 11, 2007, pp. 1438–1440.

[263] Winkler, A. M., et al., "Fluorescent and Scattering Contrast Agents in a Mouse Model of Colorectal Cancer," *Proceedings of the SPIE*, Vol. 6851, 2008, 68510L.

[264] Kotaidis, V., and Plech, A., "Cavitation Dynamics on the Nanoscale," *Applied Physics Letters*, Vol. 87, No. 21, 2005, 213102.

[265] Vogel, A., et al., "Mechanisms of Femtosecond Laser Nanosurgery of Cells and Tissues," *Applied Physics B: Lasers and Optics*, Vol. 81, No. 8, 2005, pp. 1015–1047.

[266] Sun, T., and Diebold, G. J., "Generation of Ultrasonic Waves from a Layered Photoacoustic Source," *Nature*, Vol. 355, No. 6363, 1992, pp. 806–808.

[267] Wang, X., et al., "Noninvasive Laser-Induced Photoacoustic Tomography for Structural and Functional *in Vivo* Imaging of the Brain," *Nature Biotechnology*, Vol. 21, No. 7, 2003, pp. 803–806.

[268] Ku, G., and Wang, L. V., "Deeply Penetrating Photoacoustic Tomography in Biological Tissues Enhanced with an Optical Contrast Agent," *Optics Letters*, Vol. 30, No. 5, 2005, pp. 507–509.

[269] Zhang, H. F., et al., "Functional Photoacoustic Microscopy for High-Resolution and Noninvasive in Vivo Imaging," *Nature Biotechnology*, Vol. 24, No. 7, 2006, pp. 848–851.

[270] Eghtedari, M., et al., "High Sensitivity of in Vivo Detection of Gold Nanorods Using a Laser Optoacoustic Imaging System," *Nano Letters*, Vol. 7, No. 7, 2007, pp. 1914–1918.

[271] Chao-Kang, L., et al., "Nanorod-Based Flow Estimation Using a High-Frame-Rate Photoacoustic Imaging System," *Journal of Biomedical Optics*, Vol. 12, No. 6, 2007, 064006.

[272] David, L. C., et al., "Photoacoustic Tomography of Joints Aided by an Etanercept-Conjugated Gold Nanoparticle Contrast Agent-an Ex Vivo Preliminary Rat Study," *Nanotechnology*, Vol. 19, No. 9, 2008, 095101.

[273] Wang, Y., et al., "Photoacoustic Tomography of a Nanoshell Contrast Agent in the in Vivo Rat Brain," *Nano Letters*, Vol. 4, No. 9, 2004, pp. 1689–1692.

[274] Yang, X., et al., "Photoacoustic Tomography of a Rat Cerebral Cortex in Vivo with Au Nanocages as an Optical Contrast Agent," *Nano Letters*, Vol. 7, No. 12, 2007, pp. 3798–3802.

[275] Pitsillides, C. M., et al., "Selective Cell Targeting with Light-Absorbing Microparticles and Nanoparticles," *Biophysical Journal*, Vol. 84, No. 6, 2003, pp. 4023–4032.

[276] Hirsch, L. R., et al., "Nanoshell-Mediated Near-Infrared Thermal Therapy of Tumors under Magnetic Resonance Guidance," *Proceedings of the National Academy of Sciences*, Vol. 100, No. 23, 2003, pp. 13549–13554.

[277] O'Neal, D. P., et al., "Photo-Thermal Tumor Ablation in Mice Using Near Infrared-Absorbing Nanoparticles," *Cancer Letters*, Vol. 209, No. 2, 2004, pp. 171–176.

[278] Takahashi, H., et al., "Gold Nanorod-Sensitized Cell Death: Microscopic Observation of Single Living Cells Irradiated by Pulsed Near-Infrared Laser Light in the Presence of Gold Nanorods," *Chemistry Letters*, Vol. 35, No. 5, 2006, pp. 500–501.

[279] Tong, L., et al., "Gold Nanorods Mediate Tumor Cell Death by Compromising Membrane Integrity," *Advanced Materials*, Vol. 19, No. 20, 2007, pp. 3136–3141.

[280] Pissuwan, D., et al., "A Golden Bullet? Selective Targeting of *Toxoplasma Gondii* Tachyzoites Using Antibody-Functionalized Gold Nanorods," *Nano Letters*, Vol. 7, No. 12, 2007, pp. 3808–3812.

[281] Pissuwan, D., et al., "Targeted Destruction of Murine Macrophage Cells with Bioconjugated Gold Nanorods," *Journal of Nanoparticle Research*, Vol. 9, No. 6, 2007, pp. 1109–1124.

[282] Norman, R. S., et al., "Targeted Photothermal Lysis of the Pathogenic Bacteria, *Pseudomonas Aeruginosa,* with Gold Nanorods," *Nano Letters*, Vol. 8, No. 1, 2008, pp. 302–306.

[283] Takahashi, H., Niidome, Y., and Yamada, S., "Controlled Release of Plasmid DNA from Gold Nanorods Induced by Pulsed Near-Infrared Light," *Chemical Communications*, No. 17, 2005, pp. 2247–2249.

[284] Chen, C. C., et al., "DNA-Gold Nanorod Conjugates for Remote Control of Localized Gene Expression by Near Infrared Irradiation," *Journal of the American Chemical Society*, Vol. 128, No. 11, 2006, pp. 3709–3715.

[285] Horiguchi, Y., et al., "Expression of Plasmid DNA Released from DNA Conjugates of Gold Nanorods," *Chemistry Letters*, Vol. 36, No. 7, 2007, pp. 952–953.

[286] Shiotani, A., et al., "Stable Incorporation of Gold Nanorods into *N*-Isopropylacrylamide Hydrogels and Their Rapid Shrinkage Induced by Near-Infrared Laser Irradiation," *Langmuir*, Vol. 23, No. 7, 2007, pp. 4012–4018.

[287] Gorelikov, I., Field, L. M., and Kumacheva, E., "Hybrid Microgels Photoresponsive in the Near-Infrared Spectral Range," *Journal of the American Chemical Society*, Vol. 126, No. 49, 2004, pp. 15938–15939.

[288] Das, M., et al., "Microgels Loaded with Gold Nanorods: Photothermally Triggered Volume Transitions Under Physiological Conditions," *Langmuir*, Vol. 23, No. 1, 2007, pp. 196–201.

[289] Karg, M., et al., "Nanorod-Coated PNIPAM Microgels: Thermoresponsive Optical Properties," *Small*, Vol. 3, No. 7, 2007, pp. 1222–1229.

[290] Kumar, V. R. R., et al., "Gold Nanorods Grown on Microgels Leading to Hexagonal Nanostructures," *Langmuir*, Vol. 23, No. 17, 2007, pp. 8667–8669.

[291] Wei, Q., Ji, J., and Shen, J., "Synthesis of Near-Infrared Responsive Gold Nanorod/PNIPAMm Core/Shell Nanohybrids Via Surface Initiated ATRP for Smart Drug Delivery," *Macromolecular Rapid Communications*, Vol. 29, No. 8, 2008, pp. 645–650.

[292] Huang, Y. F., Lin, Y. W., and Chang, H. T., "Control of the Surface Charges of Au-Ag Nanorods: Selective Detection of Iron in the Presence of Poly(Sodium 4-Styrenesulfonate)," *Langmuir*, Vol. 23, No. 25, 2007, pp. 12777–12781.

[293] Nakashima, H., et al., "Anisotropic Assembly of Gold Nanorods Assisted by Selective Ion Recognition of Surface-Anchored Crown Ether Derivatives," *Chemical Communications*, No. 10, 2007, pp. 1080–1082.

[294] Rex, M., Hernandez, F. E., and Campiglia, A. D., "Pushing the Limits of Mercury Sensors with Gold Nanorods," *Analytical Chemistry*, Vol. 78, No. 2, 2006, pp. 445–451.

[295] Niidome, Y., et al., "Immobilization of Gold Nanorods on the Glass Substrate by the Electrostatic Interactions for Localized Plasmon Sensing," *Chemistry Letters*, Vol. 33, No. 4, 2004, pp. 454–455.

[296] Marinakos, S. M., Chen, S., and Chilkoti, A., "Plasmonic Detection of a Model Analyte in Serum by a Gold Nanorod Sensor," *Analytical Chemistry*, Vol. 79, No. 14, 2007, pp. 5278–5283.

[297] Wang, C., et al., "Synthesis, Assembly, and Biofunctionalization of Silica-Coated Gold Nanorods for Colorimetric Biosensing," *Advanced Functional Materials*, Vol. 16, No. 13, 2006, pp. 1673–1678.

[298] Mayer, K. M., et al., "A Label-Free Immunoassay Based Upon Localized Surface Plasmon Resonance of Gold Nanorods," *ACS Nano*, Vol. 2, No. 4, 2008, pp. 687–692.

[299] Nusz, G. J., et al., "Label-Free Plasmonic Detection of Biomolecular Binding by a Single Gold Nanorod," *Analytical Chemistry*, Vol. 80, No. 4, 2008, pp. 984–989.

[300] Huang, X., et al., "Cancer Cells Assemble and Align Gold Nanorods Conjugated to Antibodies to Produce Highly Enhanced, Sharp, and Polarized Surface Raman Spectra: A Potential Cancer Diagnostic Marker," *Nano Letters*, Vol. 7, No. 6, 2007, pp. 1591–1597.

[301] Qian, X., et al., "In Vivo Tumor Targeting and Spectroscopic Detection with Surface-Enhanced Raman Nanoparticle Tags," *Nature Biotechnology*, Vol. 26, No. 1, 2008, pp. 83–90.

CHAPTER 10

Magnetic Nanoparticles in Biomedical Applications

Jinwoo Cheon, PhD and Jae-Hyun Lee

10.1 Introduction

Magnetic nanoparticles not only possess interesting nano-size phenomena and properties including superparamagnetism, they have begun to show promise in a variety of technological applications [1–3]. In recent decades, magnetic nanoparticles have shown potential applicability in the biomedical fields. They are becoming important tools for the diagnosis and treatment of diseases, and for the separation of specific pathogens and biological species. In this chapter, we will briefly cover nanoscale magnetism and describe several important applications that have leveraged this pheonomena, including magnetic resonance imaging (MRI) contrast agents, biomagnetic separation, and drug delivery.

10.2 Nanoscale Magnetic Properties

In bulk magnetic materials, the composition, crystalline structure, anisotropic energy, and crystalline defects are the crucial parameters that determine magnetic properties [4]. However, in the nanoscale regime, size is a significant parameter in determining its magnetic properties [5, 6]. One of the interesting size-dependent phenomena of nanoparticles is superparamagnetism. The main characteristics of superparamagnetism, contrary to its bulk counterpart, ferromagnetism, are shown in Figure 10.1(a, b). In bulk ferromagnetic materials, once the magnetic spins of the material are aligned along the external magnetic field (B_0), the net magnetization (M) is conserved even after B_0 is removed. An additional reverse external magnetic field referred to as the coercive field (coercivity, H_c) is required to drive the net magnetization to zero. In superparamagnetism, however, M becomes zero immediately after B_0 is removed (Figure 10.1(b)).

The origin of this phenomenon is deeply related to the magnetic anisotropy energy, the energy required for a spin flip, and it is proportional to the product of the magnetic anisotropic constant (K_u) and the volume (V) of the magnet [4]. In bulk materials the magnetic anisotropy energy (K_uV) is much larger than the thermal energy (kT) (Figure 10.1(c), blue line), whereas in a nanoparticle this energy is com-

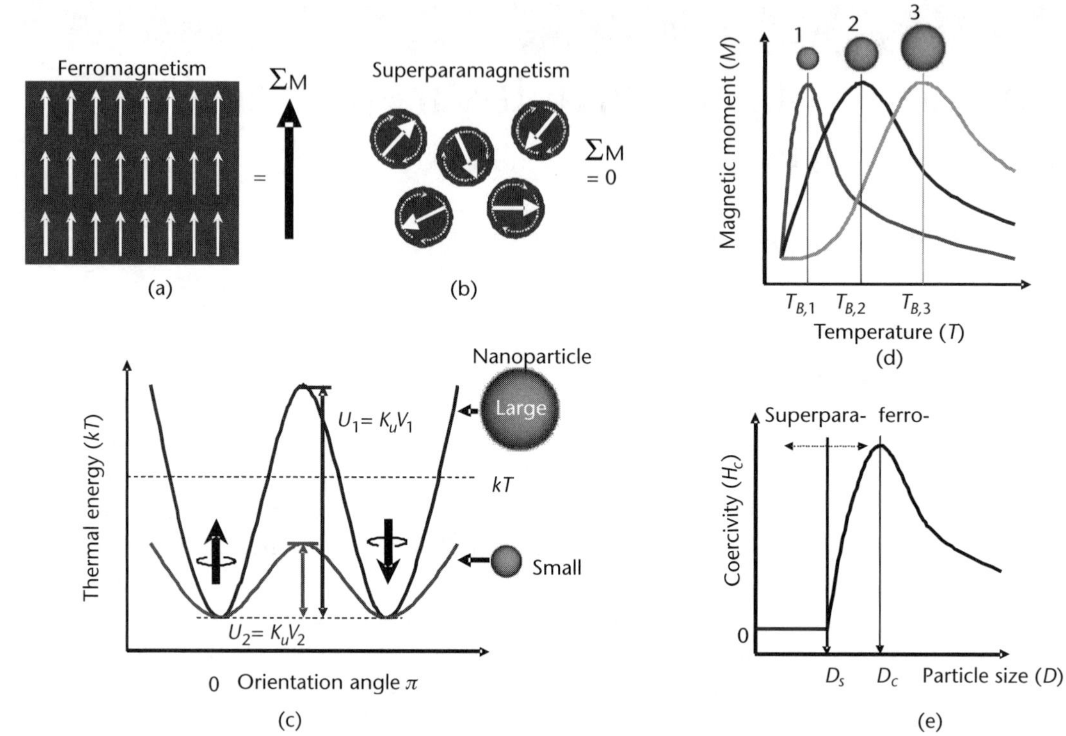

Figure 10.1 The main characteristics of nanoscale magnetism. Magnetic spin structures of (a) ferromagnetism which has a significant amount of net magnetization (*M*) after the external magnetic field (B_0) has disappeared and (b) superparamagnetism in which the net magnetization (M) becomes zero. (c) Energy diagram of magnetic nanoparticles of different particle sizes. In large particle, anisotropy energy (U_1) is higher than thermal energy (*kT*) which results in ferromagnetism (top), and in a small particle, anisotropy energy (U_2) is lower than *kT* which results in superparamagnetism (bottom). (d) Size-dependent zero-field cooling curves indicating changes in the blocking temperature (T_B). (e) Size-dependent coercivity (H_c) curve, in which magnetic domain structures changes from multidomain ferromagnetism to single-domain and superparamagnetism. (See Color Plate 20.)

parable to kT and is sufficient to readily invert the magnetic spin direction (Figure 10.1(c), red line). The magnetic spin fluctuation in nanoparticles that results in a net magnetization of zero is referred to as superparamagnetism.

In superparamagnetism, the blocking temperature (T_B) is defined as the transition temperature from ferromagnetism to superparamagnetism. Below T_B, nanoparticles remain ferromagnetic since the thermal energy (kT) is smaller than K_uV, whereas above T_B, kT is comparable to K_uV so they are easily demagnetized and become superparamagnetic. T_B can be expressed by the size-dependent relationship

$$T_B = \frac{K_u V}{25k} \tag{10.1}$$

which results in a lower T_B for smaller nanoparticles (Figure 10.1(d)) [4d].

The magnetic coercivity (H_c) also exhibits the size-dependent characteristics in nanoparticles (Figure 10.1(e)). Contrary to bulk magnets with multidomain magnetic structures, nanoparticles possesses a single-domain magnetic structure in which all spins are unidirectional below a critical size (D_c). In this stage, H_c decreases as the size of the nanoparticle decreases following the relationship

$$H_c = \frac{2K_u}{m_s}\left[1-5\left(\frac{kT}{K_u V}\right)^{1/2}\right] \tag{10.2}$$

in which m_s is the saturation magnetization of a nanoparticle [4d]. Further, the nanoparticle enters into the superparamagnetic stage of zero H_c below D_s.

Another size-dependent property observed in magnetic nanoparticles is the saturation magnetization (m_s). Magnetically disordered-spin glasslike layers exist on the surface of magnetic materials due to the thermally reduced spin-spin exchange coupling energy, which is referred to as surface spin canting. In bulk materials, the surface spin canting effect is negligible due to the relatively small surface area compared to the total volume of magnet. However, this effect becomes prominent in nanoparticle and can be described as

$$m_s = M_s\left[\frac{(r-d)}{r}\right]^3 \tag{10.3}$$

where M_s is the saturation magnetization of the bulk, r is the size of the nanopartile, and d is the thickness of the disordered surface layer [7].

Understanding these nanoscale properties of magnetic nanoparticles is critical for the design of optimized magnetic nanoparticles for their enhanced applicability in the biomedical science as contrast enhancement agents for magnetic resonance imaging (MRI), for translational vectors for magnetophoretic separation and sensing of biological species, and for magnetic drug delivery.

10.3 Magnetic Resonance Imaging (MRI) Contrast Agent

Superparamagnetic nanoparticles are emerging as next generation molecular imaging probes for observing and tracking molecular events via MRI, which is one of the most powerful medical diagnostic tools available due to its noninvasive nature and multidimensional tomographic capability coupled with its high spatial resolution [8]. Although MRI lags in sensitivity compared to other imaging modalities [9], this disadvantage can be overcome using magnetic nanoparticle-based contrast agents [10]. Under an applied magnetic field, nanoparticles are magnetized with a moment of μ and generate induced magnetic fields, which can perturb the magnetic relaxation processes of the proton in water molecules surrounding the magnetic nanoparticles.

Figure 10.2 depicts the basic concept of how a magnetic nanoparticle influences the spin-spin ($T2$) relaxation time of a proton and the resulting $T2$-weighted MRI contrast [8]. $T2$ relaxation refers to the temporal decay of the transverse magnetization ($\boldsymbol{m}_{xy}$) of the proton that is perpendicular to the external magnetic field (B_0) upon the excitation by a radiofrequency (RF) pulse. Before the excitation, the pre-

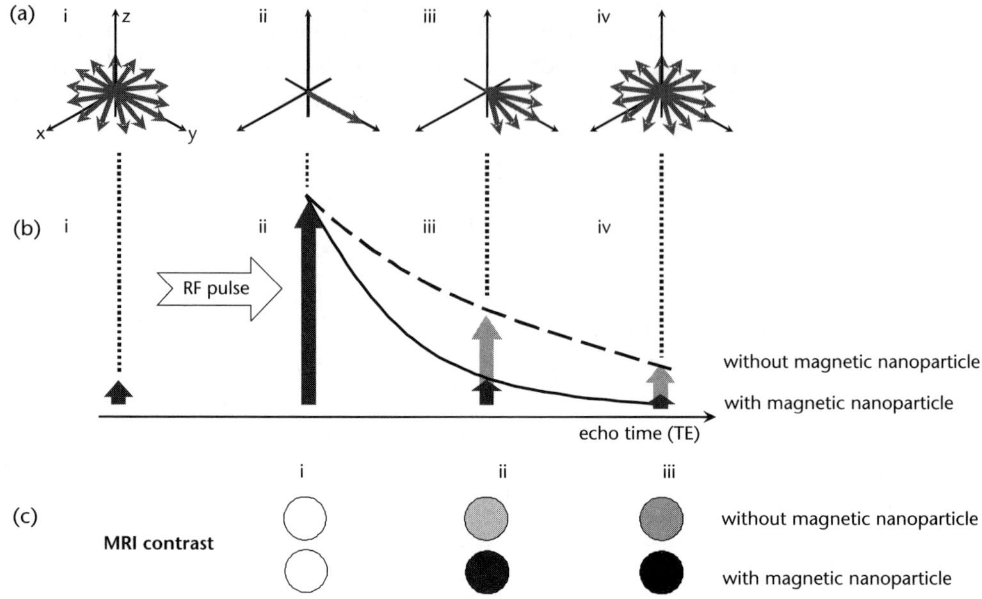

Figure 10.2 Conceptual figure of spin-spin (*T2*) relaxation processes of proton and *T2*-weighted MRI contrast. (a) Temporal decays of transverse magnetization ($\boldsymbol{m}_{xy}$) in Cartesian coordinates: (a (i)) before radiofrequency (RF) excitation, and (a (ii–iv)) after excitation along with echo time (TE). (b) The magnitude changes of transverse magnetization ($\boldsymbol{m}_{xy}$) changes in proton with TE: (b (i)) before RF excitation, and (b (ii–iv)) after excitation, with magnetic nanoparticle (black arrows) or without magnetic nanoparticles (gray arrows). (c (i–iii)) MRI contrast changes along with TE, with magnetic nanoparticle (lower circles) or without magnetic nanoparticles (upper circles).

cession of $\boldsymbol{m}_{xy}$ has nearly zero phase coherency (Figure 10.2(a) i, (b) i). However, when the RF pulse changes both the orientation of the protons and their magnetization with respect to the external magnetic field, it generates strong phase coherency of $\boldsymbol{m}_{xy}$ (Figure 10.2(a) ii, (b) ii). After that the magnetization relaxes back to the initial dephased state within a certain echo time (Figure 10.2(a) ii–iv, (b) ii–iv). MRI records this relaxation process and then reconstructs them to obtain grayscale images. In *T*2-weighted MRI, faster relaxation results in a darker MRI signal. An induced magnetic field generated by a magnetic nanoparticle can make the *T*2 relaxation much faster and result in an even darker MRI signal (Figure 10.2(c), i–iii) [10].

For conventional MRI contrast agents, superparamagnetic iron oxide (SPIO) nanoparticles are synthesized through the precipitation of iron oxide in an aqueous solution containing ferrous salts by adding an alkaline solution [11]. Such iron oxide nanoparticles are usually insoluble as-is, and a coating material is required for them to be soluble in aqueous media. For this purpose, nanoparticles with a surface coating of dextran are commonly used, including the SPIO products Feridex (Endorem), the ultrasmall superparamagnetic iron oxide (USPIO) Combidex (Sinerem), and MION (monocrystalline iron oxide nanocomposite) or CLIO (cross-linked iron oxide), which present the amine functional group on the outer surface for further bioconjugation [12]. Since these nanoparticles are relatively small in size, have a long blood half life time, and have bioconjugation capabilities, they are useful for in vivo MRI of biological targets. These agents have been used to assist in the identification of not only liver tumors, blood vessel angiography, and malignant lymph nodes, but also for target-specific molecular and cellular imaging such as small sized tumors, monitoring of gene expression in specially engineered cells that overexpress a given gene, detection of amyloid β plagues for Alzheimer's disease diagnosis, and imaging of apoptosis, which is an active process in the programmed self-destruction of cells [13]. Weissleder and coworkers demonstrated that MRI detection of transgene expression of engineered transferring receptor (ETR) in tumors is possible by using MION-trasnferrin contrast agents [13d]. Also, Bogdanov and coworkers successfully imaged angiogenesis with MRI as selectively targeting the E-selectin markers that involve angiogenesis by CLIO-anti-human E-selectin antibody conjugates [13h]. Figure 10.3 shows the scheme and in vivo MRI of apoptosis, the programmed cell death where the redistribution of phosphatidylserine in the cell membrane occurs (Figure 10.3(a)). Representative binding proteins to phosphatidylserine are annexin V and synaptotagmin I. Although imaging of apoptosis using these proteins has already been performed through radioisotope techniques, the spatial resolution is only 1~3 mm and needs improvement [14]. Brindle and coworkers have shown that conjugates of the SPIO and C2 domain of synaptotagmin I (SPIO-C2) can detect apoptotic cells through MRI with ~0.1-mm resolution [13g]. MR images were taken before and after the injection at several time intervals in a tumor-bearing mouse. The SPIO-C2s are able to detect apoptotic regions with significant MRI signal changes exhibiting as dark contrasts (Figure 10.3(b)).

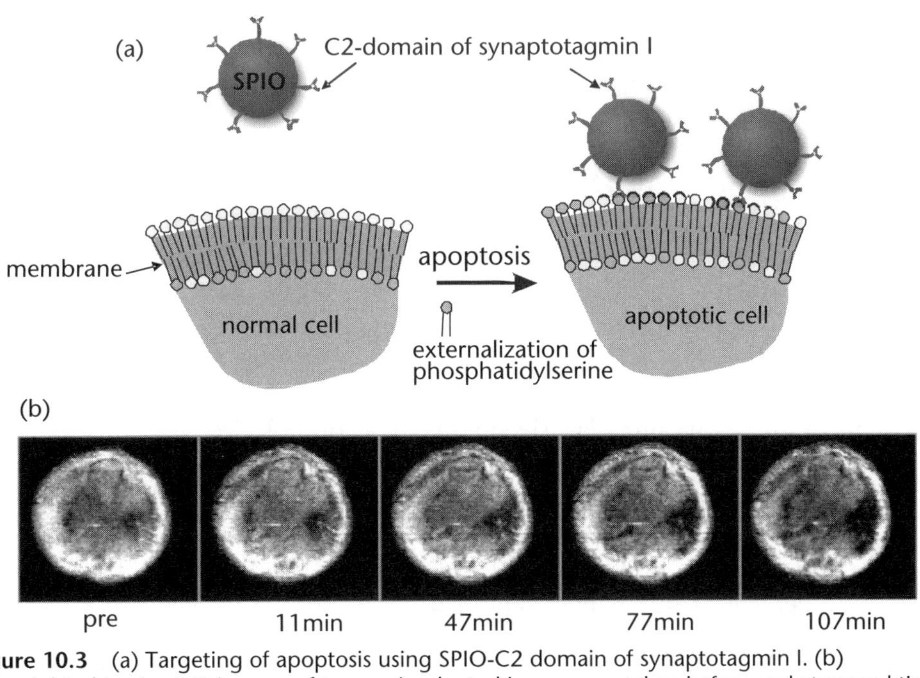

Figure 10.3 (a) Targeting of apoptosis using SPIO-C2 domain of synaptotagmin I. (b) T2-weighted in vivo MR images of tumors implanted in a mouse taken before and at several time points after the injection of SPIO-C2 domain of synaptotagmin I nanoparticles. (Reproduced with permission from [13g]. © 2001 Nature Publishing Group.)

One important issue in the MRI contrast effect using magnetic nanoparticles is the attainment of a high $R2$ value (spin-spin relaxivity, $R2 = 1/T2$), a determining factor for increasing MRI detection sensitivity. According to the outer sphere relaxation model of water protons by solute magnetic nanoparticles, $R2$ of the proton is given by

$$R2 = \frac{1}{T2} = \left(\frac{32\pi}{405}\right)\gamma_1^2 \mu^2 \frac{N_A}{1000}\left(\frac{[M]}{rD}\right)\{6.5 j_2(\omega_S) + 1.5 j_1(\omega_1) + 2 j_1(0)\} \tag{10.4}$$

where M is molarity of the magnetic nanoparticle; r is nanoparticle size; D is relative diffusion; $j_n(\omega)$ is the spectral density function; μ is the magnetic moment of the nanoparticle; γ_1 is the gyromagnetic ratio of protons; N_A is Avogadro's number; and ω_S and ω_I are the Larmor angular precession frequencies of the nanoparticle and water proton magnetic moments, respectively [15]. According to this equation, spin-spin relaxivity ($R2$) is roughly proportional to the square of the magnetic moment (μ) of the nanoparticle that has a linear relationship with saturation magnetization (m_s) [4a]. From (10.3) and (10.4), it can be shown that particle size (r) is proportional to $R2$. Recently, Cheon, Suh, and coworkers developed magnetism engineered iron oxide (MEIO) nanoparticles and empirically demonstrated their size effect on m_s and $R2$, which increase along with increasing particle size from 4 to 6, 9, and 12 nm [16].

In addition to the size effects, magnetic dopant effects of MEIO nanoparticles are also significant. For example, MEIO (Fe_3O_4) nanoparticles have ferromagnetic spin structures where Fe^{2+} and Fe^{3+} occupying O_h sites align parallel to the external magnetic field, and Fe^{3+} in T_d sites align antiparallel to the field [4d]. Incorporation of a magnetic dopant M^{2+} (M = Mn, Co, Ni) to replace O_h Fe^{2+} leads to a change in the net magnetization. MnMEIO (Mn^{2+} ion doped magnetism engineered iron oxide) nanoparticles show the highest magnetization values (110 emu/g(Mn+Fe)) and exhibit the better MR signal enhancement effects than the other metal-doped MEIO nanoparticles, including MEIO, CoMEIO, and NiMEIO with diminished mass magnetization values of 101 emu/g(Fe), 99 emu/g(Co+Fe), and 85 emu/g(Ni+Fe), respectively. One item of note is that the $R2$ coefficient ($r2$) of 12-nm MnMEIO nanoparticle (358 $mM^{-1}s^{-1}$) is ~5.8 times higher than that of a conventional molecular MR imaging contrast agent such as CLIO nanoparticles (62 $mM^{-1}s^{-1}$) [17]. Such MR signal enhancement effects of MnMEIO nanoparticles enable successful ultrasensitive in vivo detection of biological targets (Figure 10.4). When these nanoparticles are conjugated with the cancer-targeting antibody, Herceptin, and intravenously injected into a mouse bearing a small HER2/neu receptor positive cancer (<50 mg of cancer weight), they selectively detect the small cancer after 2 hr with strong MR signals (shown in blue), which represents high $R2$ (~34 percent of $R2$ change) (Figure 10.4(a–c, g)). However, under the same conditions, conventional CLIO-Herceptin probes do not distinguish tumors in MR images (shown in red) without a noticeable $R2$ change (Figure 10.4(d–g)) [17]. Such results clearly demonstrate the significance of magnetism engineering of nanoparticles in order to increase $R2$ and MRI detection sensitivity.

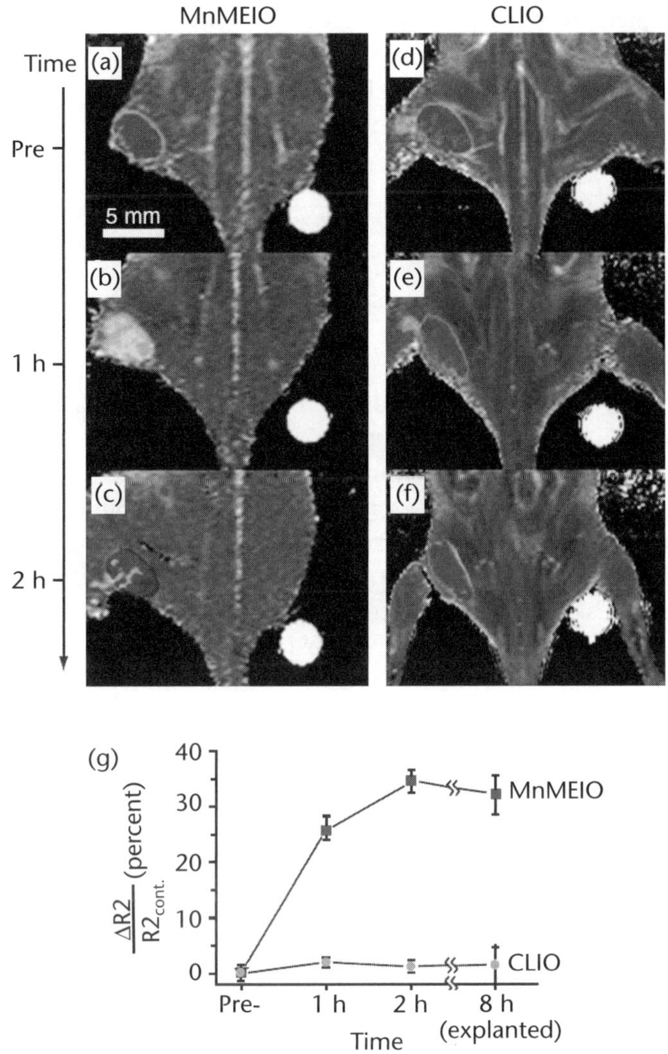

Figure 10.4 Highly sensitive in vivo cancer detection by utilization of MnMEIO-Herceptin nanoparticles. (a–c) Color mapped MRI of the tumor-bearing mouse at different temporal points following injection of MnMEIO-Herceptin nanoparticles, and (d–f) CLIO-Herceptin nanoparticles. (g) Time-dependent $\Delta R2/R2_{control}$ changes at the tumor site after injection of MnMEIO-Herceptin probes (blue square) and CLIO-Herceptin probes (red circle). (Reproduced with permission from [17]. © 2007 Nature Publishing Group.) (See Color Plate 21.)

10.4 Magnetic Separation

In biomedical applications, separation of specific biological entities from the incident solution for controlling sample concentration and subsequent analyses is important. Among the various separation techniques, magnetic separation has its merits, including fast separation time, and good separation yield and resolution, and has proven to be a very sensitive technique for separating small amounts of molecules (e.g., cells, nucleic acids, and proteins) [18].

Magnetism of the particle is a determining factor for attaining the best separation efficiency against the hydrodynamic drag force acting on the magnetic particle in the solution. The relative velocity of the particle (Δv) in the carrier fluid can be expressed as follows:

$$\Delta v = \frac{r^2 \mu}{9\varepsilon_0 \eta} \nabla\left(B^2\right) \qquad (10.5)$$

where r is particle size; μ is magnetic moment of the particle; ε_0 is permeability of free space; η is viscosity of the medium; and B is the external magnetic field [19]. According to this equation, larger particles with a large magnetic moment should be more effective in magnetic separation. Until now, magnetic beads have been widely used for such purposes, but these still have problems including low magnetic moment and magnetic inhomogeneity [20]. The use of nanoparticles with well-defined size and magnetism can be advantageous in this situation, due to the large surface areas of nanoparticles ensuring the binding of targets with very small quantities as well as high controllability and reproducibility. Furthermore, the use of nanoparticles can reduce the possibilities of the interference of targeted molecules by the magnetic particles themselves for further tests [21].

Using magnetic nanoparticles, Terstappen and colleagues devised a platform for cell analysis based on immunomagnetic selection and magnetic alignment of cells (Figure 10.5) [18b]. Whole blood is mixed with magnetic nanoparticles (SPIO) conjugated with leukocyte targeting antibodies and fluorescent probes, and placed in a magnetic field separating chamber (Figure 10.5(a)). Leukocytes selectively labeled with magnetic nanoparticles move upward by magnetic force and align between magnetic nickel lines. An epi-illumination system can optically image and measure signals obtained from the aligned cells (Figure 10.5(b)). It is notable that cell counts per unit blood volume obtained from this system are roughly 10 times larger than

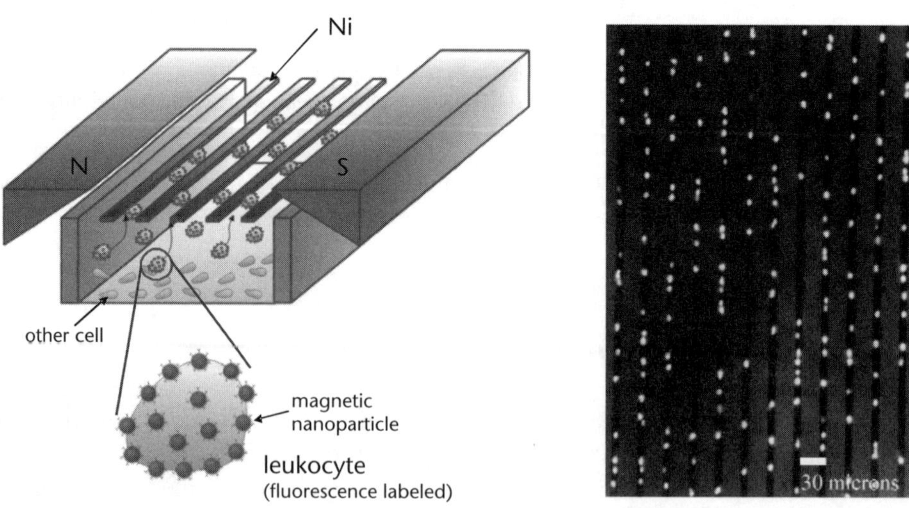

Figure 10.5 (a) Schematic representation of the cell analysis system using immunomagnetic selection. (b) Fluorescent microscopic images of leukocytes aligned between ferromagnetic nickel lines. (Reproduced with permission from [18b]. © 1999 Nature Publishing Group.)

from the standard hematology analyzer and flow cytometer, which means the magnetic separation system has significantly enhanced sensitivity with minimal complexity.

As another example, target proteins can be selectively separated out from the cell lysates. Proteins are much smaller than cells and usually have ~ 1–5 binding sites for conventional iron oxide nanoparticles with relatively low magnetic moment that do not show effective separation [18f]. Xu and coworkers used Co or $SmCo_{5.2}$ magnetic nanoparticles to resolve this problem [22]. Due to the superior magnetic moment value of Co or $SmCo_{5.2}$ to iron oxide [4b, 23], this nanoparticle can enhance the separation yield of proteins. As a feasibility test, the nanoparticles were bioconjugated with nitrilotriacetic acid (Ni-NTA) ligands that specifically bind to histidine (His) tagged proteins (Figure 10.6(a)) and successfully separate green fluorescent protein (6xHis-GFP) in whole cell lysates.

Sodiumdodecylsulfate/polyacrylamide gel electrophoresis (SDS/PAGE) show only a single intense GFP band after separation (Figure 10.6(b), lane 2), whereas numerous protein bands are observed prior to separation (Figure 10.6(b), lane 1)

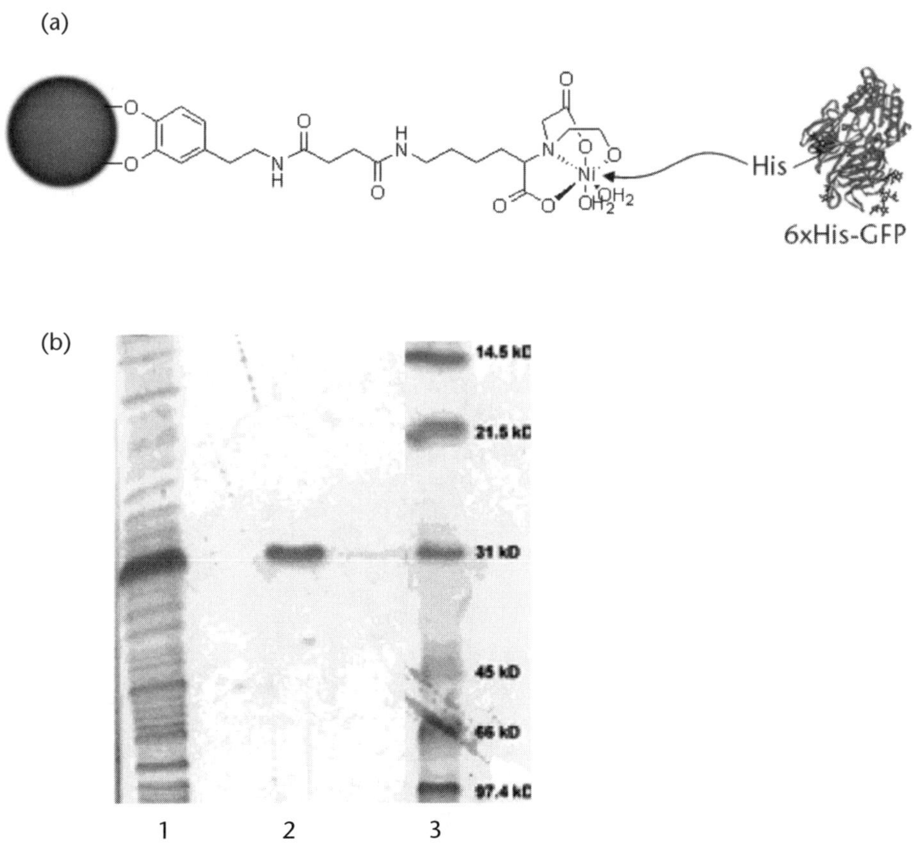

Figure 10.6 (a) Schematic of $SmCo_{5.2}$ nanoparticles conjugated with nitrilotriacetic acid (Ni-NTA) ligand for the specific separation of histidine (His) tagged green fluorescence protein (GFP). (b) SDS/PAGE analysis for the purification of the proteins. Lane 1: cell lysates; lane 2: magnetically separated GFP proteins; lane 3: molecular weight marker. (Reproduced with permission from [22a]. © 2004 Nature Publishing Group.)

[22a]. Apart from these examples, there are numerous examples of magnetic separation using magnetic nanoparticles. Recently it is shown that Fe_3O_4 nanoparticles are effective to remove arsenic from wastewater by a relatively low-gradient magnet (<100 T/m) [18g].

The magnetic separation technique can be extended to ultrasensitive and reliable target sensing and diagnostic systems. Park, Kim, Cheon, and coworkers adopted the magnetic separation to microfluidic systems for the detection of IgE, an indicator for allergy caused by a hypersensitive reaction between allergens and allergen-specific IgE antibodies [24]. For this experiment, microbeads coated with mite allergen from *Dermatophagoides farinae* are first mixed with the target IgE with varying concentrations (Figure 10.7(b)). Then antihuman IgE-coated MEIO nanoparticles with the capability to bind to the Fc region of the target IgE are further added, and the resulting solution is injected into the microfluidic channel (Figure 10.7(a)). In the microfluidic channel, the lateral velocity of IgE bound MEIO nanoparticles toward the magnetic field is carefully measured, revealing different velocities for the different concentrations of IgE. At a high concentration of the target IgE, lateral movement of the microbeads with a velocity (v_{lat}) of ~15 μm/s is observed (Figure 10.7(c)), while reduced (v_{lat} = ~2 μm/s) and negligible lateral movement is observed at lower concentrations of IgE and no IgE, respectively (Figure 10.7(d,e)). Such observations are reasonable since the higher IgE concentrations induce more binding of MEIO nanoparticles onto the microbeads. Using this sys-

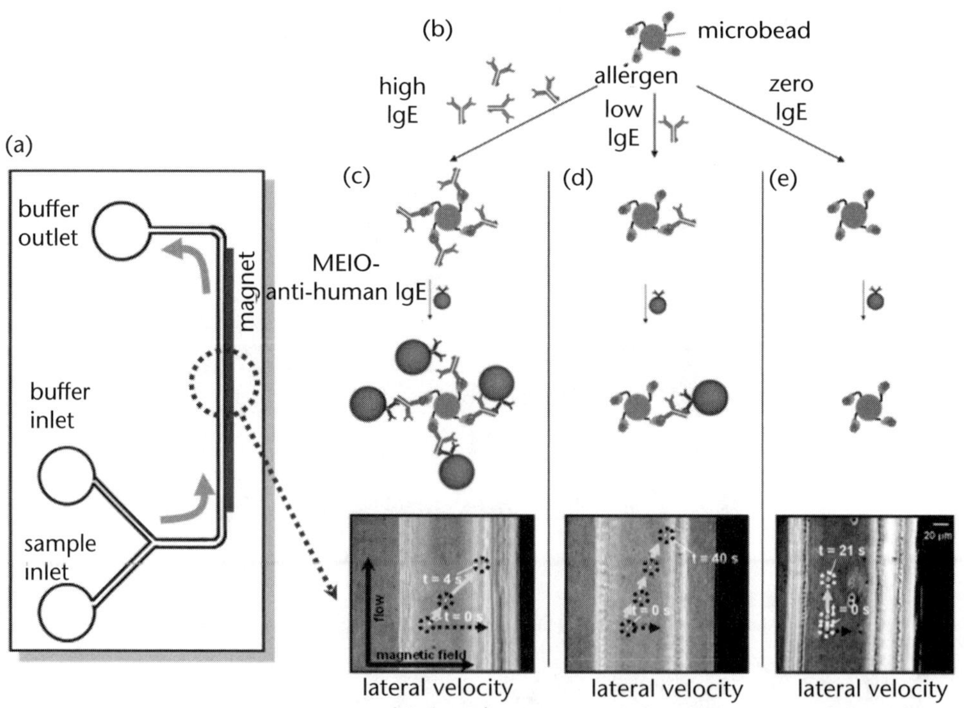

Figure 10.7 Magnetophoretic sensing of allergen-specific IgE: (a) Schematic of microfluidic channel used in these experiments; (b) microbeads coated with allergen, and detection scheme and magnetophoretic movements of the samples at (c) high, (d) low, and (e) zero concentration of the target IgE. (Reproduced with permission from [24]. © 2007 American Chemical Society.)

tem, ultrasensitive detection of IgE is possible in that the detection limit of target IgE can be lowered to subpicomolar IgE levels (~500 fM).

10.5 Magnetic Drug Delivery

The key parameters of the drug delivery system that must be optimized to overcome the current limitation of chemotherapies are (a) reducing the drug dosage level to minimize the side effects and the cytotoxic effects to normal tissues and organs, and (b) increasing the delivered dosage to a targeted region with systemic controllability [19a]. In a magnetic drug delivery system, the therapeutic drugs are conjugated to the magnetic nanoparticles, which are subsequently injected into the circulatory system and guided to the target region by an external strong magnetic. The underlying physical principles are similar to biomagnetic separation, and their efficacy is mainly determined by the magnetic field strength, particle size, and magnetic properties of particles [25]. It is known that larger particles (~1-μm microspheres or agglomerates) are more effective in resisting the counter flow dynamics of the circulatory system with magnetic flux in the range of 0.2–0.7T at the target sites [25b].

In an effort to realize this type of magnetic drug delivery system, FeRx Corporation conducted phase I/II trials with the magnetic particle bound to doxorubicin, an anticancer drug [26]. Transcatheter deliveries of the magnetic nanoparticle to the hepatic artery are guided by a 1.5T short-bore magnet, which is monitored by using intraprocedural MRI (Figure 10.8(a)), followed by interim catheter repositioning for the optimization of delivery to the tumor and minimization of delivery to nor-

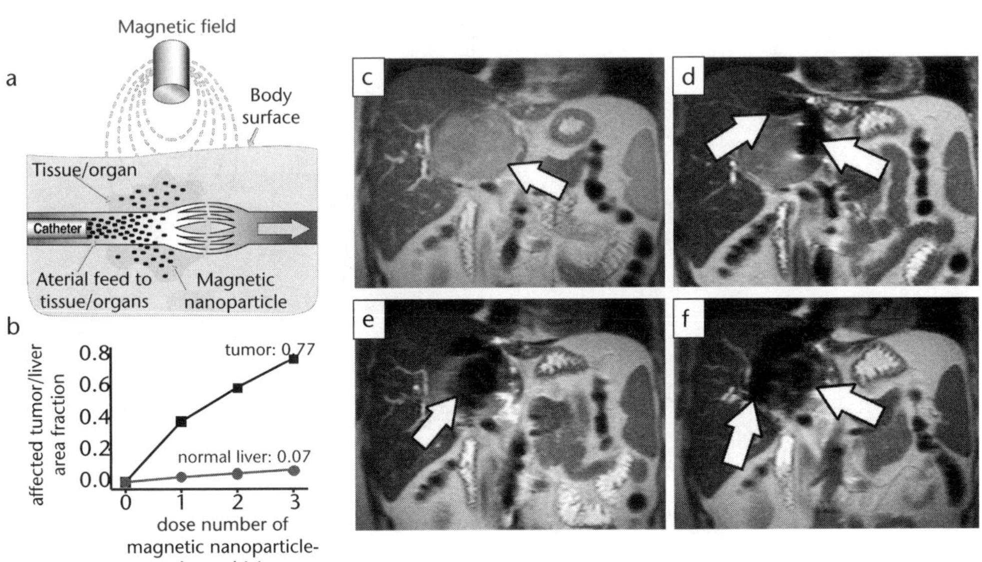

Figure 10.8 Magnetically guided transcatheter delivery of doxorubicin bound magnetic nanoparticles in a human patient: (a) Conceptual scheme and (b) cumulative nanoparticle fraction of tumor and normal liver region along with dose numbers. (c–f) MRI of magnetically guided tumor targeting (c) before, and (d) after the first, (e) the second, and (f) the third dose of the magnetically guided doxorubicin bound magnetic nanoparticles. Magnetic nanoparticle affected regions are indicated as dark MRI contrast and white arrow. (Reproduced with permission from [26c]. © 2004 The Radiological Society of North America.)

mal tissue [26c]. As can be seen in Figure 10.8(c–f), which shows MRI of hepatic tumor injected three times with magnetically guided doxorubicin bound magnetic particles, magnetic particles affect only the tumor region (white arrow) and is imaged as dark contrast not observed in the normal liver region. After the treatment, final fraction of treated tumor volume is 0.77, whereas the fraction of normal liver volume is only 0.07, which shows promise for directing magnetically targeted tumor therapies (Figure 10.8b).

As another example of the feasibility test of magnetic targeting, liposomes containing magnetic nanoparticles are used to target tumors with an extracorporeal magnet [27]. For in vivo studies, a nude mouse bearing a PC3 human prostate carcinoma tumor in each flank receives an intravenous injection of the magnetoliposomes after a small magnet with 0.3T magnetic field and a field gradient of 11 T/m is fixed to the skin above one tumor (Figure 10.9(a)). As can be seen in Figure 10.9(b), the left tumor, which is magnetically targeted for 24 hr, appears dark in *T*2-weighted MRI than the contralateral (control) tumor (right), indicating preferential accumulation of magnetoliposomes.

Despite these promising results, clinical use of magnetic drug delivery has encountered some setbacks. FeRx Corporation, one of the leading companies in magnetic targeting and drug delivery, halted operations in mid-2004 after its leading compound, doxorubicin bound magnetic particle, did not show statistical significance in clinical phase II/III compared to the products currently manufactured [28]. This failure implies the need for more efficient magnetic delivery systems that require new magnetic particles with higher magnetic moments and stronger external magnets, as discussed in (10.5). In addition, therapeutic efficacy can be improved by applying the principles described earlier and should be extended to magnetic particle-based hyperthermia and not limited to drug targeting.

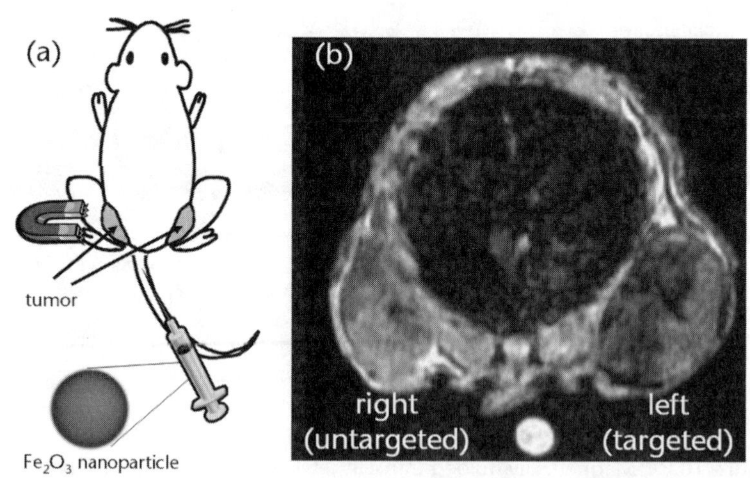

Figure 10.9 Magnetically targeted magnetoliposomes to soild tumors: (a) Conceptual scheme and (b) *T*2-weighted axial MRI of the mouse in which a magnet is attached onto the left tumors for 24 hr after intravenous injection of magnetoliposomes. (Reproduced with permission from [27]. © 2006 The Radiological Society of North America.)

10.6 Conclusions

This chapter describes the basic concepts of the interactions between magnetic nanoparticles and external magnetic fields, and shows their potential applications in the biomedical field especially for MRI contrast agents, biomagnetic separations, and magnetic drug delivery. Many other applications of magnetic nanoparticle in biomedicine are currently being explored, such as magnetic twisting cytometry, which uses cell membrane bound magnetic nanoparticles for measuring the mechanical properties of cell [29], and magnetic nanoparticle–based sensors, which uses magneto-resistance or magnetic relaxation mechanism for detecting biomolecules [30]. Some of these magnetic nanoparticle–based technologies are already commercially available (e.g., MRI contrast agent and biomagnetic separation), and there are still many possibilities for the other technologies to be transferred to clinical industries.

References

[1] (a) Zhang Q, Chen S, Winoto SH, Ong E-H, "Design of high-speed magnetic fluid bearing spindle motor," *IEEE Transac. Magn.* 2001, 37, 2647–2650. (b) Takahashi A, "Magnetic fluid sealing apparatus for a magnetic disk drive," *US Patent* 5,057,952, 1991.

[2] (a) Odenbach S., Ferrofluids: magnetically controlled suspensions. *Colloid. Surface. A* 2003, *217*, 171–178. (b) King JA, "Method for making loudspeaker with magnetic fluid enveloping the voice coil," *US Patent* 4,017,694, 1977.

[3] Raj K, Moskowitzn R. "A review of damping applications of ferrofluids," *IEEE Transac. Magn.* 1980, *16*, 358–363.

[4] (a) Cullity BD. *Introduction to Magnetic Materials.* Addison-Wesley Publishing, Reading, MA, 1972. (b) McCurrie RA. *Ferromagnetic Materials: Structure and Properties.* Academic Press, San Diego, CA, 1994. (c) Cornell RM, Schwertmann U. *The Iron Oxides.* Wiley-VCH, Weinheim, Germany, 2003. (d) Jales D. *Introduction to Magnetism and Magnetic Materials.* CRC Press, BocaRaton, FL, 1998.

[5] (a) Jun Y-W, Seo J-W, Cheon J., "Nanoscaling laws of magnetic nanoparticles and their applicabilities in biomedical sciences," *Accounts Chem. Res.* 2008, *41*, 179–189. (b) Sun SH, "Recent advances in chemical synthesis, self-assembly, and applications of FePt nanoparticles," *Adv. Mater.,* 2006, *18*, 393–403. (c) Hyeon, T., "Colloidal chemical synthsis of organic-dispersible uniform magnetic nanoparticles," Mattoussi H., Cheon J., Ed., *Inorganic Nanoprobes for Biological Sensing and Imaging,* Artech House, Norwood, 2008, Chapter 2. (d) Leslie-Pelecky, DL, Rieke RD., "Magnetic properties of nanostructured materials," *Chem. Mater.* 1996, *8*, 1770–1783.

[6] (a) Murray CB, Sun SH, Doyle H, Betley T., "Monodisperse 3d transition-metal (Co, Ni, Fe) nanoparticles and their assembly into nanoparticle superlattices," *MRS Bull.* 2001, *26*, 985–991. (b) Sun SH, Zeng H, Robinson DB, Raoux S, Rice PM, Wang SX, Li GX., "Monodisperse MFe_2O_4 (M = Fe, Co, Mn) nanoparticles," *J. Am. Chem. Soc.* 2004, *126*, 273–279. (c) Jana NR, Chen Y, Peng X, "Size- and shape-controlled magnetic (Cr, Mn, Fe, Co, Ni) oxide nanocrystals *via* a simple and general approach," *Chem. Mater.* 2004, *16*, 3931–3935. (d) Jun Y, Choi J, Cheon J., "Heterostructured magnetic nanoparticles: Their versatility and high performance capabilities," *Chem. Commun.* 2007, 1203–1214. (e) Park J, An KJ, Hwang YS, Park JG, Noh HJ, Kim JY, Park JH, Hwang NM, Hyeon T., "Ultra-large scale synthesis of monodispersed nanocrystals," *Nat. Mater.*, 2004, *3*, 891–895. (f) Cheon J, Kang N-J, Lee S-M, Yoon J-H, Oh SJ, "Shape evolution of singlecrystalline iron oxide nanocrystals," *J. Am. Chem. Soc.* 2004, *126*, 1950–1951. (g) Shevchenko EV, Talapin DV, Rogach AL, Kornowski A, Haase M, Weller H., "Colloidal

synthesis and self-assembly of $CoPt_3$ nanocrystals," *J. Am. Chem. Soc.* 2002, *124*, 11480–11485.

[7] (a) Morales MP, Veintemillas-Verdaguer S, Montero MI, Serna CJ. Surface and internal spin canting in ã-Fe_2O_3 nanoparticles. *Chem. Mater.* 1999, *11*, 3058–3064. (b) Morales MP, Serna CJ, Bødker F, Mørup S., "Spin canting due to structural disorder in maghemite," *J. Phys.: Condens. Matter* 1997, *9*, 5461–5467.

[8] Mitchell DG, *MRI Principles*, W.B.Saunders Company, Philadelphia, 1999.

[9] Massoud TF, Gambhir SS, "Molecular imaging in living subjects: seeing fundamental biological processes in a new light," *Gene. Dev.*, 2003, *17*, 545–580.

[10] (a) LaConte L, Nitin N, Bao G, "Magnetic nanoparticle probes," *Nanotoday,* 2005, *8*, 32–38. (b) Bulte JWM, Kraitchman DL. Iron oxide MR contrast agents for molecular and cellular imaging. *NMR Biomed.* 2004, *17*, 484–499. (c) Wang Y-XJ, Hussain SM, Krestin GP, "Superparamagnetic iron oxide contrast agents: Physicochemical characteristics and applications in MR imaging," *Eur. Radiol.*, 2001, *11*, 2319–2331. (d) Hamm B, Staks T, Taupitz M, Maibauer R, Speidel A, Huppertz A, Frenzel T, Lawaczeck R, Wolf KJ, Lange L., "Contrast-enhanced MR imaging of liver and spleen: First experience in humans with a new superparamagnetic iron oxide," *J. Magn. Reson. Imaging,* 1994, *4*, 659–668.

[11] (a) Sjögren CE, Johansson C, Naevestad A, Sontum PC, Briley-Saebo K, Fahlvik AK, "Crystal size and properties of superparamagnetic iron oxide (SPIO) particles," *Magn. Reson. Imaging*, 1997, *15*, 55–67. (b) Hahn PF, Stark DD, Lewis JM, Saini S, Elizondo G, Weissleder R, Fretz CJ. Ferrucci, JT, "First clinical trial of a new superparamagnetic iron oxide for use as an oral gastrointestinal contrast agent in MR imaging," *Radiology* 1990, *175*, 695–700. (c) Bach-Gansmo T., "Ferrimagnetic susceptibility contrast agents," *Acta. Radiol.,* 1993, Suppl. *387*, 1–30.

[12] (a) Weissleder R, Elizondo G, Josephson L, Compton CC, Fretz CJ, Stark DD, Ferrucci JT, "Superparamagnetic iron oxide-enhanced MR imaging: pulse sequence optimization for detection of liver cancer," *Radiology,* 1989, 171, 835–839. (b) Weissleder R, Stark DD, Engelastad BL, Bacon BR, Compton CC, White DL, Jacobs P, Lewis J., "Superparamagnetic iron oxide: pharmacokinetics and toxicity," *Am. J. Roentgenol.,* 1989, *152*, 167–173. (c) Reimer P, Rummeny EJ, Daldrup HE, Balzer T, Tombach B, Berns T, Peters PE., "Clinical results with Resovist: a phase 2 clinical trial," *Radiology,* 1995, *195*, 489–496. (d) Grubnic S, Padhani AR, Revell PB, Husband JE, "Comparative efficacy of and sequence choice for two oral contrast agents used during MR imaging," *Am. J. Roentgenol.,* 1999, *173*, 173–178. (e) Bartolozzi C, Lencioni R, Donati F, Cioni D., "Abdominal MR: liver and pancreas," *Eur. Radiol.,* 1999, *9*, 1496–1512. (f) Moore A, Marecos E, Bogdanov A, Weissleder R., "Tumoral distribution of long circulating dextran-coated iron oxide nanoparticles in a rodent model," *Radiology,* 2000, *214*, 568–574. (g) Palmacci S, Josephson L., "Synthesis of polysaccharide covered superparamagnetic oxide colloids," *US Patent*, 5,262,176, 1993. (h) Shen T, Weissleder R, Papisov M, Bogdanov A, Brady TJ., "Monocrystalline iron oxide nanocompounds (MION): Physicochemical properties," *Magn. Reson. Med.*, 1993, *29*, 599-604.

[13] (a) Weissleder R., Lee AS, Fischman AJ, Reimer P, Shen T, Wilikinson R, Callahan R, Brady TJ., "Polyclonal human immunoglobulin G labeled with polymeric iron oxide: antibody MR imaging," *Radiology,* 1991, *181*, 245–249. (b) Schmitz SA, Taupitz M, Wagner S, Wolf K-J, Beyersdorff D, Hamm B., "Magnetic resonance imaging of atherosclerotic plaques using superparamagnetic iron oxide particles," *J. Magn. Reson. Imaging* 2001, *14*, 355–361. (c) Wadghiri YZ, Sigurdsson EM, Sadowski M, Elliott JI, Li Y, Scholtzova H, Tang CY, Aguinaldo G, Pappolla M, Duff K, Wisniewski T, Turnbull DH, "Detection of Alzheimer's amyloid in transgenic mice using magnetic resonance microimaging," *Magn. Reson. Med.*, 2003, *50*, 293-302. (d) Weissleder R, Moore A, Mahmood U, Bhorade R, Benveniste H, Chiocca EA, Basilion JP. In vivo magnetic resonance imaging of transgene expression. *Nat. Med.* 2000, *6*, 351–355. (e) Tiefenauer LX, Kühne G, Andres RY, "Antibody-magnetite nanoparticles: In vitro characterization of a potential tumor-specific contrast agent for magnetic resonance imaging," *Bioconjugate Chem.* 1993, *4*, 347–352. (f) Artemov D, Mori N, Okollie B, Bhujwalla ZM. MR molecular imaging of the Her-2/neu

receptor in breast cancer cells using targeted iron oxide nanoparticles. *Magn. Reson. Med.* 2003, *49*, 403–408. (g) Zhao M, Beauregard DA, Loizou L, Davletov B, Brindle KM., "Non-invasive detection of apoptosis using magnetic resonance imaging and a targeted contrast agent," *Nat. Med.*, 2001, *7*, 1241–1244. (h) Kang HW, Josephson L, Petrovsky A, Weissleder R, Bogdanov A., "Magnetic Resonance Imaging of Inducible E-Selectin Expression in Human Endothelial Cell Culture," *Bioconugate Chem.*, 2002, *13*, 122–127. (i) Arbab AS, Frank JA. Magnetic nanoparticles assisted cellular MR imaging and their biomedical applications. Mattoussi H, Cheon J, Ed., "Inorganic Nanoprobes for Biological Sensing and Imaging," Artech House, Norwood, 2008, Chapter 11.

[14] Lahorte CM, Vanderheyden JL, Steinmetz N, Van de Wiele C, Dierckx RA, Slegers G., "Apoptosis-detecting radioligands: current state of the art and future perspectives," *Eur. J. Nucl. Med. Mol. Imaging,* 2004, *31*, 887–919.

[15] Koenig SH, Keller KE, "Theory of 1/T1 and 1/T2 NMRD profiles of solutions of magnetic nanoparticles," *Magn. Reson. Med.*, 1995, *34*, 227–233.

[16] Jun Y, Huh Y-M, Choi J-s, Lee J-H, Song H-T, Kim SJ, Yoon S, Kim K-S, Shin J-S, Suh J-S, Cheon J., "Nanoscale size effect of magnetic nanocrystals and their utilization for cancer diagnosis via magnetic resonance imaging," *J. Am. Chem. Soc.,* 2005, *127*, 5732–5733.

[17] Lee J-H, Huh Y-M, Jun Y, Seo J-w, Jang J-t, Song H-T, Kim SJ, Cho E-J, Yoon H-G, Suh J-S, Cheon J., "Artificially Engineered Magnetic Nanoparticles for Ultra-Sensitive Molecular Imaging," *Nat. Med.*, 2007, *13*, 95–99.

[18] (a) Molday RS, MacKenzie D., "Immunospecific ferromagnetic iron–dextran reagents for the labeling and magnetic separation of cells," *J. Immunol. Methods,* 1982, *52*, 353–367. (b) Tibbe A, de Grooth B, Greve J, Liberti P, Dolan G, Terstappen L., "Optical tracking and detection of immunomagnetically selected and aligned cells.," *Nat. Biotech.*, 1999, *17*, 1210–1213. (c) Kularatne BY, Lorigan P, Browne S, Suvarna SK, Smith MO, Lawry J., "Monitoring tumour cells in the peripheral blood of small cell lung cancer patients," *Cytometry,* 2002, *50* 160–167. (d) Morisada S, Miyata N, Iwahori K., "Immunomagnetic separation of scum-forming bacteria using polyclonal antibody that recognizes mycolic acids," *J. Microbiol. Methods,* 2002, *51*, 141–148. (e) Zigeuner RE, Riesenberg R, Pohla H, Hofstetter A, Oberneder R., "Isolation of circulating cancer cells from whole blood by immunomagnetic cell enrichment and unenriched immunocytochemistry in vitro," *J. Urol.* 2003, *169*, 701–705. (f) Mura CV, Becker MI, Orellana A, Wolff D., "Immunopurification of Golgi vesicles by magnetic sorting," *J. Immunol. Methods,* 2002, *260*, 263–271.

[19] (a) Pankhurst QA, Connolly J, Jones SK, Dobson J., "Applications of magnetic nanoparticles in biomedicine," *J. Phys. D: Appl. Phys.*, 2003, *36*, R167–R181. (b) Zborowski M., *Physics of magnetic cell sorting Scientific and Clinical Applications of Magnetic Carriers,* Plenum, New York, 1997.

[20] (a) Hayes MA, Polson NA, Phayre AN, Garcia AA. Flow-based microimmunoassay. *Anal. Chem.* 2001, *73*, 5896–5902. (b) Pamme N, Manz A. On-chip free-flow magnetophoresis: Continuous flow separation of magnetic particles and agglomerates. *Anal. Chem.* 2004, *76*, 7250.

[21] Hancock JP, Kemshead JT., "A rapid and highly selective approach to cell separations using an immunomagnetic colloid," *J. Immunol. Methods*, 1993, *164* 51–60.

[22] (a) Xu C, Xu K, Gu H, Zheng R, Liu H, Zhang X, Guo Z, Xu B., "Dopamine as a robust anchor to immobilize functional molecules on the iron oxide shell of magnetic nanoparticles," *J. Am. Chem. Soc.,* 2004, *126*, 9938–9939. (b) Gu H, Xu K, Xu C, Xu B., "Biofunctional magnetic nanoparticles for protein separation and pathogen detection," *Chem. Commun.*, 2006, 941–949. (c) Yavuz CT, Mayo JT, Yu WW, Prakash A, Falkner JC, Yean S, Cong L, Shipley HJ, Kan A, Tomson M, Natelson D, Colvin VL., "Low-field magnetic separation of monodisperse Fe_3O_4 nanocrystals," *Science,* 2006, *314*, 964–967.

[23] (a) Trout SR, Graham CD., "Magnetocrystalline anisotropy, magnetostriction and saturation magnetization of $SmCo_5$ single crystals," *J. Appl. Phys.,* 1979, *50*, 2361. (b) Weller D, Moser A., "Thermal effect limits in ultrahigh-density magnetic recording," *IEEE Trans. Magn.* 1999, *35*, 4423–4439.

[24] Hahn YK, Jin Z, Kang JH, Oh E, Han M-K, Kim H-S, Jang J-t, Lee J-H, Cheon J, Kim SH, Park H-S, Park J-K., "Magnetophoretic immunoassay of allergen-specific ige in an enhanced magnetic field gradient," *Anal. Chem.*, 2007, *79*, 2214–2220.

[25] (a) Lübbe AS, Bergemann C, Brock J, McClure DG., "Physiological aspects in magnetic drug-targeting," *J. Magn. Magn. Mater.*, 1999, *194*, 149–155. (b) Voltairas PA, Fotiadis DI, Michalis LK., "Hydrodynamics of magnetic drug targeting," *J. Biomech.*, 2002, *35*, 813–821. (c) Cummings LJ, Richardson G, Hazelwood L., "Drug delivery by magnetic microspheres," *Proc. Mathematics in Medicine Study Group*, University of Notingham, Nottingham, UK, 2000.

[26] (a) Goodwin S, Peterson C, Hob C, Bittner C., "Targeting and retention of magnetic targeted carriers (MTCs) enhancing intra-arterial chemotherapy," *J. Magn. Magn. Mater.*, 1999, *194*, 132–139. (b) Goodwin SC, Bittner CA, Peterson CL, Wong G., "Single-dose toxicity study of hepatic intra-arterial infusion of doxorubicin coupled to a novel magnetically targeted drug carrier," *Toxicol. Sci.*, 2001, *60*, 177–183. (c) Wilson MW, Kerlan RK, Fidleman NA, Venook AP, LaBerge JM, Koda J, Gordon RL., "Hepatocellular carcinoma: Regional therapy with a magnetic targeted carrier bound to doxorubicin in a dual MR imaging/conventional angiography suite-initial experience with four patients," *Radiology*, 2004, *230*, 287–293.

[27] Fortin-Ripoche JP, Martina MS, Gazeau F, Ménager C, Wilhelm C, Bacri J-C, Lesieur S, Clément O., "Magnetic targeting of magnetoliposomes to solid tumors with MR imaging monitoring in mice," 2006, 239, 415–424.

[28] Rittner M. Nanomagnetics: materials, devices and markets. *Business Opportunity Report: GB293*, Business Communications Company, Inc. Norwalk, CT, 2004.

[29] (a) Wang N, Butler JP, Ingber DE., "Mechanotransduction across the cell surface and through the cytoskeleton," *Science* 1993, *260*, 1124. (b) Fabry B, Maksym GN, Hubmayr RD, Butler JP, Fredberg JJ., "Implications of heterogeneous bead behavior on cell mechanical properties measured with magnetic twisting cytometry," *J. Magn. Magn. Mater.*, 1999, *194*, 120–125. (c) Fabry B, Maksym G N, Butler JP, Glogauer M, Navajas D, Fredberg JJ., "Scaling the microrheology of living cells," *Phys. Rev. Lett.*, 2001, *87*, 148102. (d) Bausch AR, Ziemann F, Boulbitch AA, Jacobson K, Sackmann E., "Local measurements of viscoelastic parameters of adherent cell surfaces by magnetic bead microrheometry," *Biophys. J.*, 1998, *75*, 2038–2049.

[30] (a) Grancharov SG, Zeng H, Sun S, Wang SX, O'Brien S, Murray CB, Kirtley JR, Held GA., "Bio-functionalization of monodisperse magnetic nanoparticles and their use as biomolecular labels in a magnetic tunnel junction based sensor," *J. Phys. Chem, B* 2005, *109*, 13030–13035. (b) Perez JM, Josephson L, O Loughlin T, Hogemann D, Weissleder R., "Magnetic relaxation switches capable of sensing molecular interactions," *Nat. Biotech.*, 2002, *20*, 816–820.

CHAPTER 11

Magnetic Nanoparticles–Assisted Cellular MR Imaging and Their Biomedical Applications

Ali S Arbab, MD, PhD and Joseph A Frank, MD, MS

11.1 Introduction

Tracking of administered cells by different imaging modalities is becoming popular among investigators. Various in vitro techniques are being used to tag these cells so that they can be detected using noninvasive imaging (see Table 11.1). Different reporter genes have been introduced into cells and are detected by optical imager/fluorescent or confocal microcopy [1–5]. Exogenous optical or fluorescent tags such as quantum dots or other near-infrared nanoparticles are being introduced into the cytoplasm of cells for optical imaging [6–10]. Nuclear medicine approaches have incorporated the sodium iodide symporter (NIS) [11–13] or herpes simplex virus thymidine kinase (HSVtk) genes into cells and have used chelated radionuclides or positron emitters to track cells [14–17]. Indium-^{111}-oxine and Technicium^{99m} chelates [18, 19] have been used to label and track by single photon emission computed tomography (SPECT) [20–23]. Positron-emitting radioisotope 2-[18F]-fluoro-2-deoxy-D-glucose (18F-FDG) and Copper 64 pyruvaldehyde-bis (N4-methylthiosemicarbazone) have been used in the in vitro labeling and subsequent tracking of labeled cells [24, 25] by positron emission tomography (PET). Labeling cells with superparamagnetic iron oxide nanoparticles (SPIO) or a paramagnetic contrast agent (gadolinium or manganese) allows for the possibility of detecting single cells or clusters of labeled cells within target tissues following either direct implantation or intravenous injection [26–32]. Various approaches have been developed to label cells with SPIO nanoparticles or soluble paramagnetic MR contrast agents [26, 27, 33–48]. This chapter will focus on how different types of cells can be labeled with different magnetic nanoparticles for cellular magnetic resonance imaging (CMRI) and how it can be used to translate from bench to bedside.

11.2 Characterization of MRI Contrast Agents or Magnetic Nanoparticles Used in Cell Labeling for CMRI

MR contrast agents used to label cells can either exhibit properties of being paramagnetic or superparamagnetic. These agents alter the nuclear magnetic resonance relaxation (NMR) times of the water protons in solution or tissue known as T1, T2, and T2*. The spin-lattice, or longitudinal relaxation time, or T1 represents the exponential recovery of the proton spine to align with the external magnetic field. The spin-spin, or transverse relaxation time, or T2 is the exponential loss of coherence among the spins oriented at an angle to the static magnetic field due to interactions of the spins. The T2* (T2 star) is the loss of phase coherence of the spins in the external magnetic field and is a combination of magnetic field in-homogeneities and T2.

11.2.1 Paramagnetic Agents

Paramagnetism refers to the ability of a metal such as manganese, gadolinium, or iron to interact with water protons through dipole-dipole interaction with direct inner sphere effects resulting in a shortening of NMR relaxation times and is usually associated with enhancement (increase in signal intensity) on T1-weighted images (T1W). Gadolinium chelates (i.e., GdDTPA, GdDOTA, or GdDO3A) and manganese chloride are paramagnetic contrast agents used in experimental and clinical studies. These agents tend to shorten T1 relaxation time greater than the T2 and T2* of tissues.

Gadolinium (Gd) chelate–based contrast agents for cell labeling have been used to label cells ex vivo with limited results. Reports indicate modest T1 enhancement or in some cases no T1 enhancement when gadolinium chelate–based agents are used for cell labeling [49–55]. Thus the need remains to identify an agent that will exert a strong T1 effect, allowing detection of cells in disease models, where the cells need to be conspicuous, versus surrounding tissues, where labeled cell numbers are low or when concentration of gadolinium is low. Giesel et al. [52] were able to label mesenchymal stem cells (MSC) using a bifunctional gadoflurine M-Cy3.5 for both MRI and optical imaging. Gadoflurine M-Cy3.5 is designed with a hydrophilic tail that allows the agent to insert itself in the cell wall and then gets internalized into cytosol. Intracerebral implantation of 10^6 gadoflurine M-Cy3.5 labeled MSC allowed for clear visualization of cells in the rat brain on T1-weighted imaging at clinically relevant 1.5 Tesla that could be confirmed by fluorescent microscopy. Anderson et al. used gadolinium fullerenol, which has higher relaxivities than conventional gadolinium chelates, to label MSCs [45]. Gadolinium fullerenol–labeled MSCs could be detected on 7T MRI following direct injection of 10^6 cells into the rat thigh. Gadolinium fullerenol–labeling decreased the stem cell proliferation initially suggesting that the agent may be altering mitochondrial function. Brekke et al. used a combination gadolinium chelate with fluorescent tag to label cells and noted a significant decrease in proliferation and increase in reactive oxygen species after 24 hr of incubation [56]. The transient negative effect on cell proliferation of a gadolinium-based agent used for cellular and molecular imaging warrants further evaluation of this agent on long-term toxicity or the ability of the cells to repair damage.

Manganese (Mn) chloride was the first paramagnetic contrast agent used in MRI. It has been shown that it can be taken up by cells in vivo through calcium channels in the cell membrane [48, 57, 58]. Aoki et al. have recently reported that lymphocytes could be labeled following incubation with manganese chloride [48]. MRI of cells in gelatin demonstrated increased signal intensity on T1W images; however, it is not clear if there would be sufficient contrast enhancement to detect Mn-labeled cells in vivo by MRI. Recently, cells have been labeled with paramagnetic manganese oxide nanoparticles, and the enhancement could be detected using standard T1-weighted imaging, although further work is needed to fully understand the uptake and safety of this agent in stem cells [59]. The major drawback when using Mn as an MR contrast agent is its narrow therapeutic window and potential toxicity.

11.2.2 Superparamagnetic Agents

Superparamagnetic iron oxide nanoparticles are a family of MRI contrast agents that are presently being used to efficiently label cells for cellular imaging. Various methods are in use for preparing SPIO nanoparticles, resulting in a wide range of physiochemical differences, including core size (e.g., ultrasmall (U)SPIO), shape, mono, or oligocrystalline composition, and outer coating, that may alter the ability to use these agents to label cells. The basic chemistry behind the formation of SPIO nanoparticles is a mixture of ferrous and ferric iron salts at alkaline pH with a coating (dextran or other types of coatings) that is actively stirred or sonicated, resulting in magnetite containing various ratios of Fe_3O_4 to Fe_2O_3 in the crystals [60, 61]. The typical synthesis of SPIO nanoparticles is represented by the chemical formula

$$Fe^{2+} + Fe^{3+} + OH^{-} + [\text{Coating}] \rightarrow \text{Magnetite} + \text{coat}$$

The size of the (U)SPIO nanoparticles depends on the surface coating used that determines if the particle is monocrystalline (Ferumoxtran) or consists of multiple or oligocrystalline such as ferumoxides [61]. Surface coatings on (U)SPIO nanoparticles may be variously sized and surface charged molecules, including dextran and modified cross-linked dextran, dendrimers, starches, citrate, or viral particles [40, 61–80]. The coating is usually added during formation of the Fe_3O_4 to Fe_2O_3 crystals and allows the SPIO nanoparticles to exist in a colloidal suspension in aqueous solutions. For several clinically approved SPIO nanoparticles (e.g., ferumoxides, ferumoxtran, and ferucarbotran), the coating is dextran, which is attached through electrostatic interaction to the iron core by hydrogen bonds between some of the dextran hydroxyl groups and the surface oxide groups of the iron core [61]. The unattached dextran tails cover the rest of the iron crystals and contribute to most of the hydrodynamic diameter of the (U)SPIO nanoparticles [61]. Figure 11.1 is a scanning electron micrograph of ferumoxides with its oligocrystal structure and dextran coating. For SPIO nanoparticles (e.g., ferumoxides or ferucarbotran), through electrostatic interactions, the dextran links or clusters multiple single iron oxide crystals together, making the nanoparticle hydrodynamic diameter range between 60 and 200 nm [61]. A discussion of chemical synthesis of magnetic nanoparticles can be found in Chapter 2.

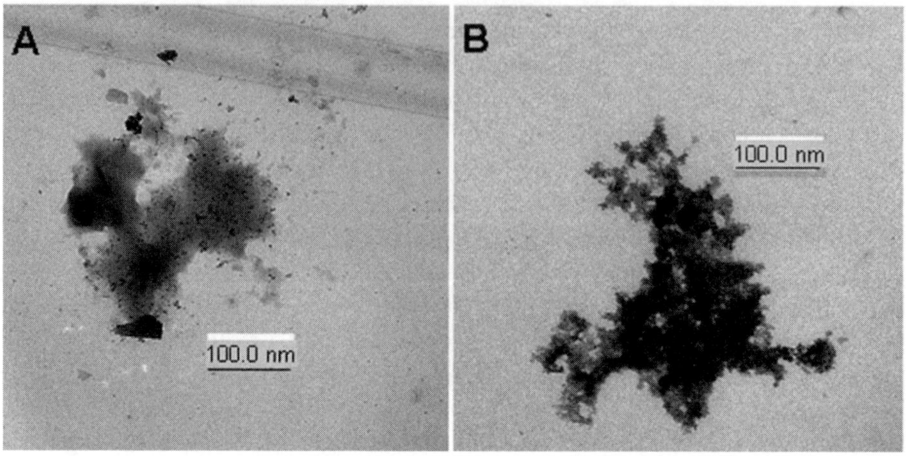

Figure 11.1 Transmission electron micrographs of ferumoxides and ferumoxides-protamine sulfate complexes. All images were taken at a magnification of 9300. (a) Ferumoxides alone; (b) ferumoxides with protamine sulfate (100 μg:2 μg).

The coating molecules (i.e., dextran) will contribute to the surface charge or zeta potential of the (U)SPIO in water. The zeta potential or the average potential difference in millivolts exists between the surface of the (U)SPIO nanoparticles immersed in a conduction liquid (water) and the bulk of the liquid. Dextran-coated ferumoxides have a zeta potential of -32 millivolts, while ferumoxtran coated with a shorter chain dextran has a measured zeta potential of -2.0–0 millivolts [81]. Ferumoxtrans near neutral surface charge and size contribute to long blood half life, compared to the larger SPIO nanoparticles. Zeta potentials have not been reported for other (U)SPIO nanoparticles characterized as having either anionic or cationic charges. Cationic (U)SIPO nanoparticles have been used to label primary and cloned cell populations in cultures because of surface chanrge of cell membrane, such as human cervical cancer cells (HeLa). HeLa cells have a negative zeta potential [82] and the (U)SPIO agent initially interacts with the plasma membrane through electrostatic interactions followed by endocytosis.

In the absence of an external magnetic field, the magnetic domains in the iron oxide crystals are randomly oriented and have zero net magnetic moment. Superparamagnetism occurs when the crystals are placed in the presence of an external magnetic field. The magnetic domains will reorient and tend to align, resulting in a large magnetic moment due to magnetic ordering exceeding the one that would occur with paramagnetic ions, such as manganese, iron, and gadolinium in aqueous solution. This induced magnetic moment causes a distortion of the local magnetic fields when the SPIO nanoparticles are MR imaged, which results in signal loss (hypointensity) compared to surrounding tissue because of magnetic susceptibility and a blooming artifact on the T2*-weighted image [63, 64, 83, 84]. The SPIO nanoparticles do not retain the residual magnetization once the external field is removed, and therefore cells labeled intracellularly with SPIO nanoparticles will not aggregate. The SPIO labeled cells can be separated from unlabeled cells using external magnetic field [28]. SPIO nanoparticles shorten the T1, T2, and T2* relaxation times of water or tissue when present in high enough concentrations [61, 85]. In general, (U)SPIO nanoparticles will alter the T2/T2* of the surrounding tissue in part due to the field gradients surrounding the nanoparticles, resulting in a rapid dephasing of the protons in the environment. (U)SPIO nanoparticles' effect on MRI signal intensities depends on various factors including particle size, hydrodynamic radius, concentration of particles within the voxel (i.e., an image volume element), image acquisition parameters, and whether the MR contrast agent is in solution or compartmentalized within a cell [30, 32, 86]. Table 11.1 summarizes the various physiochemical characteristics of (U)SPIO nanoparticles that have been used for labeling cells. Long echo time T2 weighted (T2W) spin echo pulse sequences or T2*W gradient echo MR pulse sequences are commonly used to detect the presence of (U)SPIO nanoparticles within tissues. For MR cellular imaging, (U)SPIO nanoparticles are usually compartmentalized within endosomes or macropinosomes within the cytoplasm of cells.

Table 11.1 Comparison of Different Imaging Modalities with Respect to Resolution, Imaging Depth, Acquisition Time, Available Contrast Agents, Application, and Clinical Applicability

Technique	*Resolution*	*Depth*	*Time*	*Imaging Agents*	*Application*	*Main Characteristics*	*Clinically Relevant*
MRI	10–100 μm	No limit	μsec to hours	Gadolinium, manganese, iron oxides nanoparticles	Anatomy, physiology, metabolic, cellular, molecular	Versatile, high soft tissue contrast	Yes
CT	25–50 μm	No limit	Sec to min	Iodine	Anatomy, physiology cellular?	Lung and bone	Yes?
Ultrasound	50 μm	mm-cm	Sec to min	Microbubbles	Anatomy, physiology	Vascular, interventional	Yes
PET	1–2 mm (dedicated small animal scanner) 3–5 mm for clinical system	No Limit	Min	^{18}F, ^{11}C, ^{15}O, ^{64}Cu	Physiology metabolism, molecular, cellular	Versatile, receptor studies, cyclotron needed	Yes
SPECT	1–2 mm (dedicated small animal scanner) 5 mm for clinical system	No limit	Min	^{99m}Tc, ^{111}In, ^{128}I	Physiology metabolism, molecular, cellular	Commonly used for MoAb imaging	Yes
Fluorescence reflectance imaging	2–3 mm	<1 cm	Min	GFP, NIR fluorochrome	Physiology, molecular, cellular	Rapid screening of molecular events	No
Bioluminescence imaging	2–3 mm	cm	Min	Luciferins	Cellular molecular, cellular	Gene expression	No
Intravital microscopy	1 μm	400 μm	Sec to min	Fluorochromes	Physiology, molecular, cellular	Limited depth	Limited

11.3 Methods for Labeling Cells with Magnetic Nanoparticles for CMRI

As mentioned in the earlier section, the surface of most of the commercially available (U)SPIO nanoparticles is negatively charged. On the other hand, electric charge of cell surface is also negative. Investigators have modified the surface charge of the nanoparticles by coating it with cationic materials or modified the coating by attaching membrane penetrable peptides. Commercially available transfection agents have also been used to modify negatively charged SPIO to facilitate uptake by cells.

11.3.1 Endocytosis of Contrast Agents

Cells use a variety of modes to regulate their internal environment and allow for the uptake of nutrients, cell-to-cell communication and the internalization of macromolecules and particles across the plasma membrane. *Endocytosis* is a global term used to describe the various mechanisms that cells use to internalize macromolecules and particles within vesicles that derived from the cell membrane and that are located in the cytoplasm. Endocytosis by definition includes phagocytosis (cell eating), pinocytosis (cell drinking), clathrin-mediated endocytosis, caveolin mediated endocytosis, and clathrin and caveolin independent endocytosis [87–89]. Specialized or professional phagocytic cells such as neutrophils, monocytes, macrophages, and microglia use phagocytosis to clear large particulate debris and bacteria. Phagocytosis is an active process involving specific cell surface receptors and signaling cascades, energy metabolites, and regulation of actin as part of cell cytoskeleton.

In contrast to phagocytosis, all cells exhibit pinocytosis or fluid phase uptake from the surrounding environment. The amount of uptake of a macromolecular MR contrast agent is directly proportional to the concentration in the media and the volume of the intracellular vesicles. In general, nonspecific binding of an agent to cell surfaces results in pinocytosis. A highly efficient method of intracellular incorporation of contrast agents into cells is through clathrin-mediated endocytosis (also referred to as receptor-mediated endocytosis), which would concentrate the contrast agent within clathirin-coated vesicles. The receptor binding typically triggers the local accumulation of clathrin structures on the cytoplasmic surface of the plasma membrane as it begins to invaginate, forming clathrin-coated pits. Clathrin-mediated endocytosis requires specific receptor-ligand interactions to stimulate pinocytosis, such as binding of transferrin to its receptor or the high or low density lipoprotein (HDL or LDL) particles to their respective cell surface receptors [90, 91].

MRI contrast agents can be incorporated into cells through nonspecific phagocytosis or the various endocytic pathways that nonphagocytic cells use, such as pinocytosis, clathrin-mediated endocytosis, caveolin-mediated endocytosis, and clathrin- and caveolin-independent endocytosis [87–89]. Incubating cells in high concentrations of MR contrast agents in media is a slow and inefficient method of intracytoplasmic incorporation by pinocytosis and does not usually result in high concentrations of the agent in cells [26, 27, 39, 50]. MR contrast agents with ligands or site-specific antibodies covalently bound to the nanoparticles would attach to the specific receptor on the cell surface and start the formation of the complex into a coated pit on the plasma membrane [62, 84, 92–96]. For example, transferrin receptor (TfR) has been primarily used to shuttle SPIO nanoparticles into cells either by attaching transferrin to the surface coat or by covalently attaching a monoclonal antibody directly to the rat TfR present on rat progenitor oligodendrocytes [84]. By genetically engineering tumor cells to express high levels of TfR, uptake of the transferrin-USPIO contrast agent has been used to monitor gene expression in flank tumors in experimental models, leading to the possibility of using this labeling approach to tag cells in vivo with MR contrast agents in preclinical studies [62, 92–94, 97]. Macropinocytosis allows for the uptake of larger particles from the extracellular space and is an active process starting as a membrane extension from the plasma membrane. After encompassing the particles, the extension collapses into the plasma membrane, forming irregular-sized marcopinosomes. Macropinocytosis is the presumed mechanism for which arginine containing protein transduction domains including polyarginine, HIV-transactivator transcription (Tat) proteins, peptides, polycationic transfection agents, and liposomes get incorporated into the cell [89, 98, 99]. Depending on its contents, the macropinosomes may or may not fuse with deep lysosomes in the cells, and the contents would then undergo digestion by lysosomal enzymes and buffers.

Caveolea-mediated endocytosis is primarily used by endothelial cells for extensive transcellular shuttling of serum proteins from the blood stream into tissue; however, other cells in culture may also use this method of endocytosis [88, 89]. Caveolea are flask-shaped invagination in the plasma membrane enriched in cholesterol and sphingolipods and marked by integral membrane protein, caveolin. Caveolea internalize large molecular complexes, toxins, and some viruses. For most cells, caveolea formation is a slow process and the vesicles are relatively small in size (50-60 nm) and volume when compared to clathrin-coated vesicles that can rapidly form and are about 120nm in diameter [89]. Further experiments need to be performed to determine what role caveolea-mediated endocytosis plays in the uptake of viral coated SPIO contrast agents [40] or other SPIO complexes in cell culture.

Clathrin- and caveolea-independent endocytosis tend to occur in neurons and neuroendocrine cells and are primarily the mechanisms of the reuptake following post-synaptic release of vesicles. This method of endocytosis is probably not involved in the uptake of SPIO nanoparticles into neuronal stem cells (NSC) or neuronal progenitor cells [88, 89].

11.3.2 Modified Nanoparticles for Cell Labeling

Superparamagnetic iron oxide nanoparticles are being used to efficiently label cells for cellular MRI. Dextran-coated SPIO nanoparticles such as ferumoxides, ferucarbotran, or ferumoxtran are clinically approved MR contrast agents for use as hepatic imaging or have been used in clinical trials as blood pool agent or for lymphangiography [100–104]. They are also being used to label cells. Experimental (U)SPIO nanoparticles have also been used for labeling cells. The cationic-coated USPIO nanoparticles, carboxypropyl trimethyl ammonium (i.e., WSIO), and citrate (i.e., VSOP C184) were designed so that they would attach to the negative surface charge of plasma membranes through electrostatic interactions and then get incorporated into endosomes of macrophages [70]. A discussion on the biomedical applications of magnetic nanoparticles can be found in Chapter 10.

Dendrimers are branched synthetic polymers with layered architecture that can be of various sizes or generations and have multiple applications including transfecting oligonucleotides into cells by binding to the plasma membrane and stimulating endocytosis [105–108]. Adding generation 4.5 polyamindoamine (i.e., PAMAM) dendrimer as a coating for iron oxide nanoparticles resulted in the synthesis of magnetodendrimers (e.g., MD-100) [64]. Incubating mammalian cells with MD-100 for 1–2 days resulted in a wide variety of cells demonstrating on Prussian blue staining a remarkably high degree of intracellular labeling, with the cytoplasm containing large numbers of iron-containing vesicles or endosomes. Labeling cells with MD-100 did not alter their proliferation capacity, viability, or toxicity as compared to unlabeled cells. MD-100–labeled oligodendroglial progenitors derived from neural stem cells were transplanted into the ventricles of neonatal dysmyelinated Long Evans Shaker rats, and the migration of labeled cells into the brain parenchyma could be observed by cellular MRI up to 42 days following implantation. On histology, there were areas of new myelin formation demonstrated using antimyelin basic protein stains that corresponded to areas on MRI, proving that the MD-100 did not interfere with the functioning of the labeled cells.

Modification of the dextran coating of USPIO nanoparticles by cross-linking the dextran strands (CLIO) and then covalently attaching HIV-1 Tat proteins to the surface has allowed for efficient and effective labeling of nonphagocytic cells, presumably through macropinocytosis [38]. CLIO-Tat labeled HIV-1 could be recovered following their homing to bone marrow, and could be visualized ex vivo by MR imaging. Using MR imaging, homing of CLIO-Tat labeled lymphocytes could be visualized in the liver and spleen in normal mice [109]. CLIO-Tat–labeled T-cells have been used as adoptive transfer in autoimmune diabetes mouse models, and labeled cells have been shown to selectively home to specific antigens in B16 melanoma in a mouse model by in vivo MRI [37, 110, 111]. Selective homing of antigen-sensitized CLIO-Tat–labeled T-cells to tumors can be detected using CMRI within targeted tumors 12 hr following infusion of labeled cells, and it has been reported that as few as three labeled T-cells/voxel could be detected by MRI. There are no reported differences in CLIO-Tat labeled and unlabeled cells as far as function, viability, or ability to home to target tissues [37, 112]. CLIO-Tat or a slight modification that includes attaching optical imaging agents (i.e., FITC, CY5.5) to the dextran coat, are very efficient in labeling cells ex vivo [113]. CLIO-Tat use is relatively limited since it is a custom synthesized agent and not commercially available.

Conjugating antigen-specific internalizing monoclonal antibodies (mAb) to the dextran coat of USPIO nanoparticles has facilitated the magnetic labeling of cells by clathrin-mediated endocytosis. [84, 92, 93, 114–116]. The monoclonal antibody (OX-26) to the rat TfR was covalently attached to USPIO nanoparticles (MION-46L) and used to label rat progenitor oligodendrocytes (CG-4). Iron oxide particles were observed in the CG-4 cells using transmission electron microscopy and by histology using Prussian blue staining. MION-46L-OX -26 labeled rat CG-4 cells were directly implanted into spinal cords of myelin-deficient rats and ex vivo MR images, obtained 10–14 days after implantation. They demonstrated excellent correlation between the hypointense regions and blooming artifacts caused by the presence of labeled cells and the degree of myelination in the spinal cord detected on immuno-histochemistry. The results indicated that magnetically labeled cells would not interfere with the cell differentiation, migration along area of pathology, or the formation of myelin wraps around axons. Ahrens et al. labeled dendritic cells by biotinylating anti-CD-11 mAb in conjunction with strepavidin attached to dextran coated iron oxide nanoparticles [115]. The advantage of this two-stage labeling approach is that the CD 11 mAb is commercially available, and biotin-strepavidin interaction is a commonly used molecular biology procedure resulting in the SPIO being incorporated in endosomes. While the use of target-specific mAb attached to SPIO provides for efficient cellular labeling, a major drawback of this approach is the need for a specific mAb for each cell type and species.

Viruses and viral shells are being explored as carriers for MRI contrast agents. A hemagglutinatin virus of Japan (HVJ) envelope that encapsulated SPIO nanoparticles was found to label microglial cells in culture [40, 117, 118]. The HVJ SPIO–labeled cells were intracardially injected, and clusters of cells could be seen within one day following transplantation in the brains of mice. The HVJ SPIO particles were reportedly more efficient at labeling cells than combining dextran-coated SPIO with transfection agent lipofectamine [40]; however, since HVJ envelopes are not commercially available, the use of this agent for labeling cells is limited.

Commercially available micron-sized iron oxide particles (MPIO) are also being used to label cells for cellular MRI studies in experimental models. These agents are from 0.3 to >5 microns in size, containing greater than 60 percent magnetite in a polymer coating that can include a fluorescent marker that allows for dual detection of labeled cells by MRI and fluorescent microscopy. MPIOs can be purchased with either terminal amines or carboxyl groups on the surface, thus allowing for chemical modification to attach peptides, ligands, or monoclonal antibodies to the specific targets and receptors on cells. MPIOs have been used to track macrophage infiltration in transplantation rejection, to monitor single cell migration in tissues, and to locate implanted stem cells in an area of myocardial infarction [42, 73, 119–121]. Hinds et al. [119] demonstrated that MPIOs did not alter viability, proliferation, or differential capacity of labeled hematopoietic stem cells and MSCs compared to unlabeled cells and MRI and confocal microscopy could detect these labeled cells. Recently, Shapiro et al. [42] reported uptake of very large MPIO of 5.8 microns in size in cultured hepatocytes and have been able to visualize single cells at 7 Tesla on $T2^*$-weighted images. Heyn et al. [122] have shown that following IC injection of enhanced green fluorescent protein (EGFP) transfected breast cancer cells (231BR) labeled with MPIO in mice, the number of hypointense regions detected on a balance steady state gradient echo image (e.g., FIESTA) decreased with time. Approximately 1–3 percent of original hypointense regions in the brain could be detected 28 days following IC injection of labeled cells as either remaining unchanged or becoming hyperintense tumors. The authors indicated that metastatic breast cancer detected at the end of the study reportedly originated from the hypointense voxel seen on postinfusion MRI. To date, no studies have been performed specifically addressing how the micron-sized particles are removed from the cells or whether the endosome/lysosome can digest the polymer coating.

11.3.3 Transfection Agent Mediated Cell Labeling

SPIO nanoparticles are used to magnetically label and track these cells using T2W or T2*W images [28, 30, 64, 84, 97, 110, 119, 123–134]. Although several approaches for labeling cells with SPIO nanoparticles have been explored, most of the agents used were proprietary compounds, involved unique or complex synthesis, or included biochemical modification of the dextran coat of the SPIO nanoparticles to stimulate endocytosis by cells. In 2002, a relatively straightforward approach was developed combining (U)SPIO with commonly available polycationic transfection agents to effectively label cells. Different commercially available transfection agents have been tried with varying results [26, 27, 29, 31, 33, 35, 135, 136]. However, most of the commercially available transfection agents are toxic to the cells at relatively low doses. Moreover, these transfection agents are not FDA approved to be used in the clinics. Mixing two FDA approved agents, ferumoxides (Feridex IV, Berlex, NJ) and protamine sulfate together form a complex that efficiently and effectively labels stem cells [29, 34, 35, 137–139]. Ferumoxides are dextran-coated colloidal iron oxide nanoparticles that magnetically saturate at low fields and have an extremely high NMR T2 relaxivity. Changes in R2 (R2=1/T2) are linear with respect to iron concentration. Protamine sulfate is an FDA-approved drug containing >60 percent arginine and is used for treatment of heparin anticoagulation overdose. Cells are labeled with the ferumoxides-protamine sulfate (FE-Pro) complex via macropinocytosis and can be imaged at clinically relevant MRI fields using standard imaging techniques.

The concentration of iron in cells is dependent on nuclear to cytoplasma ratio, the iron concentration in the nano- or micron-sized particles, iron content in media, incubation times, and method of endocytosis of the particles [33–35, 42]. Unlabeled stem cells usually contain less that 0.1 picogram of iron per cell, whereas labeled cells grown in suspension (i.e., HSCs, T-cells) contain 1–5 picograms of iron per cell and cells that adhere to culture dish (i.e., MSCs, HeLa, macrophages) can take up from 5 to >20 picograms of iron per cell [29, 34, 35]. Labeling cells with ferumoxides does not alter the viability and functional capability of cells or the differentiation capacity of stem cells [34, 140]. FE-Pro labeled embryonic, MSCs, HSC, and NSC showed similar rates of differentiation to different lineages, in comparison with unlabeled cells [34, 135, 140–142]. Recent articles showed the safe handling of SPIO nanoparticles by the cells [143, 144]. Soon after phagocytosis, iron particles remain within endosomes, and by days 3 to 5 these endosomes fuse with lysosomes and the iron oxides particles start to disintegrate [144]. Eddy et al. have shown that iron oxide labeling of HeLa and MSCs resulted in a transient decrease in transferrin receptor-1 (TfR-1) mRNA and protein levels. In contrast, iron oxides labeling of primary macrophages resulted in an increase in TfR-1 messenger ribonucleic acid (mRNA) but not in TfR-1 protein levels. Ferritin mRNA and protein levels increased transiently in labeled HeLa and macrophages but were sustained in MSCs [143].

11.3.4 Other Methods of Cell Labeling

Mechanical approaches such as the gene gun or electroporation have been used to effectively introduce MRI contrast agents into cells. The gene gun fires nanoparticles or magnetic beads directly into cells in culture, driving the particles through the cell membrane or directly into the nucleus; however, it is unknown what the long-term effects are on functional, metabolic, and differential capabilities of the cell [145]. Moreover the technique using particles has its own limitations with respect to efficiency, potential tissue damage created by the impact of the particles, and small area of coverage [146]. Since there are less traumatic methods to label cells with MR SPIO nanoparticles, it is unlikely that the gene gun approach will be used in the future. Direct injection of high concentrations of gadolinium chelates into Xenopus laevis eggs enable successful tracking of the labeled cell proliferation and migration during development using MRI and optical imaging [147]. However, this approach is not a practical or efficient method for labeling mammalian cells with MR contrast agents.

Electroporation has recently been used to label cells with gadolinium chelates and SPIO nanoparticles [39, 50]. Electroporation is commonly used to introduce DNA into the cell genome and well known to be associated with cell stress due to chemical imbalances and efflux or influx of chemicals from within the cell and surrounding media altering the cells viability and survival. There is relatively little experience using this approach with MRI contrast agents to label cells and it is unclear as to the long-term effects on reactive oxygen species or cell viability when using this method. Recently it has been shown that significant amount of cell lysis and death occurred during electroporation and following labeling of contrast agents [148]. It has been reported that magnetic labeling of embryonic stem cells using electroporation resulted in significant decrease in the percentage of viable cells compared to labeling cells with transfection agents complexed to ferumoxides [135]. In addition, by labeling embryonic stem cell (ESC) with ferumoxides by electroporation method, the ability of these cells to differentiate into cardiac progenitor cells was impaired, indicating that this method may not be clinically useful [135].

Magnetofection is a technique that utilizes strong magnetic force to introduce magnetic nanoparticle- or oligonucleotide- (i.e., DNA or RNA) coated SPIO nanoparticles into the cell, resulting in effective incorporation of the DNA into the cell genome [149–154]. However, direct delivery to the cell cytoplasm could be a deterrent for magnetic cell labeling because of possible toxicity following the release of iron into the nucleus. This technique is useful for rapid labeling only in adherent cells. Its utility for suspension cells or cells with small cytoplasm to nuclear ratio (such as T-cells and hematopoietic stem cells) has not been verified. Moreover, details on toxicity and nuclear uptake have not been described yet.

11.4 Methods to Monitor the Functional Status of Labeled Cells or Toxicity Following Labeling

Magnetic labeling of cells can be assessed qualitatively using Prussian blue stain for iron by identifying electron-dense material in endosomes by electron microscopy or by the using T2*W magnetic resonance imaging for determining the presences of iron in cells. Confocal microscopy is another method that can be utilized to determine the localization of magnetic particles that are tagged with fluorescent dye or proteins. Multiphoton confocal microscopy can determine the depth as well as location of iron particles in the cytoplasm or nucleus. Quantitative approaches commonly used to determine the amount of iron taken up by the cells include NMR relaxometery, spectrophotometric assays, and inductively coupled plasma mass spectrometry. Determination of intracellular iron is important in order to validate magnetic resonance imaging (MRI) techniques used to semiquantitate the number of labeled cells in a region of interest [33, 127, 130, 155]. The preservation of cell viability, cell function, and differential capacity of cells are the important measures that need to be monitored following labeling cells with MRI contrast agents because soluble iron (intracellular) is toxic to the cells and may damage DNA.

11.4.1 Determination of Cell Viability

Ionic or the transfection agents, which are used to label cells, are toxic to the cells. Ferrous forms in the cytoplasmic iron can stimulate the increased production of hydroperoxide and increase the amount of nascent hydroxyl free radicals that can cause denaturation of DNA [156–158]. Therefore, it is essential to determine the short- and long-term toxicity of labeling cells with iron in order to translate from bench to bedside. Cell viability is usually determined at time of cell counting using the trypan blue dye exclusion test. Propidium iodide (PI) can also be used to detect dead cells by fluorescent microscope or by flow cytometry. Changes in the rate of apoptosis, a long-term indication of (U)SPIO labeling of cells, can be accomplished by using incubating cells with fluorescent-labeled annexin V and PI, and analyzed using flow cytometry. Investigators have found that cell viability or rate of apoptosis is not different from unlabeled control cells when cells are labeled using any of the methods described earlier. Short- and long-term proliferation capacity of the labeled cells can be assessed by tritiated-thymidine uptake, BRDU incorporation, or MTT (3-[4,5-dimethylthiazol-2-yl]-2,5-diphenyl tetrazolium bromide) assay (Roche Molecular Biochemicals, Indianapolis, IN). Proliferative assays are usually preformed as a pulse chase labeling experiment with the (U)SPIO and determinations made at different time points [33]. The dissolving of (U)SPIO nanoparticles releasing ferrous ions in the cells or nucleus could initiate a Fenton reaction through Haber-Weiss chemistry [156] and result in the development of free radicals that could cause damage to DNA. Reactive oxygen species (ROS) can be detected by using the fluorescent probe CM-H_2DCFDA (Molecular Probes Inc., Eugene, OR). CM-H_2DCFDA is a nonfluorescent agent that forms fluorescent esters when reacted with reactive oxygen species (ROS) inside cells that can be detected by flow cytometry, fluorescent, or confocal microscopy. Pawelczyk et al. has demonstrated that following labeling of MSCs and macrophages with FE-Pro resulted in a transient decrease in gene and protein expression of the transferrin receptor while gene and protein levels of ferritin either remained stable or increased in response to the iron load [143]. These results indicate that FE-Pro labeling of cells elicited appropriate and expected physiological changes of iron metabolism or storage. To date, little or no alterations in cells viability, proliferative capacity, metabolic activity, apoptotic rate, reactive oxygen species (ROS) formation, and functional and differential capacity were reported for cells labeled with clinically approved (U)SPIO MR contrast agents when compared to unlabeled cells. Although previous studies

[159–161] indicated toxicity of TAT protein in cells, a recent publication indicated no short-term loss of cell viability or accumulation of CLIO-Tat in the nucleus [71].

11.4.2 Determination of Cell Function

It is also important that labeled cells should not deviate from their original function or get activated (in case of T-cells). Cellular functional assays should be performed after labeling and compared with that of control cells. Cell activation markers as well as phenotypic expression should be assessed for primary cell populations. Labeling lymphocytes (T-cells) with SPIO nanoparticles may change one population of T-cells (such as T helper cells) to another (such as cytotoxic T-cells). Analysis of different phenotypic cell surface marker expression (i.e., CD markers, CD4, CD8, CD11a, CD19, CD25) of T-cells and production of cytokines (interferons, interleukins, and so on) should be performed before and after labeling immune cells. For stem cells, primary as well as lineage markers should be assessed before and after labeling with MR contrast agents.

11.4.3 Determination of Cell Differentiation Capacity

Determination of differentiation capacity of labeled cells is especially important for nonhematopoietic stem cells such as MSCs and NSCs. MSC should be differentiated to adipogenic, chondrogenic, and osteogenic lineages. For HSC, differentiation to colony-forming units (CFUs) should be determined for labeled and unlabeled cells. Endothelial progenitor cells (EPC) can be differentiated to colony-forming units, endothelial cells, and cord-like structures in matrigel system. NSC should be differentiated to neuronal and/or glial cell lineages. Differentiation capacity of magnetically labeled cells can also be determined by tracking the in vivo migration and targeted incorporation or labeled stem cells in different organs [162].

11.5 MRI Techniques to Detect Cells Labeled with Superparamagnetic Iron Oxides

A variety of conventional MR imaging techniques can be used to determine the presence of iron in various tissues over a wide range of magnetic field strengths. In general, MRI methods for the detection of SPIO labeled cells usually consist of T2 or T2* imaging sequences because of the significant signal dephasing due to the magnetic field (B_0) in-homogeneities induced in water molecules in and near the cells. Differentiation between signal loss caused by the intracellular SPIO nanoparticles and native low signal in tissue can be a challenging risk. In addition, partial volume effects, motion, blood flow, or hemorrhage can all mask the presence of the magnetically labeled cells within tissues. To improve the sensitivity to track magnetically labeled stem cells or other cells, several positive contrast or white marker pulse sequences have been developed [163–166]. The signal intensities on MRI surrounding the SPIO nanoparticles have a characteristic barbell pattern and have been theoretically derived for a single dipole in a homogeneous magnetic field [167]. The off-resonance positive contrast pulse sequences allow for visualization of high signal intensities against a suppressed background in regions containing SPIO labeled cells [163–167].

The development of a post-processing positive contrast technique called susceptibility gradient mapping (SGM) has allowed for the detection of magnetically labeled cells in tissues [167, 168]. The SGM method is based on the theory that an object with a magnetic susceptibility deviates from its surroundings, thereby creating a local magnetic gradient that leads to an echo shift in k-space with gradient echo imaging. The SGM method determines the amount of the shift of the echo for every voxel in all three spatial dimensions by local one-dimensional fast Fourier transform used in generating a vector map of the susceptibility gradient. The SGM avoids the use of dedicated positive contrast pulse sequences and does not require a priori knowledge about the local SPIO nanoparticle's concentration. Comparison of the gradient compensation–based approach "white marker technique" [165–166] and an off-resonance based approach inversion recovery ON-resonance water suppress (IRON) technique [164] with the SGM method was performed in a SPIO-labeled flank tumor model in rats. The SGM, white marker, and IRON positive contrast images were acquired when the labeled tumors were between 5–20 mm in diameter to evaluate their sensitivity to the dilution of the SPIO nanoparticles as the tumor cells proliferated [167]. For small and medium-sized tumors, quantitation of the number of positive pixels (NPP) detected within the tumor for the SGM was significantly larger for the other two techniques. For large tumors, SGM resulted in similar NPP as the white marker technique, whereas the IRON method failed to generate positive contrast images. These results indicate that post-processing approaches can be useful in detecting a localized focus of magnetically labeled cells in vivo. However, when the number of SPIO labeled cells was low in a region of interest or if labeled cells were diffusely spread throughout the tissue, all three techniques were unreliable in displaying positive contrast enhancement.

Quantifying the number of labeled stem cells in target tissues is of great importance to optimize dose and timing of cellular therapy. T2 spin echo imaging has been used to quantify the amount of iron within tissue. By determining the T2 relaxation times at 0.5 Tesla and 1.5 Tesla using a multiple spin echo technique, Bulte et al. [169] demonstrated a linear relationship between the T2 relaxation rates and iron content obtained from marmosets with hemosiderosis an iron storage disease. However, T2 is sensitive to both concentration and distribution of SPIO nanoparticles, which greatly complicates its use for quantifying iron-oxide concentration. To achieve high sensitivity for the detection of intracellular SPIO nanoparticles, the T2* relaxation rate of the tissue should be measured [170, 171]. Multigradient echo pulse sequence can be used to determine the T2* relaxation times of the magnetically labeled cells in phantoms and tissues, and that can be used to approximate the number of labeled cells within a voxel [172]. Unfortunately, T2* relaxation rate is influenced not only by SPIO nanoparticles in labeled cells, but also by macroscopic susceptibilities due to differing tissues types. Several other methods have been proposed to correct for the macroscopic magnetic susceptibility [173–177]. It is also possible that the use of ultrashort echo time pulse sequences samples the water protons magnetization at <100 microseconds prior to the dephasing of the water proton spins due to the presence of directly implanted SPIO labeled cells in tissues, and this should allow for the ability to produce more accurate T2* maps for quantifying the number of iron-containing cells in tissues. The development of new MRI scanner hardware and pulse sequences, along with analysis and segmentation software, may improve the sensitivity and delineate various iron-containing pathologies from magnetically labeled cells in tissues.

11.6 Animal Studies That Have Utilized CMRI

Since the start of cell labeling with SPIO, there is great interest in and enthusiasm to use the labeled cells to track the migration and homing in different disease conditions in animal models using clinically relevant or high magnetic field MR scanners. Investigators have labeled various types of cells in order to track the administered cells by MRI for the purposes of diagnosing the disease conditions or for monitoring therapeutic effects. In this section we will discuss various reports on tracking labeled cells in different disease models.

11.6.1 Stem Cell Tracking

Cell labeling with iron oxide and cellular MRI techniques has enabled investigators to follow implanted cells in vivo and to monitor their effects in experimental animal models. Neural stem cells or neural progenitor cells have been labeled with various SPIO nanoparticles and the fate of labeled, implanted cells was tracked in normal brains of neonatal or adult animals [142, 145], in stroke [178], in traumatic brains, or in spinal cord injuries [179, 180]. Investigators have shown the migration of magnetically labeled oligodendrocyte progenitor cells (CG-4) away from the sites of implantation in the spinal cord in myelin-deficient rats by MRI, and the areas covered by the migratory CG-4 cells were correlated with the myelination of pathology in the spinal cord [84]. In the subsequent study, these investigators also showed the utility of magnetic labeling in a long-term followup of implanted neural progenitor cell derived oligodendroglial progenitor cells in rat models using clinical strength MRI system [64]. Investigators have also used cellular MRI to follow the implanted stem cells (both locally and systemically administrated) in stroke, traumatic brain injury, and spinal cord injury models. In a recent paper, Guzman et al. labeled NSCs with ferumoxides to monitor the migration and site-specific differentiation of these implanted cells in neonatal and adult rodent brains and in a brain injury models with CMRI imaging [142]. The authors concluded than implementation of noninvasive stem cell tracking might help to improve the design of future clinical NSC transplantation trends. Labeled NSCs, MSCs, or other stem cells have also been used in various brain or spinal cord injury models to track the migration and homing of these labeled cells by cellular MRI [179–183].

11.6.2 Intracranial Tumor Studies

Glioma is a central nervous system neoplasm that typically exhibits hypervascularity, especially in grade III and IV tumors, with marked heterogeneity in histological markers and vascular density. Malignant gliomas are among the most devastating tumors, with the survival of only one to three years after diagnosis. Surgery and radiation therapy (followed by adjuvant chemotherapy) very often fail due to uncertainty in delineating the tumor margins [184]. Moreover, due to the infiltrative nature of glioblastoma multiforme (GBM), it is impossible to remove 100 percent of tumor mass during surgery, and the left over tumor cells might be more aggressive and resistant to future therapies. Therefore, as pointed out by Hentschel and Sawaya, successful therapeutic approaches would depend on developing high-quality imaging modalities [185]. Chopp et al. have shown that magnetically labeled MSC can identify the sites of angiogenesis at the margin of the tumor and normal brain tissues [186]. The same group has used NSC in a rodent brain tumor model and tracked the implanted cells by MRI using magnetic labeling techniques. Magnetically labeled exogenous monocyte/macrophages have also been tracked migrating into an implanted rat glioma model [187]. We also observed (unpublished data) the migration of magnetically labeled dendritic cells to the sites of U-251 implanted glioma in rats (Figure 11.2), which was detected by 3-Tesla clinical MRI systems.

11.6.3 Tumor Angiogenesis

Angiogenesis is essential for tumor growth and the development of metastasis [188]. Migration and proliferation of endothelial cells originating from local capillaries is thought to be the primary mechanism for angiogenesis in the adults in the presence of pro-angiogenic stimuli. There are reports suggesting that bone marrow–derived EPCs also contribute to the endothelial lining of adult neovasculature in both physiological and pathological angiogenesis [189, 190]. The incorporation of EPCs from the circulation into newly formed vessels is termed *vasculogenesis*. It has been shown that genetically modified EPCs can selectively deliver a cytotoxic gene to

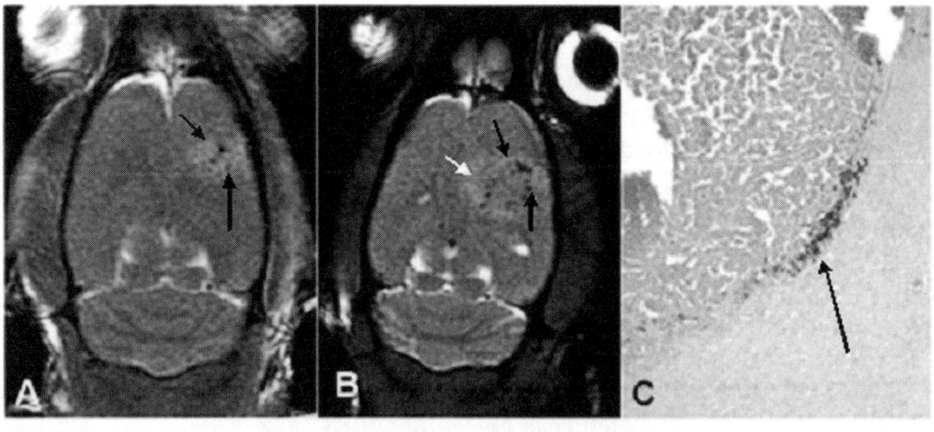

Figure 11.2 Representative case of magnetically labeled dendritic cell tracking in an implanted brain tumor in a rat model by a clinical 3T MRI system. Tumors were created in nude rats by implanting U251 glioma cell line. (a) MRI obtained using FIESTA sequence 14 days after implantation of tumor cells but before administration of magnetically labeled dendritic cells shows the margin of the tumor (arrows). Note the small low signal intensity foci in the center of the tumor due to bleeding during implantation of tumor cells. (b) MRI obtained from the same animal three days after intravenous administration of magnetically labeled dendritic cells shows multiple low signal intensity foci around the tumor (black arrows). Note the growth of the tumor beyond the accumulated dendritic cells (tumor margin, white arrow). (c) DAB-enhanced Prussian blue staining shows iron positive cells at the margin of the tumor (arrow).

tumor-induced neovasculature [191, 192]. To determine if MRI could be used to monitor the vasculogenesis associated with tumor growth, Anderson et al. intravenously infused 5×10^5 ferumoxides –poly-l-lysine FE-PLL–labeled bone marrow–derived HSC (Sca1+) into mice with implanted RT2 rat glioma in the brain [125]. Animals were implanted with tumors and ferumoxides –poly-l-lysine (FE-PLL)–labeled Sca1+ cells infused on day three post implantation or mice were sublethally irradiated and labeled cells were infused followed by implantation of tumor in the brains of SCID mice. MRI was performed at 7 Tesla and, 5 to 12 days after labeled Sca1+ cells were given intravenously to mice. T2*-weighted MRI in mice receiving labeled cells demonstrated hypointense regions within the tumor that evolved over time. In addition, a hypointense ring at the periphery of the tumor was observed by days 10–13 post infusions of labeled Sca1+ cells. Histological examination revealed Prussian blue (PB) positive cells around the tumor rim in mice that received labeled Sca1+ cells. These PB positive cells were CD31 and von Willebrand factor (vWF) positive, indicating that the infused labeled Sca1+ cells detected in the tumor have differentiated into endothelial cells and became part of neovasculature. These results demonstrate that MRI can detect the incorporation of magnetically labeled bone marrow–derived EPCs into tumor vasculature as part of ongoing angiogenesis and neovascularization. This was the first report to demonstrate high-resolution noninvasive MRI of EPC's incorporation into tumor neovasculature. Figure 11.3 shows the utilization of human endothelial progenitor cells as MRI probe to identify the margin of implanted human glioma (U-251 tumor) based on active angiogenesis.

In 2006, Arbab et al. [123] performed a study in which FE-Pro labeled human HSCs (i.e., CD34 CD 133 cells) were administered to nude mice with rapidly growing RT2 glioma in their flanks. Animals received 3×10^6 FE-Pro labeled or unlabeled CD 34 CD 133 cells synchronously when a tumor was implanted or when a tumor reached 2 mm in size. In vivo MR at 7 Tesla demonstrated linear hypointense regions within the flank tumors that had grown to = 1 cm (i.e., = day seven post implantation) in animals receiving the intravenous injection of FE-Pro labeled cells, as compared to animals that received unlabeled cells. This linear feathering-type pattern observed in mice that received labeled cells was easily differentiated as small and well-defined dark features, compared to the changes in signal intensity in large tumors of either labeled or unlabeled mice, some of which developed amorphous dark areas in the tumor images indicative of necrosis in tumors (=1.5 cm). MRI detected the presence of FE-Pro labeled CD 34 CD 133 cells in the flank tumors as early as three days post infusion of cells. Histological examination revealed positive human endothelial markers (e.g., CD 31, KDR1, vWF, and CD106) indicating endothelial transformation of the administered FE-Pro labeled or unlabeled cells and incorporation into the tumor neovasculature. Corresponding consecutive sections revealed PB positive cells in the same region as cells with positive markers for human endothelial cells. A few PB cells at the periphery of the tumor were positive for human macrophage marker (hCD68 positive cells), indicating that some of the administered FE-Pro labeled CD 34 CD 133 cells differentiated toward the macrophage lineage. These results demonstrate that HSC could be labeled with FE-Pro in a clinical good manufacturing practice (cGMP) facility and

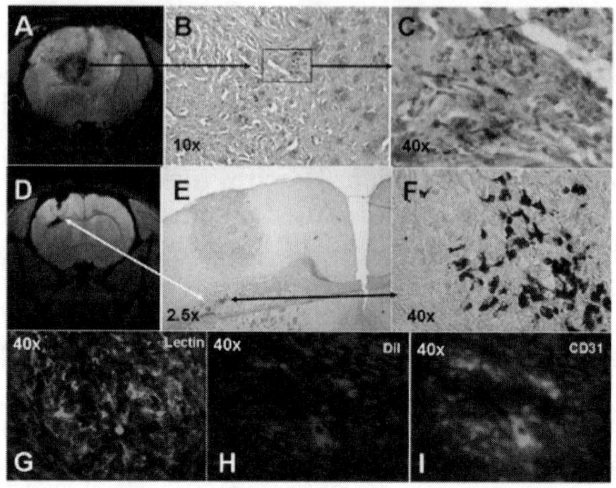

Figure 11.3 Representative cases of magnetically labeled endothelial progenitor cells' (EPCs) tracking in an implanted brain tumor in a rat model by 7 Tesla MR system. Tumors were created in nude rats by implanting U251 glioma cell line. Double-labeled (iron plus dye DiI) EPCs were administered on day seven after tumor implantation, and MRI was obtained on day 14 (seven days after intravenous administration of magnetically labeled EPCs). Panels A to C: T2*-weighted MRI image shows low signal intensity areas surrounding the tumor, indicating accumulation of magnetically labeled cells (A), which are confirmed by Prussian blue staining in the corresponding histological section (10x, B) and (40x, C). Note the blue cells within the box in the B and in C panels. Panels D to F: T2*W images show hypointense voxels around and in the tumor extension in the corpus callosum (white arrows in D and E). DAB-enhanced Prussian blue staining shows iron positive cells (E and F). Panels G to I: The section stained for endothelial lining (G, FITC-labeled tomato lectin) shows extensive formation of new vessels within the tumor, and the corresponding area (shown in the consecutive section) also shows DiI positive cells (H, red cells), which are also positive for endothelial cell marker CD31 (I, green cells). Nuclei of the cells are stained with DAPI (blue). (See Color Plate 22.)

used to detect by MRI the incorporation of magnetically labeled bone marrow–derived HSCs into tumor vasculature as part of ongoing angiogenesis.

11.6.4 Stroke and Trauma Models

There have been several studies demonstrating in rodent stroke models the ability to monitor the migration of labeled stem cells following implantation in the contralateral hemisphere to the cerebral pathology or intravenous infusion [193–199]. Hoehn et al. [200] were the first to demonstrate the transcallosal migration of 3×10^4 intracerebrally implanted sinerem (USPIO) fugene (transfection agent)–labeled embryonic stem cells over a period of eight days by MRI in a rat stroke model. The embryonic stem cells were also tagged with green fluorescent protein and the authors were able to correlate immunohistochemial results to hypointense voxels in the subventricular zone and surrounding the infracted hemisphere. Zhang et al. [178] observed on T2*W MRI that magnetically labeled neural stem cells injected into a cistern were able to enter into the cerebral parenchyma into an area of cerebral ischemia at a rate of 65 μm/hr. In a followup study, Jiang et al.

[194] labeled subventricular zone neural stem cells with SPIO nanoparticles in a rat stroke model and tracked the cells into area of cerebral infarction by MRI. Based on dynamic contrast enhanced cerebral perfusion studies, the authors were able to demonstrate an increase in angiogenesis in the area of cerebral infarction as a result of infusion of NSCs. These results indicate that magnetic labeling of stem cells does not interfere with the ability to assess cerebral physiology in a stroke model. Jendelova et al. [198] intravenously injected rat MSCs colabeled with ferumoxides and bromodeoxyuridine (BrdU) following the infusion of Bengal rose and light to induce photochemical lesions. In vivo MRI was used to track the fate of the cells with PB staining and transmission electron microscopy confirmed the presence of iron-oxide nanoparticles inside the cells. One week after infusion of the magnetically labeled MSCs, hypointense voxels were detected on T2*-weighted MRI at the lesion site and populated the border zone of the damaged cortical parenchyma. Labeled cells were identified on histology at one month post injection of rat MSCs. The results of these studies indicate the potential of cellular MRI to track labeled stem cells to areas of cerebral ischemia and stroke independent of route of administration. Figure 11.4 shows the migration of NSCs in a rat stroke model.

Magnetic labeling of endothelial precusor cells is possible during the cell separation process using immunomagnetic beads. The immunomagnetic beads are clinical grade material similar to the MPIOs used for positive or negative selection of cells. Jendelova et al. [199] selected CD34 HSCs and found that these cells inefficiently endocytosed the beads. After direct implantation of the CD 34 into a contralateral hemisphere to a photochemically injured rat cortex, the migration of these cells by MRI into the subventricular zone and around the cortical lesion by PB stain was shown. The same group demonstrated the migration of ferumoxide-labeled human MSCs in a spinal cord injury model [201]. However, since the model is associated with hemorrhage, it was difficult for these investigators to clearly demonstrate differences between endogenous iron (i.e., hemosiderin) and SPIO labeled cells by T2*W MRI. Dunning et al. [202] evaluated the migration patterns of SPIO-labeled schwann cells or olfactory ensheathing cells (OEC), following a demylenation injury model in the rat spinal cord. These authors noted in animals that received unlabeled OECs that there were PB positive cells present in area of lesion similar to animals that received magnetically labeled cells. MRI at the center of the lesions from the three groups of rats were similar demonstrating hypointense regions on T2*W images; however, it was possible to track the migration of the labeled cells further in the spinal cord in animals that received magnetically labeled schwann cells and OECs. These results underscore one of the limitations in tracking SPIO labeled cells and the inability to distinguish areas of endogenous iron due to hemorrhage or hemosiderin from infused or implanted cells.

11.6.5 Myocardial Infarction and Vascular Models

There have been several excellent reviews on the monitoring by MRI of magnetically labeled stem cells in experimental animals for the treatment of myocardial ischemia and infarction with the goal of improving cardiac function, angiogenesis and perfusion, and limiting or decreasing the size of damage [203–206]. The reader is encouraged to seek out many of these reviews. One of the first studies to monitor

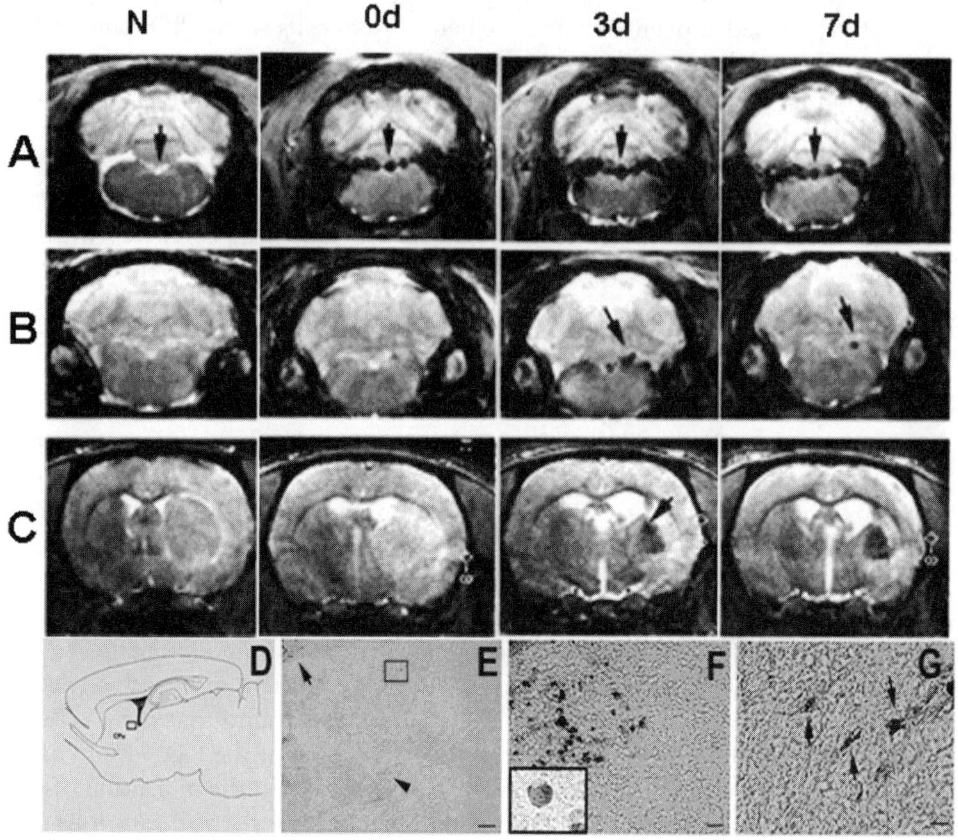

Figure 11.4 Dynamic migration of iron labeled transplanted subventricular zone (SVZ) neural stem cells in ischemic brain in a representative ischemic rat. MRI signals (dark areas) were not detected before transplantation of labeled SVZ cells (A, N to C, N). In contrast, the same rat exhibited MRI signals at the fourth ventricle on the day of injection of ferromagnetic particle–labeled cells into the cistern (A, 0d, arrow). MRI signals moved forward along the fourth ventricle and reached the ipsilateral striatum nearby the ipsilateral lateral ventricle two to three days after transplantation (C, 3d, arrow). MRI signal in the ipsilateral striatum increased during three to seven days after transplantation (C, 7d). MRI signals were not detected in the contralateral hemisphere at any time point after transplantation (C, 0d to 7d). Panels A to C represent different levels of coronal sections from the posterior to anterior brain (A, bregma –13.3 mm; B, bregma –11.8 mm; and C, bregma –1.3 mm). N represents one day before transplantation and 0d to 7d indicate days after transplantation from a representative rat. To identify ferromagnetic particle–labeled cells on sagittal or coronal sections, Prussian blue staining was performed. Panel D is a schematic representation of a sagittal section from the ipsilateral hemisphere at lateral 1.40 mm. Panels E to G are microphotography of Prussian blue–stained sections from the same rat in which MRI images were presented. Panel E is from the boxed area in panel D. The arrow in panel E indicates transplanted cells around the ischemic boundary. Higher magnification revealed that these cells had round morphology (F and insert). A box and an arrowhead in panel E show transplanted cells at a distance from the ischemic boundary, and these cells exhibited bipolar morphology (G), indicating that these cells migrate. (Courtesy of Dr. Zheng Gang Zhang of Neurology, Henry Ford Hospital, used with the permission of *Annals of Neurology*.) For details, please see [178].

migration of MPIO-labeled MSC in a myocardial infarction model was performed at the National Heart Lung and Blood Institute at the National Institutes of Health. MPIO-labeled swine MSCs were implanted through an intra-arterial catheter placed in the heart and injected directly into and around the myocardial infarction using MRI guidance [119, 120]. T2*-weighted MRI [207] was used to monitor the migration of cells in a myocardium that was correlated with histology. These studies illustrated the need in testing and evaluating the different routes of administration of labeled cells and the importance of determining viability following passage through an arterial catheter. Similar results have been observed in MI models in which stem cells improved cardiac function and decreased infarction size (Figure 11.5) [208]. Recently, Kraitchman et al. [209] infused MSCs labeled with indium^{111} oxine and ferumoxides and reported focal and diffuse uptake of MSC in the infarcted myocardium by single photon emission tomography (SPECT/CT) at seven days post injection of cells. However, ferumoxide-labeled MSCs that were detected

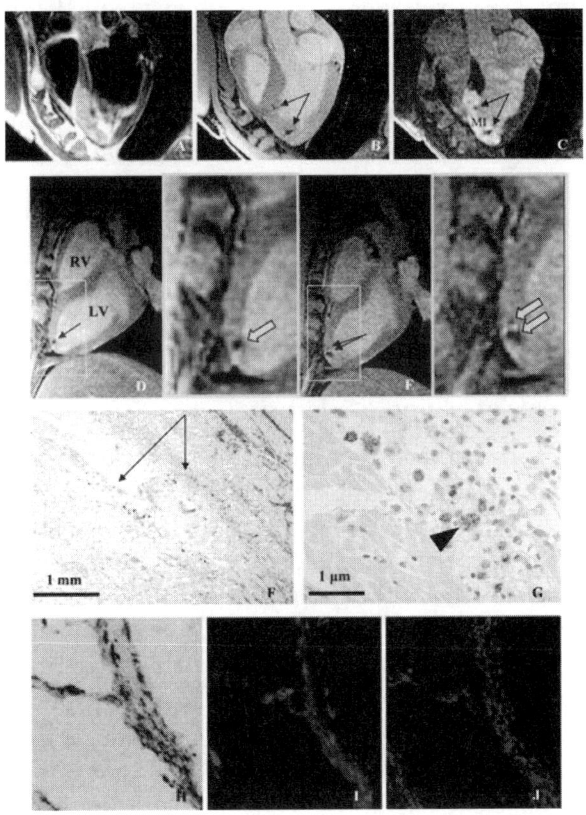

Figure 11.5 Representative hypointense lesions in FSE (A), FGRE (B), and DE-MRI (C) of MR-MSC injection sites (arrows) within 24 hr of injection. MR-MSCs were injected in the infarct (MI, hyperintense region in C). Long-axis MRIs showing hypointense lesions (arrows) caused by MR-MSCs acquired within 24 hr (D) and one week (E) of injection, with inset at right demonstrating expansion of lesion over one week. Needle tract (arrow) of MR-MSCs is demonstrated in the histological section at one week after injection with Prussian blue staining (F) as cells with blue iron inclusions (arrowhead) that are excluded from nucleus (G). Iron inclusion from DAB-enhanced Prussian blue staining (H) matches colabeling with DiI (I) and DAPI fluorescent dyes (J) on adjacent histological sections at ×20 magnification at 24 hr after MSC injection in another animal, indicating Feridex is still contained within original MSCs. LV indicates left ventricle; RV, right ventricle. (See Color Plate 23.) (Used with permission of *Circulation.*)

by PB staining around the rim of the infarction were not observed on MRI at 1.5 Tesla using gradient echo pulse sequence with a short echo time. The authors concluded that MRI has lower sensitivity to detect dual-labeled MSC in comparison to radionuclide approaches. This study demonstrated the need to develop novel MRI techniques to detect the presence of distributed magnetically labeled cells within target tissues.

There are a number of studies suggesting that circulating macrophages will endocytosis magnetic nanoparticles that are intravenously given [139]. Wu et al. infused MPIOs in a rat model of cardiac rejection [121] and visualized that "single" labeled macrophage in the rejected heart. These authors did not demonstrate whether the MPIOs were taken up by circulating monocytes or possibly in regional lymph nodes or by macrophages resident with rejected organ. It should be possible by obtaining tissue or blood samples or MRI to figure out where the MPIO particles were endocytosed by macrophages in this model. In vivo tagging of macrophages with SPIO nanoparticles may also be useful for characterizing organ rejection [73]. Focal hypointense voxels were detected on ex vivo MRI that could be differentiated from the infiltration of USPIO into extravascular spaces in the rejected heart. These results suggested the possibility of monitoring organ transplantation rejection using magnetic nanoparticles and noninvasive imaging techniques.

MRI has also been able to detect the migration of intravenously injected ferumoxide-labeled bone marrow stem cells into areas of sites of injured arteries [210] or trafficking to areas of atherosclerotic plaques [211]. Labeled cells could be detected in thickened adventitia injured arteries by MRI on T2*W images, Imaging results were correlated to histology suggesting the use of cellular MRI in assessing vascular damage.

11.6.6 Models of Multiple Sclerosis

Multiple Sclerosis (MS) is an inflammatory and demyelinating disease of the central nervous system that affects approximately 350,000 young adults in North America. The theories behind the development of MS lesions are based primarily upon studies performed in an experimental allergic encephalomyelitis (EAE) model in the [212] mouse and more recently the marmoset [213]. The adoptive transfer (AT) of sensitized T-cells into SJL WCE results in a relapsing-remitting (RR) EAE disease course that is similar RRMS patients. Trafficking of T-cells across the blood-brain barrier is considered an essential component in the development of the inflammatory process in the CNS in the EAE mouse model and in MS. In 2004, Anderson et al. [124] labeled encephalitogenic T-cells with FE-PLL and adoptively transferred 2×10^7 labeled or unlabeled cells into mice to induce EAE. Labeled T-cells containing an average of 1–3 picograms of iron per cell were PB positive on histology. In vivo MR microscopy was performed on days 8–15 post-AT EAE according to clinical score. FE-PLL labeled T-cells were viable and demonstrated strong proliferative recall response to myelin. Flow cytometric analysis of unlabeled and FE-PLL–labeled cells showed similar numbers of CD4 T-cells in each population expressing similar T-cell phenotypes. In vivo MR microscopy demonstrated FE-PLL–labeled T-cells within EAE lesions as either focal hypointense areas within the white matter or areas of diffuse hypointensities suggesting an infiltrative process. MR microscopy correlated well with histology, and PB positive cells were detected in spinal cord of mice [124]. This was the first demonstration of the migration of sensitized T-cells into an EAE lesion into the spinal cord of a mouse on in vivo MR microscopy. Magnetic cell labeling studies in MS and other diseases could be used to monitor specific cellular phenotypes (CD 4 or CD 8 T-cells, tumor infiltrating lymphocytes, or dendritic cells) or pharmacologically or genetically engineered cells by MRI, advancing the understanding and potential of directing cell therapy to specific sites of disease.

Stem cell therapy is being explored as a potential new treatment for demyelinating diseases. Pluchino, et al. demonstrated the homing of synergenic adult neural stem cells into lesions and saw improvement in the disease course following intravenous injection into an EAE mouse model [214]. Recent studies have shown the potential of either MSCs or NSCs in attenuating or modulating the immune response of EAE [215–217]. Intravenous administration of single or multiple doses of MSCs prior to or at the start of the first neurological event were shown to be effective in causing a significantly milder EAE course compared to control animals. However, when MSCs were given after the first exacerbation, there was no significant alteration in clinical course. Bulte et al. administered ferumoxide-labeled neuronal pluripotent stem cells at the peak of the EAE disease in rats that were allowed to recover and subsequently euthanized one week later [218]. Ex vivo MR microscopy demonstrated clear migration of labeled stem cells into the white matter, as compared to control animals in which minimal dissemination of cells was observed. Ben-Hur et al. [219] transplanted ferumoxide-labeled NSC into mice with chronic EAE and were able to monitor the rate of migration of the cells over time. There was a linear correlation between the distance of cell migration with clinical severity of disease and the number of microglia in the white matter tracts, supporting the notion that inflammatory signals promote transplanted cell migration. These authors could not clearly demonstrate a beneficial effect of the NSCs on a clinical course. Recently, Politi et al. [220] infused SPIO-labeled NSC 17 days after induction of EAE and detected hypointense regions developing in areas of blood-brain barrier disruption on MRI. These imaging findings were consistent with inflammation in the mouse brain. The hypointense regions contained PB positive neurons on histology and demonstrated that most of the infused labeled NSCs were located in areas of periventricular white matter lesions. In addition, EAE mice that received the neural stem cells had lower clinical scores compared to control animals, suggesting that this type of cellular therapy may play a role in patients with multiple sclerosis.

11.7 Translation to the Clinic

11.7.1 Human Studies

There are only two early-phase clinical trials in the literature using MRI to monitor the migration of ferumoxide-labeled cells. de Vries et al. investigated on a phase I clinical trial the biodistribution of magnetically labeled dendritic cells [221]. The dendritic cells were first transformed from monocytes that were labeled with ferumoxides for 2 days and intubated in appropriately conditioned media. They were then transplanted directly into lymph nodes of patients with melanoma, and the temporal spatial migration of these cells were serially monitored by MRI through lymphatic vessels into adjacent lymph nodes. This was the first clinical trial to demonstrate the utility of labeling cells with ferumoxides for monitoring cellular therapy. These investigators were able to delineate whether labeled cells were actually implanted into lymph nodes or surrounding subcutaneous fat. In this study, the authors indicated that MRI could detect approximately 2,000 ferumoxide-labeled dendritic cells per voxel. Improvements in MRI techniques should allow for the detection of fewer numbers of labeled cells within a region of interest.

Zhu et al. [222] reported a study in a small group of patients who had suffered traumatic brain injury with open head trauma. They had cells extracted and were place in cultures and labeled with ferumoxides. In this early phase trial, patients received intracerebral injections of ferumoxide-labeled or -unlabeled "neuronal cells" around the area of injured brain based on T2-weighted images. Serial MRIs over 21 days demonstrated the migration of ferumoxide-labeled NSCs from injections sites into white and gray matter that was not observed in patients receiving unlabeled cells. The authors did not report any neurological complications as a result of implanting cells into patients with brain trauma (Figure 11.6).

11.7.2 Regulatory Issues

The translation of novel superparamagnetic iron oxide nanoparticles from experimental studies to clinical applications will require a significant amount of preparation and perseverance by the investigator in order to successfully evaluate the agent in a phase I clinical trial. It is crucial that investigators to establish an early dialogue with the appropriate regulatory agencies such as the Food and Drug Administration (FDA) to discuss the preclinical experimental studies that would be needed to finally perform clinical trials with the novel magnetic nanoparticles. Unfortunately, labeling cells with novel SPIO nanoparticles for cellular MRI does not fall under the guidelines provided by the FDA for exploratory investigative new drugs (IND), and therefore preparation by the investigator will be required so that these agents can be used for labeling cells [223]. The FDA will require certification and possible reformulation of the novel SPIO nanoparticles in a good laboratory practice (GLP) facility in addition to the preclinical evaluation before filing an IND as part of an early phase clinical trial. Research groups planning on using novel SPIO nanoparticles to label cells will need to demonstrate the following: (1) the novel SPIO nanoparticles are nontoxic to the cells or experimental animals (i.e., mice, rats, or larger animals); (2) the agent has a large therapeutic window (i.e., lethal dose 50 percent level) for the product; (3) the agent does not alter cell proliferation and viability, change differentiation capacity, or result in an increase in reactive oxygen species or apoptosis compared to control unlabeled cells; and (4) there is standardization of the composition of the contrast agent, along with the ability to reproducibly manufacture the agent. In addition, in order to use the novel SPIO agent in clinical trials, the investigator will need to demonstrate the following: (1) all products and instrumentation used in making the agent are approved for clinical use or an exemption from the FDA will be required to use these products for clinical use in cell labeling; (2) cell labeling with the novel agent can be performed using good manufacturing practices in an approved facility; (3) the cGMP facility should follow approved standard oper-

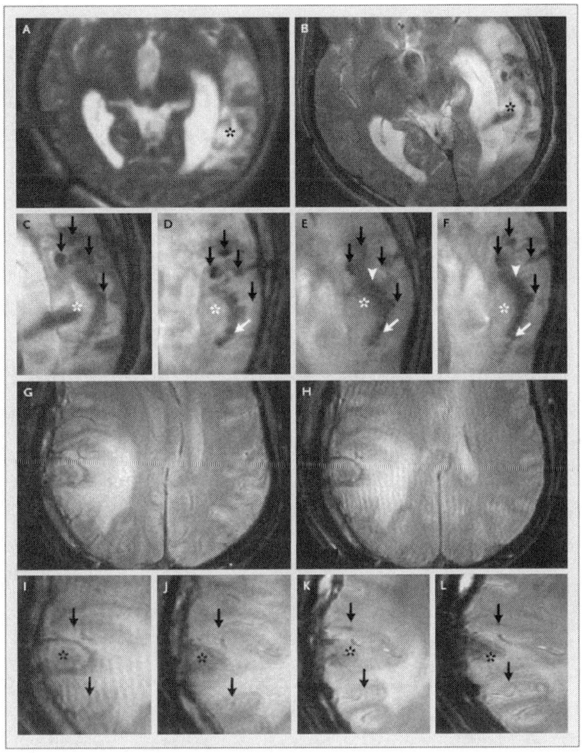

Figure 11.6 MRI scans from the patient who received neural stem cells labeled with iron oxide nanoparticles (panels A through F) and the patient who received unlabeled cells (panels G through L). The scan obtained before the implantation of the labeled neural stem cells (panel A) did not show a pronounced hypointense signal around the lesion (asterisk) in the left temporal lobe, whereas circular areas of hypointense signals were visible at the injection sites one day after implantation (panel B). Magnified images are shown in panels C through F. Four hypointense signals (black arrows) were observed at injection sites around the lesion on day 1 (panel C), day 7 (panel D), day 14 (panel E), and day 21 (panel F). On day 7 (panel D), we observed dark signals (white arrow) posterior to the lesion, a finding that was consistent with the presence of the labeled cells. By day 14 (panel E), the hypointense signals at the injection sites had faded, and another dark signal (white arrowhead) had appeared and spread along the border of the damaged brain tissue. By day 21 (panel F), the dark signal had thickened and extended further along the lesion (white arrow). The scans in Panels G and H, from the patient who underwent implantation of unlabeled cells, were obtained on days 0 and 1, respectively, and the magnified views in Panels I, J, K, and L were obtained on days 1, 7, 14, and 21, respectively. A slightly hypointense signal is present around the injection sites in panels I, J, K, and L. In these panels, the black arrows indicate the hypointense signal, and the asterisks indicate the lesion. (Used with the permission of the *New England Journal of Medicine.*)

ating procedures for handling, processing, and evaluating stem cells or other cells and be able to perform labeling on large scale; (4) the cGMP facility would be required to maintain an audit trail of the cells obtained from the subject that will be used for transplantation; (5) the labeled cells have similar viability as unlabeled cells without significant loss during the labeling process; (6) the phenotype of the cells is unaltered as result of the labeling with magnetic nanoparticles; and (7) there are no toxins or infectious (viral) agents present in the resulting product that would be released to the subjects in a clinical trial.

Preclinical studies performed in experimental disease models will probably include the infusion of magnetically labeled and unlabeled cells, along with sham controls and assessment of toxicity. Serum chemistries and complete blood count evaluations will probably be required. MRI studies of the experimental animals can be performed using either clinical scanners or higher field strength scanners routinely used for MRI in rodents. MRI results should be correlated to histology. Of note, prior to the study it will be important to identify and validate the immuno-histochemical techniques that will be used to assess the presence of magnetically labeled cells in tissues. An approved Intramural Review Board clinical protocol will be required for each cell type and potential patient population that would receive labeled cells. Developing methods of tracking of magnetically labeled cells should involve a multidisciplinary approach and teams of clinicians and scientists working together on cells in the evaluation of novel cellular therapies.

References

[1] Brazelton, T.R. and Blau, H.M., "Optimizing techniques for tracking transplanted stem cells in vivo," *Stem Cells*, Vol. 23, No. 9, 2005, pp. 1251–1265.

[2] Blits, B., et al., "Lentiviral vector-mediated transduction of neural progenitor cells before implantation into injured spinal cord and brain to detect their migration, deliver neurotrophic factors and repair tissue," *Restor Neurol Neurosci*, Vol. 23, No. 5-6, 2005, pp. 313–324.

[3] Tanaka, M., et al., "In vivo visualization of cardiac allograft rejection and trafficking passenger leukocytes using bioluminescence imaging," *Circulation*, Vol. 112, No. 9 Suppl, 2005, pp. I105–110.

[4] Paulmurugan, R. and Gambhir, S.S., "Novel fusion protein approach for efficient high-throughput screening of small molecule-mediating protein-protein interactions in cells and living animals," *Cancer Res*, Vol. 65, No. 16, 2005, pp. 7413–7420.

[5] Paulmurugan, R. and Gambhir, S.S., "Firefly luciferase enzyme fragment complementation for imaging in cells and living animals," *Anal Chem*, Vol. 77, No. 5, 2005, pp. 1295–1302.

[6] Bruchez, M.P., "Turning all the lights on: quantum dots in cellular assays," *Curr Opin Chem Biol*, Vol. 9, No. 5, 2005, pp. 533–537.

[7] Akerman, M.E., et al., "Nanocrystal targeting in vivo," *Proc Natl Acad Sci U S A*, Vol. 99, No. 20, 2002, pp. 12617–12621.

[8] Michalet, X., et al., "Quantum dots for live cells, in vivo imaging, and diagnostics," *Science*, Vol. 307, No. 5709, 2005, pp. 538–544.

[9] Potapova, I.A., et al., "Mesenchymal stem cells support migration, extracellular matrix invasion, proliferation, and survival of endothelial cells in vitro," *Stem Cells*, Vol. 25, No. 7, 2007, pp. 1761–1768.

[10] Rosen, A.B., et al., "Finding fluorescent needles in the cardiac haystack: tracking human mesenchymal stem cells labeled with quantum dots for quantitative in vivo three-dimensional fluorescence analysis," *Stem Cells*, Vol. 25, No. 8, 2007, pp. 2128–2138.

[11] Dingli, D., et al., "Combined I-124 positron emission tomography/computed tomography imaging of NIS gene expression in animal models of stably transfected and intravenously transfected tumor," *Mol Imaging Biol.*, Vol. 8, No. 1, 2006, pp. 16–23.

[12] Kim, D.E., et al., "Near-infrared fluorescent imaging of cerebral thrombi and blood-brain barrier disruption in a mouse model of cerebral venous sinus thrombosis," *Journal of Cerebral Blood Flow & Metabolism*, Vol. 25, No. 2, 2005, pp. 226–233.

[13] Chung, J.K., "Sodium iodide symporter: its role in nuclear medicine," *J Nucl Med*, Vol. 43, No. 9, 2002, pp. 1188–1200.

[14] Yaghoubi, S.S., et al., "Imaging progress of herpes simplex virus type 1 thymidine kinase suicide gene therapy in living subjects with positron emission tomography," *Cancer Gene Ther*, Vol. 12, No. 3, 2005, pp. 329–339.

[15] Buursma, A.R., et al., "18F-FEAU as a radiotracer for herpes simplex virus thymidine kinase gene expression: in-vitro comparison with other PET tracers," *Nucl Med Commun*, Vol. 27, No. 1, 2006, pp. 25–30.

[16] Hustinx, R., et al., "Imaging in vivo herpes simplex virus thymidine kinase gene transfer to tumour-bearing rodents using positron emission tomography and," *Eur J Nucl Med*, Vol. 28, No. 1, 2001, pp. 5–12.

[17] Cao, F., et al., "In vivo visualization of embryonic stem cell survival, proliferation, and migration after cardiac delivery," *Circulation*, Vol. 113, No. 7, 2006, pp. 1005–1014.

[18] Zhang, H., et al., "Synthesis and evaluation of bombesin derivatives on the basis of pan-bombesin peptides labeled with indium-111, lutetium-177, and yttrium-90 for targeting bombesin receptor-expressing tumors," *Cancer Res*, Vol. 64, No. 18, 2004, pp. 6707–6715.

[19] Love, C., et al., "Diagnosing infection in the failed joint replacement: a comparison of coincidence detection 18F-FDG and 111In-labeled leukocyte/99mTc-sulfur colloid marrow imaging," *J Nucl Med*, Vol. 45, No. 11, 2004, pp. 1864–1871.

[20] Botti, C., et al., "Comparison of three different methods for radiolabelling human activated T lymphocytes," *Eur J Nucl Med*, Vol. 24, No. 5, 1997, pp. 497–504.

[21] Read, E.J., et al., "In vivo traffic of indium-111-oxine labeled human lymphocytes collected by automated apheresis," *J Nucl Med*, Vol. 31, No. 6, 1990, pp. 999–1006.

[22] Griffith, K.D., et al., "In vivo distribution of adoptively transferred indium-111-labeled tumor infiltrating lymphocytes and peripheral blood lymphocytes in patients with metastatic melanoma," *J Natl Cancer Inst*, Vol. 81, No. 22, 1989, pp. 1709–1717.

[23] Fisher, B., et al., "Tumor localization of adoptively transferred indium-111 labeled tumor infiltrating lymphocytes in patients with metastatic melanoma," *J Clin Oncol*, Vol. 7, No. 2, 1989, pp. 250–261.

[24] Adonai, N., et al., "Ex vivo cell labeling with 64Cu-pyruvaldehyde-bis(N4-methylthiosemicarbazone) for imaging cell trafficking in mice with positron-emission tomography," *Proc Natl Acad Sci U S A*, Vol. 99, No. 5, 2002, pp. 3030–3035.

[25] Hofmann, M., et al., "Monitoring of bone marrow cell homing into the infarcted human myocardium," *Circulation*, Vol. 111, No. 17, 2005, pp. 2198–2202.

[26] Frank, J.A., et al., "Magnetic intracellular labeling of mammalian cells by combining (FDA-approved) superparamagnetic iron oxide MR contrast agents and commonly used transfection agents," *Acad Radiol*, Vol. 9 Suppl 2, No. 2002, pp. S484–487.

[27] Frank, J.A., et al., "Clinically applicable labeling of mammalian and stem cells by combining superparamagnetic iron oxides and transfection agents," *Radiology*, Vol. 228, No. 2, 2003, pp. 480–487.

[28] Arbab, A.S., et al., "In vivo trafficking and targeted delivery of magnetically labeled stem cells," *Human Gene Therapy*, Vol. 15, No. 4, 2004, pp. 351–360.

[29] Arbab, A.S., et al., "Intracytoplasmic tagging of cells with ferumoxides and transfection agent for cellular magnetic resonance imaging after cell transplantation: methods and techniques," *Transplantation*, Vol. 76, No. 7, 2003, pp. 1123–1130.

[30] Modo, M., Hoehn, M., and Bulte, J.W., "Cellular MR imaging," *Mol Imaging*, Vol. 4, No. 3, 2005, pp. 143–164.

[31] Bulte, J.W., et al., "Preparation of magnetically labeled cells for cell tracking by magnetic resonance imaging," *Methods in Enzymology*, Vol. 386, No. 2004, pp. 275–299.

[32] Bulte, J.W. and Kraitchman, D.L., "Iron oxide MR contrast agents for molecular and cellular imaging," *NMR in Biomedicine*, Vol. 17, No. 7, 2004, pp. 484–499.

[33] Arbab, A.S., et al., "Characterization of biophysical and metabolic properties of cells labeled with superparamagnetic iron oxide nanoparticles and transfection agent for cellular MR imaging," *Radiology*, Vol. 229, No. 3, 2003, pp. 838–846.

[34] Arbab, A.S., et al., "Efficient magnetic cell labeling with protamine sulfate complexed to ferumoxides for cellular MRI," *Blood*, Vol. 104, No. 4, 2004, pp. 1217–1223.

[35] Arbab, A.S., et al., "Comparison of transfection agents in forming complexes with ferumoxides, cell labeling efficiency, and cellular viability," *Molecular Imaging: Official Journal of the Society for Molecular Imaging*, Vol. 3, No. 1, 2004, pp. 24–32.

[36] Kircher, M.F., et al., "A multimodal nanoparticle for preoperative magnetic resonance imaging and intraoperative optical brain tumor delineation," *Cancer Research*, Vol. 63, No. 23, 2003, pp. 8122–8125.

[37] Moore, A., et al., "Tracking the recruitment of diabetogenic CD8+ T-cells to the pancreas in real time," *Diabetes*, Vol. 53, No. 6, 2004, pp. 1459–1466.

[38] Josephson, L., et al., "High-efficiency intracellular magnetic labeling with novel superparamagnetic-Tat peptide conjugates," *Bioconjug Chem.*, Vol. 10, No. 2, 1999, pp. 186–191.

[39] Walczak, P., et al., "Instant MR labeling of stem cells using magnetoelectroporation," *Magn Reson Med*, Vol. 54, No. 4, 2005, pp. 769–774.

[40] Toyoda, K., et al., "Effective magnetic labeling of transplanted cells with HVJ-E for magnetic resonance imaging," *Neuroreport*, Vol. 15, No. 4, 2004, pp. 589–593.

[41] van den Bos, E.J., et al., "Improved efficacy of stem cell labeling for magnetic resonance imaging studies by the use of cationic liposomes," *Cell Transplant*, Vol. 12, No. 7, 2003, pp. 743–756.

[42] Shapiro, E.M., Skrtic, S., and Koretsky, A.P., "Sizing it up: cellular MRI using micron-sized iron oxide particles," *Magn Reson Med*, Vol. 53, No. 2, 2005, pp. 329–338.

[43] Zheng, H., et al., "Novel potential neuroprotective agents with both iron chelating and amino acid-based derivatives targeting central nervous system neurons," *Biochem Pharmacol*, Vol. 70, No. 11, 2005, pp. 1642–1652.

[44] Vuu, K., et al., "Gadolinium-rhodamine nanoparticles for cell labeling and tracking via magnetic resonance and optical imaging," *Bioconjug Chem.*, Vol. 16, No. 4, 2005, pp. 995–999.

[45] Anderson, S.A., Lee, K.K., and Frank, J.A., "Gadolinium-fullerenol as a paramagnetic contrast agent for cellular imaging," *Invest Radiol.*, Vol. 41, No. 3, 2006, pp. 332–338.

[46] Rudelius, M., et al., "Highly efficient paramagnetic labelling of embryonic and neuronal stem cells," *Eur J Nucl Med Mol Imaging*, Vol. 30, No. 7, 2003, pp. 1038–1044.

[47] Aime, S., et al., "Targeting cells with MR imaging probes based on paramagnetic Gd(III) chelates," *Curr Pharm Biotechnol*, Vol. 5, No. 6, 2004, pp. 509–518.

[48] Aoki, I., et al., "Cell labeling for magnetic resonance imaging with the T1 agent manganese chloride," *NMR Biomed*, Vol. 19, No. 1, 2006, pp. 50–59.

[49] Crich, S.G., et al., "Improved route for the visualization of stem cells labeled with a Gd-/Eu-chelate as dual (MRI and fluorescence) agent," *Magnetic Resonance in Medicine*, Vol. 51, No. 5, 2004, pp. 938–944.

[50] Crich, S.G., et al., "Visualization through magnetic resonance imaging of DNA internalized following "in vivo" electroporation," *Molecular Imaging*, Vol. 4, No. 1, 2005, pp. 7–17.

[51] Himmelreich, U., et al., "A responsive MRI contrast agent to monitor functional cell status," *Neuroimage*, Vol. 32, No. 3, 2006, pp. 1142–1149.

[52] Giesel, F.L., et al., "Gadofluorine m uptake in stem cells as a new magnetic resonance imaging tracking method: an in vitro and in vivo study," *Invest Radiol*, Vol. 41, No. 12, 2006, pp. 868–873.

[53] Modo, M., et al., "Tracking transplanted stem cell migration using bifunctional, contrast agent-enhanced, magnetic resonance imaging," *Neuroimage.*, Vol. 17, No. 2, 2002, pp. 803–811.

[54] Daldrup-Link, H.E., et al., "Cell tracking with gadophrin-2: a bifunctional contrast agent for MR imaging, optical imaging, and fluorescence microscopy," *Eur J Nucl Med Mol Imaging*, Vol. 31, No. 9, 2004, pp. 1312–1321.

[55] Su, W., et al., "Synthesis and cellular uptake of a MR contrast agent coupled to an antisense peptide nucleic acid—cell-penetrating peptide conjugate," *Contrast Media Mol Imaging*, Vol. 2, No. 1, 2007, pp. 42–49.

[56] Brekke, C., et al., "The in vitro effects of a bimodal contrast agent on cellular functions and relaxometry," *NMR Biomed*, Vol. 20, No. 2, 2007, pp. 77–89.

[57] Wolf, G.L., et al., "Contrast agents for magnetic resonance imaging," *Magn Reson Annu*, Vol. No. 1985, pp. 231–266.

[58] Mendonca-Dias, M.H., Gaggelli, E., and Lauterbur, P.C., "Paramagnetic contrast agents in nuclear magnetic resonance medical imaging," *Semin Nucl Med*, Vol. 13, No. 4, 1983, pp. 364–376.

[59] Na, H.B., et al., "Development of a T1 contrast agent for magnetic resonance imaging using MnO nanoparticles," *Angew Chem Int Ed Engl*, Vol. 46, No. 28, 2007, pp. 5397–5401.

[60] Wang, Y.X., Hussain, S.M., and Krestin, G.P., "Superparamagnetic iron oxide contrast agents: physicochemical characteristics and applications in MR imaging," *Eur Radiol*, Vol. 11, No. 11, 2001, pp. 2319–2331.

[61] Jung, C.W. and Jacobs, P., "Physical and chemical properties of superparamagnetic iron oxide MR contrast agents: ferumoxides, ferumoxtran, ferumoxsil," *Magn Reson Imaging*, Vol. 13, No. 5, 1995, pp. 661–674.

[62] Hogemann, D., et al., "Improvement of MRI probes to allow efficient detection of gene expression," *Bioconjug Chem*, Vol. 11, No. 6, 2000, pp. 941–946.

[63] Yeh, T.C., et al., "Intracellular labeling of T-cells with superparamagnetic contrast agents," *Magn Reson Med*, Vol. 30, No. 5, 1993, pp. 617–625.

[64] Bulte, J.W., et al., "Magnetodendrimers allow endosomal magnetic labeling and in vivo tracking of stem cells," *Nature Biotechnology*, Vol. 19, No. 12, 2001, pp. 1141–1147.

[65] Ittrich, H., et al., "Labeling of mesenchymal stem cells with different superparamagnetic particles of iron oxide and detectability with MRI at 3T," *Rofo*, Vol. 177, No. 8, 2005, pp. 1151–1163.

[66] Mikhaylova, M., Kim do, K, Bobrysheva, N, Osmolowsky, M, Semenov, V, Tsakalakos, T, Muhammed, M., "Superparamagnetism of magnetite nanoparticles: dependence on surface modification," *Langmuir*, Vol. 20, No. 6, 2004, pp. 2472–2477.

[67] Hawrylak, N., et al., "Nuclear magnetic resonance (NMR) imaging of iron oxide-labeled neural transplants," *Exp Neurol*, Vol. 121, No. 2, 1993, pp. 181–192.

[68] Yeh, T.C., et al., "In vivo dynamic MRI tracking of rat T-cells labeled with superparamagnetic iron-oxide particles," *Magn Reson Med*, Vol. 33, No. 2, 1995, pp. 200–208.

[69] Shen, T.T., et al., "Magnetically labeled secretin retains receptor affinity to pancreas acinar cells," *Bioconjug Chem*, Vol. 7, No. 3, 1996, pp. 311–316.

[70] Fleige, G., et al., "In vitro characterization of two different ultrasmall iron oxide particles for magnetic resonance cell tracking," *Invest Radiol*, Vol. 37, No. 9, 2002, pp. 482–488.

[71] Kaufman, C.L., et al., "Superparamagnetic iron oxide particles transactivator protein-fluorescein isothiocyanate particle labeling for in vivo magnetic resonance imaging detection of cell migration: uptake and durability," *Transplantation*, Vol. 76, No. 7, 2003, pp. 1043–1046.

[72] Koch, A.M., et al., "Uptake and metabolism of a dual fluorochrome Tat-nanoparticle in HeLa cells," *Bioconjugate Chemistry*, Vol. 14, No. 6, 2003, pp. 1115–1121.

[73] Ho, C. and Hitchens, T.K., "A non-invasive approach to detecting organ rejection by MRI: monitoring the accumulation of immune cells at the transplanted organ," *Curr Pharm Biotechnol*, Vol. 5, No. 6, 2004, pp. 551–566.

[74] Song, H., Choi, JS, Huh, YM, Kim, S, Jun, YW, Suh, JS, Cheon, J., "Surface modulation of magnetic nanocrystals in the development of highly efficient magnetic resonance probes for intracellular labeling," *J Am Chem Soc.*, Vol. 127, No. 28, 2005, pp. 9992–9993.

[75] Schulze, E., Ferrucci, JT Jr, Poss, K, Lapointe, L, Bogdanova, A, Weissleder, R., "Cellular uptake and trafficking of a prototypical magnetic iron oxide label in vitro.," *Invest Radiol.*, Vol. 30, No. 10, 1995, pp. 604–610.

[76] Bulte, J.W., et al., "Monitoring stem cell therapy in vivo using magnetodendrimers as a new class of cellular MR contrast agents," *Academic Radiology*, Vol. 9 Suppl 2, No. 2002, pp. S332–335.

[77] Smirnov, P., et al., "In vivo cellular imaging of magnetically labeled hybridomas in the spleen with a 1.5-T clinical MRI system," *Magn Reson Med*, Vol. 52, No. 1, 2004, pp. 73–79.

[78] Riviere, C., et al., "Iron oxide nanoparticle-labeled rat smooth muscle cells: cardiac MR imaging for cell graft monitoring and quantitation," *Radiology*, Vol. 235, No. 3, 2005, pp. 959–967.

[79] Brillet, P.Y., et al., "Evaluation of tumoral enhancement by superparamagnetic iron oxide particles: comparative studies with ferumoxtran and anionic iron oxide nanoparticles," *Eur Radiol*, Vol. 15, No. 7, 2005, pp. 1369–1377.

[80] Wilhelm, C., et al., "Intracellular uptake of anionic superparamagnetic nanoparticles as a function of their surface coating," *Biomaterials*, Vol. 24, No. 6, 2003, pp. 1001–1011.

[81] Kalish, H., et al., "Combination of transfection agents and magnetic resonance contrast agents for cellular imaging: relationship between relaxivities, electrostatic forces, and chemical composition," *Magn Reson Med*, Vol. 50, No. 2, 2003, pp. 275–282.

[82] Walliser, S. and Redmann, K., "Effect of 5-fluorouracil and thymidine on the transmembrane potential and zeta potential of HeLa cells," *Cancer Res*, Vol. 38, No. 10, 1978, pp. 3555–3559.

[83] Bulte, J.W., et al., "Dextran-magnetite particles: contrast-enhanced MRI of blood-brain barrier disruption in a rat model," *Magnetic Resonance in Medicine*, Vol. 23, No. 2, 1992, pp. 215–223.

[84] Bulte, J.W., et al., "Neurotransplantation of magnetically labeled oligodendrocyte progenitors: magnetic resonance tracking of cell migration and myelination," *Proceedings of the National Academy of Sciences of the United States of America*, Vol. 96, No. 26, 1999, pp. 15256–15261.

[85] Josephson, L., et al., "The effects of iron oxides on proton relaxivity," *Magn Reson Imaging*, Vol. 6, No. 6, 1988, pp. 647–653.

[86] Taupitz, M., Schmitz, S., and Hamm, B., "Superparamagnetic iron oxide particles: current state and future development," *Rofo*, Vol. 175, No. 6, 2003, pp. 752–765.

[87] Mukherjee, S., Ghosh, R.N., and Maxfield, F.R., "Endocytosis," *Physiol Rev*, Vol. 77, No. 3, 1997, pp. 759–803.

[88] Conner, S.D. and Schmid, S.L., "Regulated portals of entry into the cell," *Nature*, Vol. 422, No. 6927, 2003, pp. 37–44.

[89] Medina-Kauwe, L.K., Xie, J., and Hamm-Alvarez, S., "Intracellular trafficking of nonviral vectors," *Gene Ther*, Vol. 12, No. 24, 2005, pp. 1734–1751.

[90] Brodsky, F.M., et al., "Biological basket weaving: formation and function of clathrin-coated vesicles," *Annu Rev Cell Dev Biol*, Vol. 17, No. 2001, pp. 517–568.

[91] Schmid, S.L., "Clathrin-coated vesicle formation and protein sorting: an integrated process," *Annu Rev Biochem*, Vol. 66, No. 1997, pp. 511–548.

[92] Moore, A., et al., "Human transferrin receptor gene as a marker gene for MR imaging," *Radiology*, Vol. 221, No. 1, 2001, pp. 244–250.

[93] Moore, A., et al., "Measuring transferrin receptor gene expression by NMR imaging," *Biochim Biophys Acta*, Vol. 1402, No. 3, 1998, pp. 239–249.

[94] Kresse, M., et al., "Targeting of ultrasmall superparamagnetic iron oxide (USPIO) particles to tumor cells in vivo by using transferrin receptor pathways," *Magn Reson Med*, Vol. 40, No. 2, 1998, pp. 236–242.

[95] Ichikawa, T., et al., "MRI of transgene expression: correlation to therapeutic gene expression," *Neoplasia*, Vol. 4, No. 6, 2002, pp. 523–530.

[96] Daldrup-Link, H.E. and Brasch, R.C., "Macromolecular contrast agents for MR mammography: current status," *Eur Radiol*, Vol. 13, No. 2, 2003, pp. 354–365.

[97] Daldrup-Link, H.E., et al., "Targeting of hematopoietic progenitor cells with MR contrast agents," *Radiology*, Vol. 228, No. 3, 2003, pp. 760–767.

[98] Nakase, I., et al., "Cellular uptake of arginine-rich peptides: roles for macropinocytosis and actin rearrangement," *Mol Ther*, Vol. 10, No. 6, 2004, pp. 1011–1022.

[99] Kaplan, I.M., Wadia, J.S., and Dowdy, S.F., "Cationic TAT peptide transduction domain enters cells by macropinocytosis," *J Control Release*, Vol. 102, No. 1, 2005, pp. 247–253.

[100] Bluemke, D., Weber, TM, Rubin, D, de Lange, EE, Semelka, R, Redvanly, RD, Chezmar, J, Outwater, E, Carlos, R, Saini, S, Holland, GA, Mammone, JF, Brown, JJ, Milestone, B, Javitt, MC, Jacobs, P., "Hepatic MR imaging with ferumoxides: multicenter study of safety and effectiveness of direct injection protocol.," *Radiology*, Vol. 228, No. 2, 2003, pp. 457–464.

[101] Harisinghani, M., Barentsz, J, Hahn, PF, Deserno, WM, Tabatabaei, S, van de Kaa, CH, de la Rosette, J, Weissleder, R., "Noninvasive detection of clinically occult lymph-node metastases in prostate cancer.," *N Engl J Med.* , Vol. 343, No. 25, 2003, pp. 2491–2499.

[102] Harisinghani, M.G., et al., "Differentiation of liver hemangiomas from metastases and hepatocellular carcinoma at MR imaging enhanced with blood-pool contrast agent Code-7227," *Radiology*, Vol. 202, No. 3, 1997, pp. 687–691.

[103] Harisinghani, M., Saini, S, Weissleder, R, Hahn, PF, Yantiss, RK, Tempany, C, Wood, BJ, Mueller, PR., "MR lymphangiography using ultrasmall superparamagnetic iron oxide in patients with primary abdominal and pelvic malignancies: radiographic-pathologic correlation," *AJR Am J Roentgenol.* , Vol. 172, No. 5, 1999, pp. 1347–1351.

[104] Mack, M.G., et al., "Superparamagnetic iron oxide-enhanced MR imaging of head and neck lymph nodes," *Radiology*, Vol. 222, No. 1, 2002, pp. 239–244.

[105] Sato, N., et al., "Pharmacokinetics and enhancement patterns of macromolecular MR contrast agents with various sizes of polyamidoamine dendrimer cores," *Magn Reson Med.*, Vol. 46, No. 6, 2001, pp. 1169–1173.

[106] Yan, G.P., et al., "Synthesis and evaluation of gadolinium complexes based on PAMAM as MRI contrast agents," *J Pharm Pharmacol.*, Vol. 57, No. 3, 2005, pp. 351–357.

[107] Bryant, L.H., Jr., et al., "Synthesis and relaxometry of high-generation (G 5, 7, 9, and 10) PAMAM dendrimer-DOTA-gadolinium chelates," *Journal of Magnetic Resonance Imaging*, Vol. 9, No. 2, 1999, pp. 348–352.

[108] Kobayashi, H., et al., "Macromolecular MRI contrast agents with small dendrimers: pharmacokinetic differences between sizes and cores," *Bioconjug Chem.*, Vol. 14, No. 2, 2003, pp. 388–394.

[109] Dodd, C.H., et al., "Normal T-cell response and in vivo magnetic resonance imaging of T cells loaded with HIV transactivator-peptide-derived superparamagnetic nanoparticles," *Journal of Immunological Methods*, Vol. 256, No. 1-2, 2001, pp. 89–105.

[110] Moore, A., et al., "MRI of insulitis in autoimmune diabetes," *Magn Reson Med*, Vol. 47, No. 4, 2002, pp. 751–758.

[111] Kircher, M.F., et al., "In vivo high resolution three-dimensional imaging of antigen-specific cytotoxic T-lymphocyte trafficking to tumors," *Cancer Research*, Vol. 63, No. 20, 2003, pp. 6838–6846.

[112] Lewin, M., et al., "Tat peptide-derivatized magnetic nanoparticles allow in vivo tracking and recovery of progenitor cells," *Nature Biotechnology*, Vol. 18, No. 4, 2000, pp. 410–414.

[113] Josephson, L., et al., "Near-infrared fluorescent nanoparticles as combined MR/optical imaging probes," *Bioconjugate Chemistry*, Vol. 13, No. 3, 2002, pp. 554–560.

[114] Bulte, J.W., et al., "Specific MR imaging of human lymphocytes by monoclonal antibody-guided dextran-magnetite particles," *Magnetic Resonance in Medicine*, Vol. 25, No. 1, 1992, pp. 148–157.

[115] Ahrens, E.T., et al., "Receptor-mediated endocytosis of iron-oxide particles provides efficient labeling of dendritic cells for in vivo MR imaging," *Magnetic Resonance in Medicine*, Vol. 49, No. 6, 2003, pp. 1006–1013.

[116] Berry, C.C., et al., "The influence of transferrin stabilised magnetic nanoparticles on human dermal fibroblasts in culture," *Int J Pharm*, Vol. 269, No. 1, 2004, pp. 211–225.

[117] Miyoshi, S., Flexman, JA, Cross, DJ, Maravilla, KR, Kim, Y, Anzai, Y, Oshima, J, Minoshima, S., "Transfection of Neuroprogenitor Cells with Iron Nanoparticles for Magnetic Resonance Imaging Tracking: Cell Viability, Differentiation, and Intracellular Localization," *Mol Imaging iol*, Vol. 4, No. 2005, pp. 1–10.

[118] Song, Y., et al., "Magnetic resonance imaging using hemagglutinating virus of Japan-envelope vector successfully detects localization of intra-cardially administered microglia in normal mouse brain," *Neurosci Lett*, Vol. 395, No. 1, 2006, pp. 42–45.

[119] Hinds, K.A., et al., "Highly efficient endosomal labeling of progenitor and stem cells with large magnetic particles allows magnetic resonance imaging of single cells," *Blood*, Vol. 102, No. 3, 2003, pp. 867–872.

[120] Hill, J.M., et al., "Serial cardiac magnetic resonance imaging of injected mesenchymal stem cells," *Circulation*, Vol. 108, No. 8, 2003, pp. 1009–1014.

[121] Wu, Y.L., et al., "In situ labeling of immune cells with iron oxide particles: an approach to detect organ rejection by cellular MRI," *Proc Natl Acad Sci U S A*, Vol. 103, No. 6, 2006, pp. 1852–1857.

[122] Heyn, C., et al., "In vivo MRI of cancer cell fate at the single-cell level in a mouse model of breast cancer metastasis to the brain," *Magn Reson Med*, Vol. 56, No. 5, 2006, pp. 1001–1010.

[123] Arbab, A.S., et al., "Magnetic resonance imaging and confocal microscopy studies of magnetically labeled endothelial progenitor cells trafficking to sites of tumor angiogenesis," *Stem Cells*, Vol. 24, No. 3, 2006, pp. 671–678.

[124] Anderson, S.A., et al., "Magnetic resonance imaging of labeled T-cells in a mouse model of multiple sclerosis," *Annals of Neurology*, Vol. 55, No. 5, 2004, pp. 654–659.

[125] Anderson, S.A., et al., "Noninvasive MR imaging of magnetically labeled stem cells to directly identify neovasculature in a glioma model," *Blood*, Vol. 105, No. 1, 2005, pp. 420–425.

[126] Oweida, A.J., Dunn, E.A., and Foster, P.J., "Cellular imaging at 1.5 T: detecting cells in neuroinflammation using active labeling with superparamagnetic iron oxide," *Molecular Imaging: Official Journal of the Society for Molecular Imaging*, Vol. 3, No. 2, 2004, pp. 85–95.

[127] Daldrup-Link, H.E., et al., "Migration of iron oxide-labeled human hematopoietic progenitor cells in a mouse model: in vivo monitoring with 1.5-T MR imaging equipment," *Radiology*, Vol. 234, No. 1, 2005, pp. 197–205.

[128] Evgenov, N.V., et al., "In vivo imaging of islet transplantation," *Nat Med*, Vol. 12, No. 1, 2006, pp. 144–148.

[129] Tai, J.H., et al., "Imaging islets labeled with magnetic nanoparticles at 1.5 Tesla," *Diabetes*, Vol. 55, No. 11, 2006, pp. 2931–2938.

[130] Foster-Gareau, P., et al., "Imaging single mammalian cells with a 1.5 T clinical MRI scanner," *Magnetic Resonance in Medicine*, Vol. 49, No. 5, 2003, pp. 968–971.

[131] Heyn, C., et al., "In vivo magnetic resonance imaging of single cells in mouse brain with optical validation," *Magn Reson Med*, Vol. 55, No. 1, 2006, pp. 23–29.

[132] Shapiro, E.M., et al., "Magnetic resonance imaging of the migration of neuronal precursors generated in the adult rodent brain," *Neuroimage*, Vol. 32, No. 3, 2006, pp. 1150–1157.

[133] Shapiro, E.M., et al., "MRI detection of single particles for cellular imaging," *Proc Natl Acad Sci U S A*, Vol. 101, No. 30, 2004, pp. 10901–10906.

[134] Shapiro, E.M., et al., "In vivo detection of single cells by MRI," *Magn Reson Med*, Vol. 55, No. 2, 2006, pp. 242–249.

[135] Suzuki, Y., et al., "In vitro comparison of the biological effects of three transfection methods for magnetically labeling mouse embryonic stem cells with ferumoxides," *Magn Reson Med*, Vol. 57, No. 6, 2007, pp. 1173–1179.

[136] Neri, M., et al., "Efficient In Vitro Labeling Of Human Neural Precursor Cells With Superparamagnetic Iron Oxide Particles: Relevance For In Vivo Cell Tracking," *Stem Cells*, 2007.

[137] Montet-Abou, K., et al., "Transfection agent induced nanoparticle cell loading," *Mol Imaging*, Vol. 4, No. 3, 2005, pp. 165–171.

[138] Reynolds, F., Weissleder, R., and Josephson, L., "Protamine as an efficient membrane-translocating peptide," *Bioconjug Chem*, Vol. 16, No. 5, 2005, pp. 1240–1245.

[139] Wu, Y.J., et al., "In Vivo Leukocyte Labeling with Intravenous Ferumoxides/Protamine Sulfate Complex and in vitro Characterization for Cellular Magnetic Resonance Imaging," *Am J Physiol Cell Physiol*, Vol. No. 2007, pp. 00215.02007.

[140] Arbab, A.S., et al., "Labeling of cells with ferumoxides-protamine sulfate complexes does not inhibit function or differentiation capacity of hematopoietic or mesenchymal stem cells," *NMR Biomed.*, Vol. 18, No. 8, 2005, pp. 553–559.

[141] Arbab, A.S., et al., "Ferumoxides-protamine sulfate labeling does not alter differentiation of mesenchymal stem cells.," *Blood*, Vol. 104, No. 10, 2004, pp. 3412–3413.

[142] Guzman, R., et al., "Long-term monitoring of transplanted human neural stem cells in developmental and pathological contexts with MRI," *Proc Natl Acad Sci U S A*, Vol. 104, No. 24, 2007, pp. 10211–10216.

[143] Pawelczyk, E., et al., "Expression of transferrin receptor and ferritin following ferumoxides-protamine sulfate labeling of cells: implications for cellular magnetic resonance imaging," *NMR Biomed*, Vol. 19, No. 5, 2006, pp. 581–592.

[144] Arbab, A.S., et al., "A model of lysosomal metabolism of dextran coated superparamagnetic iron oxide (SPIO) nanoparticles: implications for cellular magnetic resonance imaging," *NMR Biomed.*, Vol. 18, No. 6, 2005, pp. 383–389.

[145] Zhang, R.L., et al., "Migration and differentiation of adult rat subventricular zone progenitor cells transplanted into the adult rat striatum," *Neuroscience*, Vol. 116, No. 2, 2003, pp. 373–382.

[146] Davidson, J.M., Krieg, T., and Eming, S.A., "Particle-mediated gene therapy of wounds," *Wound Repair Regen*, Vol. 8, No. 6, 2000, pp. 452–459.

[147] Jacobs, R.E. and Fraser, S.E., "Magnetic resonance microscopy of embryonic cell lineages and movements," *Science*, Vol. 263, No. 5147, 1994, pp. 681–684.

[148] Terreno, E., et al., "Effect of the intracellular localization of a Gd-based imaging probe on the relaxation enhancement of water protons," *Magn Reson Med*, Vol. 55, No. 3, 2006, pp. 491–497.

[149] Bhattarai, S.R., et al., "Laboratory formulated magnetic nanoparticles for enhancement of viral gene expression in suspension cell line," *Journal of Virological Methods*, 2008.

[150] Scherer, F., et al., "Magnetofection: enhancing and targeting gene delivery by magnetic force in vitro and in vivo," *Gene Ther*, Vol. 9, No. 2, 2002, pp. 102–109.

[151] Plank, C., et al., "Magnetofection: enhancing and targeting gene delivery with superparamagnetic nanoparticles and magnetic fields," *J Liposome Res*, Vol. 13, No. 1, 2003, pp. 29–32.

[152] Gersting, S., et al., "Gene delivery to respiratory epithelial cells by magnetofection," *The Journal of Gene Medicine*, Vol. 6, No. 8, 2004, pp. 913–922.

[153] Huth, S., et al., "Insights into the mechanism of magnetofection using PEI-based magnetofectins for gene transfer," *The Journal of Gene Medicine*, Vol. 6, No. 8, 2004, pp. 923–936.

[154] Mykhaylyk, O., et al., "Generation of magnetic nonviral gene transfer agents and magnetofection in vitro," *Nat. Protocols*, Vol. 2, No. 10, 2007, pp. 2391–2411.

[155] Rad, A.M., et al., "Measurement of quantity of iron in magnetically labeled cells: comparison among different UV/VIS spectrometric methods " *Biotechniques*, Vol. 43, No. 5, 2007, pp. 627–636.

[156] Emerit, J., Beaumont, C., and Trivin, F., "Iron metabolism, free radicals, and oxidative injury," *Biomed Pharmacother.*, Vol. 55, No. 6, 2001, pp. 333–339.

[157] Gutteridge, J.M. and Halliwell, B., "The role of the superoxide and hydroxyl radicals in the degradation of DNA and deoxyribose induced by a copper-phenanthroline complex," *Biochem Pharmacol.*, Vol. 31, No. 17, 1982, pp. 2801–2805.

[158] Gutteridge, J.M. and Toeg, D., "Iron-dependent free radical damage to DNA and deoxyribose. Separation of TBA-reactive intermediates," *Int J Biochem*, Vol. 14, No. 10, 1982, pp. 891–893.

[159] Stauber, R.H., et al., "Analysis of intracellular trafficking and interactions of cytoplasmic HIV-1 Rev mutants in living cells," *Virology*, Vol. 251, No. 1, 1998, pp. 38–48.

[160] Stauber, R.H. and Pavlakis, G.N., "Intracellular trafficking and interactions of the HIV-1 Tat protein," *Virology*, Vol. 252, No. 1, 1998, pp. 126–136.

[161] Kruman, II, Nath, A., and Mattson, M.P., "HIV-1 protein Tat induces apoptosis of hippocampal neurons by a mechanism involving caspase activation, calcium overload, and oxidative stress," *Exp Neurol*, Vol. 154, No. 2, 1998, pp. 276–288.

[162] Watson, D.J., et al., "Structure-specific patterns of neural stem cell engraftment after transplantation in the adult mouse brain," *Hum Gene Ther*, Vol. 17, No. 7, 2006, pp. 693–704.

[163] Cunningham, C.H., et al., "Positive contrast magnetic resonance imaging of cells labeled with magnetic nanoparticles," *Magn Reson Med*, Vol. 53, No. 5, 2005, pp. 999–1005.

[164] Stuber, M., et al., "Positive contrast visualization of iron oxide-labeled stem cells using inversion-recovery with ON-resonant water suppression (IRON)," *Magn Reson Med*, Vol. 58, No. 5, 2007, pp. 1072–1077.

[165] Seppenwoolde, J.H., Viergever, M.A., and Bakker, C.J., "Passive tracking exploiting local signal conservation: the white marker phenomenon," *Magn Reson Med*, Vol. 50, No. 4, 2003, pp. 784–790.

[166] Seppenwoolde, J.H., Vincken, K.L., and Bakker, C.J., "White-marker imaging—separating magnetic susceptibility effects from partial volume effects," *Magn Reson Med*, Vol. 58, No. 3, 2007, pp. 605–609.

[167] Liu, W., et al., "In vivo MRI using positive-contrast techniques in detection of cells labeled with superparamagnetic iron oxide nanoparticles," *NMR Biomed*, Vol. No. 2007, pp.

[168] Dahnke, H., et al., "Susceptibility Gradient Mapping (SGM): A New Positive Contrast Method Applied to SPIO Labeled Cells," *Magnetic Resonance in Medicine*, Vol. No. in press.

[169] Bulte, J.W., et al., "Hepatic hemosiderosis in non-human primates: quantification of liver iron using different field strengths," *Magn Reson Med*, Vol. 37, No. 4, 1997, pp. 530–536.

[170] Bowen, C.V., et al., "Application of the static dephasing regime theory to superparamagnetic iron-oxide loaded cells," *Magnetic Resonance in Medicine*, Vol. 48, No. 1, 2002, pp. 52–61.

[171] Rad, A.M., et al., "Quantification of superparamagnetic iron oxide (SPIO)-labeled cells using MRI," *J Magn Reson Imaging*, Vol. 26, No. 2, 2007, pp. 366–374.

[172] Dahnke, H. and Schaeffter, T., "Limits of detection of SPIO at 3.0 T using T2 relaxometry," *Magn Reson Med*, Vol. 53, No. 5, 2005, pp. 1202–1206.

[173] Young, I.R., et al., "The benefits of increasing spatial resolution as a means of reducing artifacts due to field inhomogeneities," *Magn Reson Imaging*, Vol. 6, No. 5, 1988, pp. 585–590.

[174] Frahm, J., Merboldt, K.D., and Hanicke, W., "Direct FLASH MR imaging of magnetic field inhomogeneities by gradient compensation," *Magn Reson Med*, Vol. 6, No. 4, 1988, pp. 474–480.

[175] Cho, Z.H. and Ro, Y.M., "Reduction of susceptibility artifact in gradient-echo imaging," *Magn Reson Med*, Vol. 23, No. 1, 1992, pp. 193–200.

[176] Glover, G.H., "3D z-shim method for reduction of susceptibility effects in BOLD fMRI," *Magn Reson Med*, Vol. 42, No. 2, 1999, pp. 290–299.

[177] Glover, G.H., "Deconvolution of impulse response in event-related BOLD fMRI," *Neuroimage*, Vol. 9, No. 4, 1999, pp. 416–429.

[178] Zhang, Z.G., et al., "Magnetic resonance imaging and neurosphere therapy of stroke in rat," *Ann Neurol*, Vol. 53, No. 2, 2003, pp. 259–263.

[179] Sykova, E. and Jendelova, P., "In vivo tracking of stem cells in brain and spinal cord injury," *Prog Brain Res*, Vol. 161, No. 2007, pp. 367–383.

[180] Sykova, E. and Jendelova, P., "Magnetic resonance tracking of implanted adult and embryonic stem cells in injured brain and spinal cord," *Ann N Y Acad Sci*, Vol. 1049, No. 2005, pp. 146–160.

[181] Yano, S., et al., "Do bone marrow stromal cells proliferate after transplantation into mice cerebral infarct?—a double labeling study," *Brain Res*, Vol. 1065, No. 1-2, 2005, pp. 60–67.

[182] Wei, J. J., et al., "In vivo tracking of bone marrow mesenchymal stem cells labeled with superparamagnetic iron oxide after cerebral ischemia in rats by magnetic resonance imaging," *Zhongguo Yi Xue Ke Xue Yuan Xue Bao*, Vol. 29, No. 1, 2007, pp. 73–77.

[183] Sykova, E. and Jendelova, P., "Magnetic resonance tracking of transplanted stem cells in rat brain and spinal cord," *Neurodegener Dis*, Vol. 3, No. 1-2, 2006, pp. 62–67.

[184] Dhermain, F., et al., "Use of the functional imaging modalities in radiation therapy treatment planning in patients with glioblastoma," *Bull Cancer.*, Vol. 92, No. 4, 2005, pp. 333–342.

[185] Hentschel, S.J. and Sawaya, R., "Optimizing outcomes with maximal surgical resection of malignant gliomas," *Cancer Control.*, Vol. 10, No. 2, 2003, pp. 109–114.

[186] Zhang, Z., et al., "In vivo magnetic resonance imaging tracks adult neural progenitor cell targeting of brain tumor," *Neuroimage*, Vol. 23, No. 1, 2004, pp. 281–287.

[187] Valable, S., et al., "In vivo MRI tracking of exogenous monocytes/macrophages targeting brain tumors in a rat model of glioma," *Neuroimage*, Vol. 37 Suppl 1, No. 2007, pp. S47–58.

[188] Folkman, J., "Tumor angiogenesis: therapeutic implications," *N Engl J Med*, Vol. 285, No. 21, 1971, pp. 1182–1186.

[189] Asahara, T., et al., "Bone marrow origin of endothelial progenitor cells responsible for postnatal vasculogenesis in physiological and pathological neovascularization," *Circulation Research*, Vol. 85, No. 3, 1999, pp. 221–228.

[190] Asahara, T., et al., "Isolation of putative progenitor endothelial cells for angiogenesis," *Science*, Vol. 275, No. 5302, 1997, pp. 964–967.

[191] Ferrari, N., et al., "Bone marrow-derived, endothelial progenitor-like cells as angiogenesis-selective gene-targeting vectors," *Gene Therapy*, Vol. 10, No. 8, 2003, pp. 647–656.

[192] De Palma, M., et al., "Targeting exogenous genes to tumor angiogenesis by transplantation of genetically modified hematopoietic stem cells," *Nat Med*, Vol. 9, No. 6, 2003, pp. 789–795.

[193] Zhang, R., et al., "Activated neural stem cells contribute to stroke-induced neurogenesis and neuroblast migration toward the infarct boundary in adult rats," *Journal of Cerebral Blood Flow & Metabolism*, Vol. 24, No. 4, 2004, pp. 441–448.

[194] Jiang, Q., et al., "Investigation of neural progenitor cell induced angiogenesis after embolic stroke in rat using MRI," *Neuroimage.*, Vol. 28, No. 3, 2005, pp. 698–707. Epub 2005 Aug 2019.

[195] Chen, J., et al., "Intravenous administration of human bone marrow stromal cells induces angiogenesis in the ischemic boundary zone after stroke in rats," *Circulation Research*, Vol. 92, No. 6, 2003, pp. 692–699.

[196] Li, Y., et al., "Human marrow stromal cell therapy for stroke in rat: neurotrophins and functional recovery," *Neurology*, Vol. 59, No. 4, 2002, pp. 514–523.

[197] Chen, J., et al., "Intravenous bone marrow stromal cell therapy reduces apoptosis and promotes endogenous cell proliferation after stroke in female rat," *J Neurosci Res*, Vol. 73, No. 6, 2003, pp. 778–786.

[198] Jendelova, P., et al., "Imaging the fate of implanted bone marrow stromal cells labeled with superparamagnetic nanoparticles," *Magn Reson Med.*, Vol. 50, No. 4, 2003, pp. 767–776.

[199] Jendelova, P., Herynek, V, Urdzikova, L, Glogarova, K, Rahmatova, S, Fales, I, Andersson, B, Prochazka, P, Zamecnik, J, Eckschlager, T, Kobylka, P, Hajek, M, Sykova, E, "Magnetic resonance tracking of human CD34+ progenitor cells separated by means of immunomagnetic selection and transplanted into injured rat brain.," *Cell Transplant*, Vol. 14, No. 4, 2005, pp. 173–182.

[200] Hoehn, M., Kustermann, E, Blunk, J, Wiedermann, D, Trapp, T, Wecker, S, Focking, M, Arnold, H, Hescheler, J, Fleischmann, BK, Schwindt, W, Buhrle, C., "Monitoring of implanted stem cell migration in vivo: a highly resolved in vivo magnetic resonance imaging investigation of experimental stroke in rat. ," *Proc Natl Acad Sci U S A.*, Vol. 99, No. 25, 2002, pp. 16267–16272.

[201] Jendelova, P., et al., "Magnetic resonance tracking of transplanted bone marrow and embryonic stem cells labeled by iron oxide nanoparticles in rat brain and spinal cord," *J Neurosci Res.*, Vol. 76, No. 2, 2004, pp. 232–243.

[202] Dunning, M.D., et al., "Superparamagnetic iron oxide-labeled Schwann cells and olfactory ensheathing cells can be traced in vivo by magnetic resonance imaging and retain functional properties after transplantation into the CNS," *Journal of Neuroscience*, Vol. 24, No. 44, 2004, pp. 9799–9810.

[203] Rogers, W.J., Meyer, C.H., and Kramer, C.M., "Technology insight: in vivo cell tracking by use of MRI," *Nat Clin Pract Cardiovasc Med*, Vol. 3, No. 10, 2006, pp. 554–562.

[204] Sheikh, A.Y. and Wu, J.C., "Molecular imaging of cardiac stem cell transplantation," *Curr Cardiol Rep*, Vol. 8, No. 2, 2006, pp. 147–154.

[205] Zhou, R., Acton, P.D., and Ferrari, V.A., "Imaging stem cells implanted in infarcted myocardium," *J Am Coll Cardiol*, Vol. 48, No. 10, 2006, pp. 2094–2106.

[206] Kim, D., Hong, K.S., and Song, J., "The present status of cell tracking methods in animal models using magnetic resonance imaging technology," *Mol Cells*, Vol. 23, No. 2, 2007, pp. 132–137.

[207] Graham, J.J., Lederman, R.J., and Dick, A.J., "Magnetic resonance imaging and its role in myocardial regenerative therapy," *Regen Med*, Vol. 1, No. 3, 2006, pp. 347–355.

[208] Kraitchman, D.L., et al., "In vivo magnetic resonance imaging of mesenchymal stem cells in myocardial infarction," *Circulation*, Vol. 107, No. 18, 2003, pp. 2290–2293.

[209] Kraitchman, D.L., et al., "Dynamic imaging of allogeneic mesenchymal stem cells trafficking to myocardial infarction," *Circulation.*, Vol. 112, No. 10, 2005, pp. 1451–1461, Epub, 2005, Aug., 1429.

[210] Gao, F., et al., "MRI of intravenously injected bone marrow cells homing to the site of injured arteries," *NMR Biomed*, Vol. 20, No. 7, 2007, pp. 673–681.

[211] Qiu, B., et al., "In vivo MR imaging of bone marrow cells trafficking to atherosclerotic plaques," *J Magn Reson Imaging*, Vol. 26, No. 2, 2007, pp. 339–343.

[212] Martin, R. and McFarland, H.F., "Immunological aspects of experimental allergic encephalomyelitis and multiple sclerosis," *Crit Rev Clin Lab Sci*, Vol. 32, No. 2, 1995, pp. 121–182.

[213] Jordan, E.K., et al., "Serial MR imaging of experimental autoimmune encephalomyelitis induced by human white matter or by chimeric myelin-basic and proteolipid protein in the common marmoset," *AJNR Am J Neuroradiol*, Vol. 20, No. 6, 1999, pp. 965–976.

[214] Pluchino, S., et al., "Injection of adult neurospheres induces recovery in a chronic model of multiple sclerosis," *Nature*, Vol. 422, No. 6933, 2003, pp. 688–694.

[215] Zappia, E., et al., "Mesenchymal stem cells ameliorate experimental autoimmune encephalomyelitis inducing T-cell anergy," *Blood*, Vol. 106, No. 5, 2005, pp. 1755–1761.

[216] Gerdoni, E., et al., "Mesenchymal stem cells effectively modulate pathogenic immune response in experimental autoimmune encephalomyelitis," *Ann Neurol*, Vol. 61, No. 3, 2007, pp. 219–227.

[217] Einstein, O., et al., "Neural precursors attenuate autoimmune encephalomyelitis by peripheral immunosuppression," *Ann Neurol*, Vol. 61, No. 3, 2007, pp. 209–218.

[218] Bulte, J.W., et al., "MR microscopy of magnetically labeled neurospheres transplanted into the Lewis EAE rat brain," *Magn Reson Med*, Vol. 50, No. 1, 2003, pp. 201–205.

[219] Ben-Hur, T., et al., "Serial in vivo MR tracking of magnetically labeled neural spheres transplanted in chronic EAE mice," *Magn Reson Med*, Vol. 57, No. 1, 2007, pp. 164–171.

[220] Politi, L.S., et al., "Magnetic-resonance-based tracking and quantification of intravenously injected neural stem cell accumulation in the brains of mice with experimental multiple sclerosis," *Stem Cells*, Vol. 25, No. 10, 2007, pp. 2583–2592.

[221] de Vries, I.J., et al., "Magnetic resonance tracking of dendritic cells in melanoma patients for monitoring of cellular therapy," *Nat Biotechnol.*, Vol. 23, No. 11, 2005, pp. 1407–1413. Epub 2005 Oct 1430.

[222] Zhu, J., Zhou, L., and XingWu, F., "Tracking neural stem cells in patients with brain trauma," *N Engl J Med*, Vol. 355, No. 22, 2006, pp. 2376–2378.

[223] Frank, J.A., et al., "Methods for magnetically labeling stem and other cells for detection by in vivo magnetic resonance imaging," *Cytotherapy*, Vol. 6, No. 6, 2004, pp. 621–625.

About the Editors

Hedi Mattoussi is a senior research physicist at the Naval Research Laboratory (NRL), Optical Sciences Division, Washington, DC. After graduating with a B.S. degree in physics from the University of Tunis (Tunisia), he completed his Ph.D. in condensed matter physics at the University of Pierre, Marie Curie (Paris VI) in 1987, and a habilitation to direct research (also at University of Pierre and Marie Curie) in 1994. His graduate research was completed at the Laboratory of Condensed Matter Physics, College de France, Paris. Prior to joining NRL in 1997, he spent time at a few U.S.-based laboratories, including the Polymer Science and Engineering Department (University of Massachusetts, Amherst, as a postdoctoral fellow) and the Center for Materials Science and Engineering at MIT (as a visiting scientist). His interest in nano-structured materials started during his stay at MIT and has expanded at NRL to various aspects of interfacing inorganic nanocrystals with biological systems. He presently focuses on the development of inorganic nanoparticles (including semiconductor QDs and metallic nanocrystals), their structural and optical characterization, the development of effective schemes to promote their transfer to aqueous media, and the design of effective coupling chemistries to interface them with biological receptors. Recently, he has intensively worked on developing QDs as a platform for arraying a variety of biomolecules (e.g., proteins and peptides), the use of these platforms to develop live cell and tissue imaging, and on the design of several biological assays based on Förster resonance energy transfer and redox interactions. He has also worked on developing light-emitting devices and photovoltaic devices based on semiconducting and metallic nanoparticles. He has organized several international meetings (including the symposia at Materials Research Society fall meetings), and SPIE meetings. He has authored over 140 reports and book chapters and has recently been chosen as the winner of the 2008 Sigma Xi Pure Science award, sponsored by the NRL-Edison Chapter of Sigma Xi.

Jinwoo Cheon is a professor of chemistry at Yonsei University. He is also the director of Convergence Nanomaterials National Research Laboratory and the head of the Nanomaterials Division of the Nano-Medical National Core Research Center of Korea. He graduated from Yonsei University in Seoul, Korea, and received his Ph.D. from the University of Illinois, Urbana-Champaign in 1993 where he researched organometallics and materials chemistry under Prof. G. Girolami. After receiving postdoctoral training at U.C. Berkeley and also at UCLA studying inorganic materials chemistry, he joined the faculty of the Korea Advanced Institute of Science and Technology (KAIST). In 2002, he moved to Yonsei University. His current research interests include the design and property study of inorganic nanostructures, nanomagnetism, and the applications of nanomaterials for biomedical and energy-related technologies. He was elected as a fellow of the Royal Society of Chemistry (FRSC, 2008), a junior member of the Korean Academy of Science and Technology (2003), and is a recipient of awards including the Song-gok Science Award (2007), the Yonsei Research Achievement Award (2006), the Korean Chemical Society Award in Inorganic Chemistry (2004), the National Science Prize for Junior Faculty (2002), and the Korean Chemical Society-Wiley Young Chemist Award (2001). Currently, he is an editorial board member of the *Journal of Materials Chemistry* (RSC). He has given numerous seminars at international societies including plenary lectures at the 36th International Conference on Coordination Chemistry (Mexico, 2004) and 49th SPIE Annual Meeting (Denver, 2004).

List of Contributors

Sarit S. Agasti
Gradute Researcher
Department of Chemistry
University of Massachusetts
710 North Pleasant Street, Amherst, MA, U.S.A.

Ali S Arbab, MD, PhD
Associate Scientist
Director, Cellular and Molecular Imaging Laboratory
Department of Radiology
Henry Ford Hospital
1 Ford Place, 2F
Detroit, MI 48202 U.S.A.

Laurent A. Bentolila
Director, Advanced Light Microscopy
University of California at Los Angeles
Spectroscopy Laboratory
California NanoSystems Institute
Project Scientist, Department of Chemistry and Biochemistry
Los Angeles, CA 90095-1569 U.S.A.

Jinwoo Cheon
Professor of Chemistry
Yonsei University
Department of Chemistry and
Nanomedical National Core Research Center
262 Seongsanno, Seodaemun-gu, Seoul 120-749, Korea

Sören Doose
Postdoctoral Associate
Universität Bielefeld
Angewandte Laserphysik & Laserspektroskopie
Fakultät für Physik
33615 Bielefeld, Germany

Yuval Ebenstein
University of California at Los Angeles
Department of Chemistry and Biochemistry
Los Angeles, CA 90095-1569 U.S.A.

Maria H Etchehon
Graduate Student
Department of Organic Chemistry
Faculty of Exact and Natural Sciences
University of Buenos Aires
Ciudad Universitaria, Pab. II
1428, Buenos Aires, Argentina

Joseph A. Frank
Senior Investigator
Chief, Experimental Neuroimaging Section
Laboratory of Diagnostic Radiology Research
Imaging Sciences Program, Clinical Center
National Institutes of Health
Building 10 Room B1N256
Bethesda, Maryland 20892 U.S.A.

Taeghwan Hyeon
Director
National Creative Research Initiative Center for Oxide Nanocrystalline Materials and School of Chemical and Biological Engineering
Seoul National University
Seoul 151-744
Republic of Korea

Soon Gu Kwon
Graduate Student
National Creative Research Initiative Center for Oxide Nanocrystalline Materials and School of Chemical and Biological Engineering
Seoul National University
Seoul 151-744
Republic of Korea

Gopal Iyer
Postdoctoral Associate
University of California at Los Angeles
Department of Chemistry and Biochemistry
Los Angeles, CA 90095-1569 U.S.A.

Elizabeth Jares-Erijman, PhD
Associate Professor
University of Buenos Aires
Member of CONICET
Department of Organic Chemistry
Faculty of Exact and Natural Sciences
University of Buenos Aires
Ciudad Universitaria, Pab. II
1428, Buenos Aires, Argentina

Thomas M. Jovin, MD,
Director
Laboratory of Cellular Dynamics
Max Planck Institute for Biophysical Chemistry
Am Fassberg 11, 37077
Goettingen Germany

Jae-Hyun Lee
Graduate Student
Yonsei University
Department of Chemistry and
Nanomedical National Core Research Center
262 Seongsanno, Seodaemun-gu, Seoul 120-749, Korea

J. Jack Li
Postdoctoral Associate
University of California at Los Angeles
Department of Chemistry and Biochemistry
Los Angeles, CA 90095-1569 U.S.A.

Hedi Mattoussi
Senior Research Physicist
Naval Research Laboratory
Optical Sciences Division
4555 Overlook Avenue, SW
Washington, DC 20375 U.S.A.

Dusica Maysinger
Professor
Department of Pharmacology and Therapeutics
McGill University
3655 Promenade Sir-William-Osler, Room 1314
McIntyre Medical Sciences Building
Montreal, Quebec, Canada H3G 1Y6

Igor L. Medintz
Research Biologist
Naval Research Laboratory
Center for Biomolecular Science & Enginee4ring, Code 6900
4555 Overlook Avenue, SW
Washington, D.C. 20375 U.S.A.

Guillermo Menendez
Graduate Student
Department of Organic Chemistry
Faculty of Exact and Natural Sciences
University of Buenos Aires
Ciudad Universitaria, Pab. II
1428, Buenos Aires, Argentina

Xavier Michalet
University of California at Los Angeles
Project Scientist
Department of Chemistry and Biochemistry
Los Angeles, CA 90095-1569 U.S.A.

Myoung-Hwan Park
Graduate Researcher
Department of Chemistry
University of Massachusetts
710 North Pleasant Street, Amherst, MA, U.S.A.

Avishay Pelah, PhD
Formerly Postdoctoral Fellow
Laboratory of Cellular Dynamics
Max Planck Institute for Biophysical Chemistry
Am Fassberg 11, 37077
Goettingen Germany

Lia Pietrasanta, PhD
Coordinator
Center for Advanced Microscopy
Faculty of Exact and Natural Sciences
University of Buenos Aires
Ciudad Universitaria, Pab. II
1428, Buenos Aires, Argentina

Fabien Pinaud
Ecole Normale Superieure
Departement de Biologie
75005 Paris, France

Thomas Pons
Research Scientist
Institut National de la Santé et la Recherche Médicale Laboratoire Photons et Matière
Centre National de la Recherche Scientifique
UPRA005
Ecole Supérieure de Physique et Chimie Industrielle
10, rue Vauquelin
75235 Paris Cedex 5 – France

María Julia Roberti
Graduate Student
Department of Organic Chemistry
Faculty of Exact and Natural Sciences
University of Buenos Aires
Ciudad Universitaria, Pab. II
1428, Buenos Aires, Argentina

Vincent M. Rotello
Charles A. Goessmann Professor of Chemistry
Department of Chemistry
University of Massachusetts
710 North Pleasant Street,
Amherst, MA , U.S.A.

Valeria Sigot, PhD
Formerly Graduate Student
Laboratory of Cellular Dynamics
Max Planck Institute for Biophysical Chemistry
Am Fassberg 11, 37077
Goettingen, Germany

Kimihiro Susumu
Research Associate
Naval Research Laboratory
Optical Sciences Division
4555 Overlook Avenue, SW
Washington, D.C. 20375 U.S.A.

James Tsay
Postdoctoral Researcher
University of California at San Diego
Department of Physics
La Jolla, CA 92093 USA

Alexander Wei
Purdue University
Professor and University Faculty Scholar
Wetherill Laboratory of Chemistry
560 Oval Drive
West Lafayette, IN 47907-2084 U.S.A.

Qingshan Wei
Purdue University
Graduate Research Associate
Wetherill Laboratory of Chemistry
560 Oval Drive
West Lafayette, IN 47907-2084 U.S.A.

Shimon Weiss
Professor
University of California at Los Angeles
Department of Chemistry and Biochemistry and
Department of Physiology
Los Angeles, CA 90095-1569 U.S.A.

Françoise M. Winnik
Professor
Department of Chemistry and
Faculty of Pharmacy
University of Montreal
CP 6128 Succursale Centre Ville
Montreal QC H3C 3J7 Canada

Chang-Cheng You
Postdoctoral Researcher
Department of Chemistry
University of Massachusetts
710 North Pleasant Street,
Amherst, MA, U.S.A.

Index

M

N

R

S

T